D1708250

Andrew Budson and Paul Solomon, two of America's top memory ana .... experts, have packed this book with practical advice for clinicians caring for patients with dementia. Here is a single book that is equally useful to the student, the primary care provider, and the specialist. Few books provide both a comprehensive review of relevant diseases plus provide a step-by-step guide of how to diagnosis and treat patients with every stage of Alzheimer's. After reviewing just a few chapters, even nonspecialists will be able to confidently diagnose and treat patients with memory loss. The "Quick Start" sections at the beginning of each chapter provide a succinct summary and tell the reader exactly what the chapter will cover. The case studies are both educational and will allow clinicians to test their knowledge. I strongly recommend this book to all those who treat patients with memory loss—physicians, social workers, psychologists, nurses—at every level of training and experience.

P. Murali Doraiswamy, M.D.,
Professor & Head, Division of Biological Psychiatry,
Duke University, and
co-author of *The Alzheimer's Action Plan*.

Memory Loss: A Practical Guide for Clinicians provides the in-the-trenches clinician with the information critical to delivering great care to patients with memory impairment. Drs. Budson and Solomon become your personal guides to how to assess, diagnose, and treat the many complex causes of memory loss. The Guide addresses the major treatment issues and provides practical information regarding cholinesterase inhibitors, memantine, psychotropics, vitamins and supplements as well as non-pharmacologic dimensions of care. Often ignored topics such as legal and financial issues and life adjustments required of patients and caregivers are realistically discussed. Cases are described to lead the reader through real-world challenges and innovative solutions they may apply in their own practices. The Guide is a very welcome addition to our armamentarium of weapons to fight disease; it enhances our knowledge of how best to care for and comfort our patients and caregivers. In short, Memory Loss: A Practical Guide for Clinicians provides the assessment, diagnostic and therapeutic insights clinicians need to provide exemplary care to memory impaired patients. Don't go to the clinic without it.

Jeffrey L. Cummings, M.D.,
Director, Lou Ruvo Center for Brain Health,
The Andrea L. and Joseph F. Hahn MD Chair of Neurotherapeutics,
Cleveland Clinic, Las Vegas

Drs. Budson and Solomon have produced a sensible, well-crafted, manual ideally suited for frequent consultation in any primary care setting. It belongs on the shelf of every primary provider where it can be quickly and frequently consulted as a versatile aid to diagnosis and management. The subject matter is arranged in a concise, easy to access format that will encourage busy practitioners to frequently reach for it for nuggets of practical information. I'm sure this volume will be dog-eared in short order given its clear no-nonsense style. The range of topics is comprehensive—including diagnosis, drug treatment, care and financial planning, and community resources—but the content is *concise and pithy to encourage frequent use. This is not a reference volume where you will find a comprehensive list of differential diagnosis or drug treatments for memory loss rather, in its 250 pages some odd pages, you will find the distilled wisdom of two highly experienced clinicians with several decades of clinical experience gleaned by treating a wide range of patients with memory loss. As the title states, it is a practical guide designed for easy reference to satisfy the real time needs of clinicians in hectic clinical settings. Budson and Solomon provide concise step-by-step guidance on how to evaluate patients with memory loss that I am sure primary care providers will find invaluable. The case studies section is especially instructive and will help the clinician confronting the sometimes overwhelming challenge of evaluating and treating patients with memory loss.*

Neil W. Kowall, M.D.,
Professor of Neurology and Pathology, Boston University School of Medicine,
Director, Boston University Alzheimer's Disease Center,
Director, VA New England Geriatric Research Education and Clinical Center,
Chief, Neurology Service, VA Boston Healthcare System

This book serves as an invaluable resource for neuropsychologists, neurologists, and others involved in the care of older adults with dementia. It is an excellent resource for providing accurate diagnosis and effective treatment. Rarely does one find a book that summarizes the most recent knowledge on neurodegenerative disorders and treatment in a manner that is accessible to both the experienced clinician and those entering the fields of neurology and neuropsychology. It is clear that the authors are not only accomplished academics, but are also dedicated clinicians. This book summarizes complex material in a manner that benefits clinical practitioners at all levels. This is an excellent addition to the library of professionals serving older adults. This book brings together the most current state of knowledge about the diagnosis and treatment of neurodegenerative disorders. Both the seasoned professional and students in neurology and neuropsychology should be sure to add this important text to their library.

Maureen K. O'Connor, Psy.D., ABCN,
Chief, Neuropsychology Service,
Edith Nourse Rogers Memorial Veterans Hospital,
Bedford, MA

Memory Loss

Judith —

It is a pleasure working with you and learning from you.

Best, Andrew

Cover Images

Images show the electrical activity of the brain as a memory is being retrieved in young adults. In the first row, early frontal activity appears at about 400 ms, as the item observed by the subject is perceived as familiar. In the second row, parietal activity is present at about 600 ms, as rich, contextual details of the memory are being retrieved, allowing the subject to "time-travel" back to the initial viewing of the item. In the third row, late frontal activity alternates with more posterior activity from about 800 to 1500 ms as the subject purposefully recalls additional details of the memory. Patients with amnestic mild cognitive impairment and those with Alzheimer's disease show greatest dysfunction of the processes that occur in the second row (Ally et al., 2009; Budson et al., 2000). (Images were created by Joshua McKeever using data taken from Ally & Budson, 2007.)

References:

Ally, B.A., Budson, A.E., 2007. The worth of pictures: Using high-density event-related potentials to understand the memorial power of pictures and the dynamics of recognition memory. NeuroImage 35, 378–395.

Ally, B.A., McKeever, J.D., Waring, J.D., Budson, A.E., 2009. Preserved frontal memorial processing for pictures in patients with mild cognitive impairment. Neuropsychologia 47, 2044–2055.

Budson, A.E., Daffner, K.R., Desikan, R., Schacter, D.L., 2000. When false recognition is unopposed by true recognition: Gist based memory distortion in Alzheimer's disease. Neuropsychology 14, 277–287.

Commissioning Editor: *Lotta Kryhl*
Development Editor: *Poppy Garraway*
Project Manager: *Anita Somaroutu*
Designer: *Charles Gray*
Illustration Manager: *Bruce Hogarth*
Illustrator: *Robert Britton*
Marketing Managers (UK/USA): *Gaynor Jones/Carla Holloway*

Memory Loss
A Practical Guide for Clinicians

Andrew E. Budson, M.D.

Geriatric Research Education Clinical Center &
Neurology Service,
Veterans Affairs Boston Healthcare System, Boston, MA;
Alzheimer's Disease Center & Department of Neurology,
Boston University School of Medicine, Boston, MA;
Division of Cognitive & Behavioral Neurology,
Department of Neurology, Brigham and Women's Hospital,
Boston, MA;
Harvard Medical School, Boston, MA;
The Memory Clinic, Bennington, VT

Paul R. Solomon, Ph.D.

Department of Psychology, Program in Neuroscience,
Williams College, Williamstown, MA;
The Memory Clinic, Bennington, VT

ELSEVIER
SAUNDERS

ELSEVIER
SAUNDERS

SAUNDERS is an imprint of Elsevier Inc.

Notices

Knowledge and best practice in this field are constantly changing. As new research and experience broaden our understanding, changes in research methods, professional practices, or medical treatment may become necessary.

Practitioners and researchers must always rely on their own experience and knowledge in evaluating and using any information, methods, compounds, or experiments described herein. In using such information or methods they should be mindful of their own safety and the safety of others, including parties for whom they have a professional responsibility.

With respect to any drug or pharmaceutical products identified, readers are advised to check the most current information provided (i) on procedures featured or (ii) by the manufacturer of each product to be administered, to verify the recommended dose or formula, the method and duration of administration, and contraindications. It is the responsibility of practitioners, relying on their own experience and knowledge of their patients, to make diagnoses, to determine dosages and the best treatment for each individual patient, and to take all appropriate safety precautions.

To the fullest extent of the law, neither the Publisher nor the authors, contributors, or editors, assume any liability for any injury and/or damage to persons or property as a matter of products liability, negligence or otherwise, or from any use or operation of any methods, products, instructions, or ideas contained in the material herein.

Saunders

British Library Cataloguing in Publication Data

Memory loss : a practical guide for clinicians.
  1. Dementia. 2. Dementia–Diagnosis.
  I. Budson, Andrew. II. Solomon, Paul.
  616.8'3-dc22

ISBN-13: 9781416035978

Printed in China

Contents

Foreword

Memory loss is one of the most feared consequences of aging and it is becoming a bona fide epidemic. Alois Alzheimer saw the index patient, Ms. Auguste Deter, in 1901, when she was 51 years old. She had a disorder of her cognitive functions that progressed relatively rapidly and took her life. He later was able to examine her brain and, in 1906, presented his now seminal findings of plaques and neurofibrillary tangles. At the time, Alzheimer's disease, or presenile dementia, was thought to be a rare and curious disorder, distinct from the loss of cognition that had been known for centuries as simple senility. In the intervening century, it has become clearer that Alzheimer's findings were characteristic of the most common form of dementia (progressive loss of cognition) and that he had discovered the tip of an iceberg which was intensely age-dependent. The prevalence of the disease is probably about 2% in the age group 65–69; 4% in the age group 70–74; 8% in the age group 75–79; 16% in the age group 80–84; and 40% in people over 85. If these numbers are even close to correct, we are facing 14 million patients with Alzheimer's disease by 2040.

Furthermore, Alzheimer's disease is not the only form of dementia, though it is the most frequent, accounting for somewhere between half and three-quarters of all cases. Other disorders include various lobar atrophies (once called Pick's disease), the most common of which is frontotemporal dementia (the most common dementia in those younger than age 65), vascular dementia, Lewy body dementia (the second most common dementia overall), hydrocephalus, and a wide array of other syndromes.

The seminal feature of dementia is memory loss, and it is this problem that most often takes the patient to the doctor, either complaining himself or compelled to seek medical attention by his family, friends, or employers. Every type of primary care provider (internists, emergency physicians, family doctors, nurse practitioners, physician assistants) and many specialists (neurologists, psychiatrists, psychologists) are faced with patients who either believe they are losing their memory or have been told their memory is abnormal by others. Fear of dementia is a disease in its own right, fueled by widespread media attention to the problem that can be traced primarily to former President Ronald Reagan's highly publicized illness.

The medical literature has burgeoned with an overwhelming number of scientific papers on the subject, and there is almost no aspect of the problem that is not rife with controversy. At the moment, it is fair to say that the cause of Alzheimer's disease remains a mystery, and its treatments are ineffective in halting or even slowing the brain deterioration. The practitioner of medicine cannot hope to keep abreast of the scientific debates, but must still be competent to diagnose and treat patients with a memory disorder and their families. Despite the absence of a dramatically effective treatment or prevention, much can be done for patients and families coping with this complex array of disorders that cause memory problems.

It is in this context that Andrew Budson, a neurologist with special expertise in cognitive disorders, and Paul Solomon, a psychologist with a broad and deep experience in diagnosing and treating memory disorders, have collaborated to provide the practitioner with a practical, evidence-based, and expertly informed road map for dealing with virtually every aspect of this complex medical and psychosocial problem.

Memory Loss: A Practical Guide for Clinicians is divided into five major sections. The first section deals with the methods for evaluating patients with memory loss from history-taking to the use of the dizzying array of neuropsychological tests that are available. In the second section, the authors expound on the differential diagnosis of memory loss. This exposition is critical in that many of the imitators of Alzheimer's disease may well have a specific therapy that may be much more effective than the symptomatic treatments that are now available for Alzheimer's disease itself. Section III contains an excellent evidence-based approach to the treatment of memory loss, and Section IV deals with the often most difficult problem of all: the behavioral and psychosocial symptoms of dementia. Finally, in Section V the authors offer some very practical advice about the life adjustments that are required for the patients and their caregivers as well as important legal and financial issues that inevitably arise in the course of diseases which rob people of their cognition.

This volume will be a welcome aid for all of those practitioners who must diagnose and treat patients with memory loss, giving them the confidence they need to deal with one of the most challenging aspects of clinical medicine.

Martin A. Samuels, M.D.
Chairman
Department of Neurology
Brigham and Women's Hospital;
Professor of Neurology
Harvard Medical School
Boston, MA

Preface

The statistics are overwhelming (Alzheimer's Association, 2010):

- there are 5.3 million Americans living with Alzheimer's disease
- one in eight adults age 65 and older have Alzheimer's disease
- every 70 seconds someone develops Alzheimer's disease in America
- by 2050, someone will develop Alzheimer's disease every 33 seconds.

And these numbers do not include all the additional individuals who have or will be diagnosed with other causes of dementia.

This book is written for the clinicians who are and will be caring for these more than 5 million individuals with memory loss due to Alzheimer's disease and other dementias. It is written for all these clinicians, whether their degree is in medicine, psychology, nursing, social work, or therapies. It is written for the generalist and the specialist, the student and the experienced clinician. Primary care providers, nurses, psychologists, and students will find this book a very practical, clinically oriented guide that helps them know what to do when sitting in the office with a patient complaining of memory loss. Specialists, including psychiatrists, neurologists, neuropsychologists, geriatricians, and others, will find this book a wealth of up-to-date information regarding the latest diagnostic tools and treatments for their patients with memory loss.

This book is based upon the most recent peer-reviewed published studies in the literature. However, this book also reflects our opinions on how to care for patients with memory loss based upon our training and our combined experience in treating more than 3500 patients with memory loss over approximately 27,000 patient visits. Where our opinions are supported by the literature we have provided appropriate references, and where our opinions differ from the literature we have done our best to point this discrepancy out. There are, of course, large areas of clinical practice for which there are no randomized, double-blind, placebo-controlled trials to guide one. It is here that our training and experience proves most valuable. Part of the usefulness of this book, in fact, is that we did not limit ourselves to only reporting the results of randomized, double-blind, placebo-controlled trials, but instead used those trials as a basis to provide comprehensive care.

This book concentrates mainly on Alzheimer's disease for several reasons. First, Alzheimer's disease is by far the most common cause of memory loss that the clinician will encounter. Second, we know more about Alzheimer's disease than we do about any other cause of memory loss and dementia. Third, most of the principles of disease management discussed for Alzheimer's disease are also directly applicable to other dementias. And, last, treatments approved by the US Food and Drug Administration for memory loss and those currently in development are all for Alzheimer's disease.

HOW TO USE THIS BOOK

Everyone should read Chapters 1–3. Other chapters can then be read when there are relevant issues such as suspected diagnoses other than Alzheimer's disease (Section II,

Chapters 4–12), questions regarding medications for memory loss (Section III, Chapters 13–18), and issues with the behavioral and psychological symptoms of dementia as well as caring for the caregiver (Section IV, Chapters 19–22). Section V discusses life adjustments, as well as legal, financial, and other issues. Finally, Section VI provides a series of case studies. The Web appendices provide additional useful information including cognitive test and questionnaire forms that can be immediately used (Appendix A), an expanded discussion on screening for memory loss (Appendix B), and other useful information.

A note on abbreviations

Because we want this book to be accessible to a wide variety of audiences from diverse fields, each with their own standard abbreviations, we have endeavored to eliminate abbreviations. This will often make sentences longer, but we hope that these sentences will be, on the whole, more easily understood.

Reference

Alzheimer's Association, 2010. 2010 Alzheimer's disease facts and figures. Alzheimers Dement. 6, 158–194.

Acknowledgments

This manuscript is dedicated first to patients with memory loss and their caregivers; we hope that this book will lead to improvement in their lives. We also dedicate this book to our families, Danny, Leah, Jessica, Todd, and Amy, who supported us while we worked on this book during early mornings, late nights, weekends, and vacations.

We want to thank our many colleagues who were kind enough to review some or all of our manuscript, particularly Cynthia A. Murphy, Psy.D., MBA, Lisa Catapano-Friedman, M.D., Maureen K. O'Connor, Psy.D., Richard D. Budson, M.D., Daniel Z. Press, M.D., and Victoria M. Derevianko. A special thanks goes to Ann C. McKee, M.D., for providing the neuropathology figures.

Disclosures

Disclosures (current and/or during the past 5 year):

Dr. Budson receives grant support from the National Institute on Aging, National Institutes of Health (NIH). He was a former speaker for the pharmaceutical companies Eisai, Pfizer, Johnson & Johnson, Forest Pharmaceuticals, and Novartis, ending in June 2009.

Dr. Solomon receives or has received grant support from Abbott, Alzheimer's Disease Cooperative Study, Astellas, Astra Zeneca, Avid, Eisai, Elan, EnVivo EPIX, Forest, Genentech, GlaxoSmithKline, Lilly, Janssen, Novartis, Memory Pharmaceuticals Neurochem, Pfizer, Merck, Myriad, Sanofi, Sonexa, Voyager, and Wyeth. He consults or has consulted for Abbott, Astellas, Avid, Eisai, EPIX, Pfizer, and Toyoma.

Note: The content of this book has been derived from the patients that Dr. Budson and Dr. Solomon have seen separately and together in The Memory Clinic in Bennington, Vermont, along with literature reviews conducted solely for the purpose of this book. These reviews and the writing of this book have been conducted during early mornings, late nights, weekends, and vacations. Dr. Budson's contribution to this book was conducted outside of both his VA tour of duty and his Boston University/NIH research time.

About the Authors

Dr. Budson received his bachelor's degree at Haverford College, where he majored in both chemistry and philosophy. After graduating *cum laude* from Harvard Medical School, he was an intern in internal medicine at Brigham and Women's Hospital. He then attended the Harvard–Longwood Neurology Residency Program, for which he was chosen to be chief resident in his senior year. He next pursued a fellowship in behavioral neurology and dementia at Brigham and Women's Hospital, after which he joined the neurology department there. He participated in numerous clinical trials of new drugs to treat Alzheimer's disease in his role as the Associate Medical Director of Clinical Trials for Alzheimer's Disease at Brigham and Women's Hospital. Following his clinical training he spent 3 years studying memory as a postdoctoral fellow in experimental psychology and cognitive neuroscience at Harvard University under Professor Daniel Schacter. While continuing in the Neurology Department at Brigham and Women's Hospital, in 2000 he began work as Consultant Neurologist for The Memory Clinic in Bennington, Vermont. After 5 years as Assistant Professor of Neurology at Harvard Medical School, he joined the Boston University Alzheimer's Disease Center and the Geriatric Research Education Clinical Center (GRECC) at the Bedford VA Hospital. During his 5 years at the Bedford GRECC he served in several roles, including the Director of Outpatient Services, Associate Clinical Director, and later the overall GRECC Director. From March 2009 through February 2010 he served as Bedford's Acting Chief of Staff. In March 2010 he moved to Boston as the Deputy Chief of Staff of the Boston VA Healthcare System. He is also the Director of the Center for Translational Cognitive Neuroscience at the Boston VA, Associate Director for Research at the Boston University Alzheimer's Disease Center, Professor of Neurology at Boston University School of Medicine, Lecturer in Neurology at Harvard Medical School, and Consultant Neurologist at the Division of Cognitive and Behavioral Neurology, Department of Neurology, at Brigham and Women's Hospital. Dr. Budson has had continuous NIH research funding since 1998, receiving a National Research Service Award and a Career Development Award in addition to a Research Project (R01) grant. He has given over 275 local, national, and international grand rounds and other academic talks, including at the Institute of Cognitive Neuroscience, Queen Square, London, UK; Berlin, Germany; and the University of Cambridge, UK. He has published over 80 papers in peer-reviewed journals including *The New England Journal of Medicine, Brain*, and *Cortex*, and is a reviewer for more than 40 journals. He was awarded the Norman Geschwind Prize in Behavioral Neurology in 2008 and the Research Award in Geriatric Neurology in 2009, both from the American Academy of Neurology. His current research uses the techniques of experimental psychology and cognitive neuroscience to understand memory and memory distortions in patients with Alzheimer's disease and other neurological disorders. In his memory disorders clinic at the Boston VA he treats patients while teaching fellows, residents, and medical students. He continues to see patients once a month with Dr. Solomon at The Memory Clinic in Bennington, Vermont.

Dr. Solomon received his Ph.D. in Psychology from the University of Massachusetts–Amherst. He was a postdoctoral fellow in the laboratory of Richard F. Thompson in the

Department of Psychobiology at the University of California at Irvine. He is currently Professor of Psychology and founding Chairman of the Neuroscience Program, Williams College. Dr. Solomon teaches in the areas of neuropsychology and behavioral neuroscience and conducts research on the neurobiology of memory disorders. He is particularly interested in the memory deficits associated with Alzheimer's disease. He is the author of nine books, has also contributed chapters to 20 edited volumes, and has co-authored and presented more than 200 research papers. His work has been published in *Science, Scientific American, Journal of the American Medical Association,* and *The Lancet.* He has delivered more than 400 invited colloquia, symposia, grand rounds, lectures, and presentations. He has been the recipient of research grants from the National Science Foundation, the National Institute on Aging, the National Institute of Mental Health, the United States Environmental Protection Agency, as well as private foundations and pharmaceutical research divisions. Dr. Solomon has received numerous awards including a Distinguished Teaching Award from the University of Massachusetts, a National Research Service Award from the National Institutes of Health, and a National Needs Postdoctoral Fellowship from the National Science Foundation, and a clinical research award from the American Association of Family Physicians. He has been elected as a Fellow of the American Association for the Advancement of Science, the American Psychological Association and the American Psychological Society. He is listed in *Who's Who in America, American Men and Women of Science, Who's Who in Education,* and *Who's Who in Frontier Science and Technology.* Dr. Solomon has served on the Editorial Board of several journals and serves as an external reviewer for numerous journals and granting agencies. He has lectured widely at colleges and universities on age-related memory disorders and at medical centers and hospitals on the diagnosis and treatment of Alzheimer's disease. He has also appeared frequently to discuss pharmacotherapy for Alzheimer's disease on national television including the *Today Show, Good Morning America,* the *CBS Morning Show,* and CBS, ABC, and NBC evening news. His work on screening for Alzheimer's disease has been featured on *Dateline NBC.* In addition to his academic undertakings, Dr. Solomon is a licensed psychologist in Massachusetts and Vermont. He is also founder and Clinical Director of The Memory Clinic in Bennington, Vermont, and President of Clinical Neuroscience Research Associates. He has served as the first Director of Training for the Southwestern Vermont Psychology Consortium. He serves on the advisory board of the Massachusetts Alzheimer's Association and the Northeastern New York Alzheimer's Association.

CHAPTER

Why diagnose and treat?

1

QUICK START: WHY DIAGNOSE AND TREAT?

- Current treatments can help improve or maintain the patient's cognitive and functional status by "turning back the clock" on memory loss.
- Families and other caregivers are helped by treatments that maintain or improve functional status and neuropsychiatric symptoms.
- Using current treatments saves money, as shown by pharmaco-economic studies.
- New, disease-modifying treatments are being developed and may be available soon.
- Accurate diagnosis helps define prognosis, facilitating future planning.
- Improving the quality (not quantity) of life is the goal.

A 72-year-old woman comes into the clinic at the urging of her son. She has noticed some difficulties finding words for the past 6 months, but denies problems with memory or other aspects of her thinking. Her son reports that his mother has had memory problems which began 5 years ago, and have been gradually worsening. He notes that his mother used to have an excellent memory, and would keep her calendar, grocery and other lists in her head. Now she needs to write everything down or she is totally lost. She used to send out birthday cards to her grandchildren every year, but over the past 2 years has either forgotten to do this or sends them out at the wrong time. In addition to memory problems, he agrees that she also has word-finding difficulties, and often has trouble finishing sentences. From a functional standpoint, she is also having difficulty. She is living with her husband, and he has gradually been taking over household responsibilities that she used to do, such as going to the grocery store. She continues to cook, but there are now just a few meals that she prepares, and these have become much simpler than they used to be.

The first question that needs to be addressed in this book is: what should be done about this 72-year-old woman? Is it important to diagnose and treat memory loss? Although the answer to this question may seem obvious to some, in the current healthcare climate it is a very reasonable question. There are four basic answers to this question: (1) to help the patient, (2) to help the family and other caregivers, (3) to save money, and, lastly, (4) to plan for the future.

HELPING THE PATIENT

Current treatments for Alzheimer's disease have been shown to be able to "turn the clock back" on memory loss for 6–12 months (Cummings, 2004). That is, although memory loss cannot be halted or reversed to where it was prior to their developing Alzheimer's disease, current treatments are able to improve patients' memory to where it was 6–12 months ago. Although to some this may not seem worthwhile, we believe that this level of improvement can make a significant difference in the lives of our patients. Treatment can enable patients with very mild memory loss to be able to take that last trip to Europe, attend and remember their grandchild's wedding, or finish writing their memoirs. For patients with mild memory loss, treatments allow them to continue independent activities such as shopping for groceries and paying bills. For patients with moderate to severe memory loss, treatments may provide functional improvements in basic activities of daily living such as dressing, bathing, and toileting.

Perhaps most importantly, many new treatments are being developed for patients with memory loss, some of which have the potential to dramatically slow down or even stop memory loss entirely. These so-called "disease-modifying" treatments will be specific to different diseases causing dementia, and thus accurate diagnosis will be critical.

HELPING THE FAMILY OR OTHER CAREGIVER

The majority of patients diagnosed with dementia live at home and are cared for by a family member. It follows logically that, if the patient is showing improvements, life for family members and other caregivers will also improve (Grossberg, 2008). If patients with mild memory loss can do their own shopping and pay their own bills, then no one has to spend time helping them with these chores. And, of course, if activities of daily living are improved, families and other caregivers will have more time for their own activities. One study found that treatment was associated with a saving of 68 minutes per day on average for caregivers (Sano et al., 2003).

SAVING MONEY

Current pharmacological treatments for memory loss cost money, between $1500 and $2000 per year for each medication. Are the beneficial effects for patients and caregivers worth the costs? Although certain aspects of this question cannot be readily answered, an easier question to answer is whether the dollars spent on medications to treat memory loss and to improve quality of life end up saving money. This issue has been studied and the results are clear: treatment of memory loss does save money (Getsios et al., 2001; Moore et al., 2001; Wimo et al., 2003a,b). When patients are treated for their memory loss, fewer medications to control behavior need be prescribed. There is less use of home health aids. Caregivers have more time to spend in the workplace bringing in revenue to the household. And placement in nursing homes can be delayed (Lyseng-Williamson & Plosker, 2002; Geldmacher et al., 2003).

PLANNING FOR THE FUTURE

Planning for the future is absolutely essential for any patient with progressive memory loss. Documents such as a power of attorney and healthcare proxy will need to be drawn up and signed. Banking, bill paying, and driving need to be addressed. The physical environment within the home will often need changes. Usually the patient will end up moving to a new residence. Some patients move in with a family member in a room, a separate suite, or an apartment in the house. Other patients move to senior housing, retirement communities, or assisted living. (See Chapters 23: *Life adjustment* and 24: *Legal and financial issues* for more on these important topics.) Understanding the patient's prognosis in as much detail as possible is invaluable when helping families to anticipate when some of these changes will likely take place, and which options to pursue. For example, we have had a number of families inform us that they are either adding an addition onto their house or are building a new house so the patient can live with them. Whether the construction will be completed in time to be of use to the patient will often depend upon the etiology of the memory loss.

QUALITY VERSUS QUANTITY

A word on the goal of treatment. We would argue that the goal of treating memory loss is not necessarily to prolong life, but is, rather, to improve the quality of life that the patient has available to him or her. For example, if a patient has 10 years between the time of diagnosis and death, the goal of treatment is not to prolong life, but to improve the quality of life that the patient has left. Over time memory loss progresses to dementia, and dementia progresses from mild to moderate to severe. At the end of life, the goal of therapy shifts to that of allowing the patient to die with dignity and comfort. At that point we would suggest it is appropriate to withdraw treatments for memory loss, and it is our observation that withdrawal of such treatments does allow the patient to die more quickly.

References

Cummings, J.L., 2004. Alzheimer's disease. N. Engl. J Med. 351, 56–67.

Geldmacher, D.S., Provenzano, G., McRae, T., et al., 2003. Donepezil is associated with delayed nursing home placement in patients with Alzheimer's disease. J. Am. Geriatr. Soc. 51, 937–944.

Getsios, D., Caro, J.J., Caro, G., Ishak, K., 2001. Assessment of health economics in Alzheimer's disease (AHEAD): galantamine treatment in Canada. Neurology 57, 972–978.

Grossberg, G.T., 2008. Impact of rivastigmine on caregiver burden associated with Alzheimer's disease in both informal care and nursing home settings. Drugs Aging 25, 573–584.

Lyseng-Williamson, K.A., Plosker, G.L., 2002. Galantamine: a pharmacoeconomic review of its use in Alzheimer's disease. Pharmacoeconomics 20, 919–942.

Moore, M.J., Zhu, C.W., Clipp, E.C., 2001. Informal costs of dementia care: estimates from the National Longitudinal Caregiver Study. J. Gerontol. B Psychol. Sci. Soc. Sci. 56, S219–S228.

Sano, M., Wilcock, G.K., van Baelen, B., et al., 2003. The effects of galantamine treatment on caregiver time in Alzheimer's disease. Int. J. Geriatr. Psychiatry 18, 942–950.

Wimo, A., Winblad, B., Engedal, K., et al., 2003a. An economic evaluation of donepezil in mild to moderate Alzheimer's disease: results of a 1-year, double-blind, randomized trial. Dement. Geriatr. Cogn. Disord. 15, 44–54.

Wimo, A., Winblad, B., Stoffler, A., et al., 2003b. Resource utilisation and cost analysis of memantine in patients with moderate to severe Alzheimer's disease. Pharmacoeconomics 21, 327–340.

2 Evaluating the patient with memory loss

QUICK START: EVALUATING THE PATIENT WITH MEMORY LOSS

- Talking with the family (or other caregivers) is critical to obtaining an accurate history.
- Important elements of the history to investigate include:
  - Characterization of the onset and course of the disorder
  - Memory loss and memory distortions
  - Word-finding
  - Fluctuations in attention
  - Getting lost in a new or familiar environment
  - Problems with reasoning and judgment
  - Changes in behavior
  - Depression and anxiety
  - Loss of insight
  - Current functional status including basic and instrumental activities of daily living.
- Review of systems, past medical history, physical examination, and laboratory studies should evaluate for medical, neurological, and psychiatric problems that can impair cognition and memory, such as strokes, Parkinson's disease, and depression.
- Cognitive testing is essential, whether with brief tests in the office or a formal neuropsychological evaluation.
- Interpret current cognition and function in light of the patient's previous abilities.
- Routine screening for memory loss will allow patients to be diagnosed and treated earlier, which can help them to avoid a decline in function and to maintain quality of life.
- A brain CT or MRI scan is essential for evaluating possible strokes and other anatomic lesions.
- A functional imaging scan (SPECT or PET) can be helpful to confirm the diagnosis of an atypical dementia and to provide additional diagnostic information for young patients.
- Beware of diagnosing dementia in the patient hospitalized for a medical issue!

In this chapter we will discuss how to evaluate a patient with memory loss, including the history, physical examination, cognitive testing, and laboratory and imaging studies. We will illustrate this evaluation by focusing on the most common cause of memory loss, Alzheimer's disease. Elements of the evaluation are similar to other medical evaluations and should include:

1. a history of present illness
2. medical history

3. current and relevant past medications

4. allergies to medications

5. social history including education, occupation, and any possible learning disabilities

6. family history, including a history of late-life memory problems even if considered normal for age at that time

7. physical and neurological examination

8. cognitive examination

9. laboratory studies

10. neuroimaging studies.

TALKING WITH THE FAMILY

One aspect of the evaluation that is both critically important and different from most other appointments is the need to speak with the family member or other caregiver separately. The family or caregiver must be interviewed in order to obtain an accurate history. Commonly, patients with memory loss truly do not remember the various instances in which they forget things. Or patients may remember at least some of these instances, but are reluctant to share them with the clinician. This reluctance may stem from a variety of issues. Often patients find it frightening to admit—even to themselves—that they have memory problems, because in our society the label of "Alzheimer's disease" has become tantamount to what cancer was 20 years ago: synonymous with a death sentence. Sometimes patients do not want to admit their memory problems to the clinician or their families, for fear that, at best, they will be condescended to and, at worst, they will be sent to a nursing home.

The importance of interviewing the family or caregivers separately is because family members are often reluctant to give a full, accurate, and detailed history to the clinician in the presence of the patient. Sometimes this reluctance is present because the history includes inappropriate sexual behavior, aggression, driving, or other sensitive subjects that families prefer to discuss in private. More often the reluctance is present because patients will often deny that they have memory problems for the reasons mentioned above. Some patients may become upset when confronted by what they view as accusations leveled against them by their family. Other patients may become visibly depressed. Even if family members begin to give an accurate history in front of the patient, they usually stop when they see their loved one becoming angry or depressed. In addition, family members quite correctly view it as impolite to have a discussion about the patient in front of him or her as if they were not there. Lastly, talking in private can provide a comfortable atmosphere for the family or caregiver to discuss the patient candidly.

IN THE CLINIC
Setting up the appointment

There are many different ways to successfully set up a clinic appointment to evaluate the patient with memory loss. The part of the evaluation that is different from many others is the opportunity to speak with the family alone (Table 2.1). Because this takes time, the evaluation is often best divided into two or even three visits.

Table 2.1 Comparision between a typical medical evaluation and a dementia evaluation

Medical evaluation	Dementia evaluation
Self-history important	Self-history can be unreliable
Family observations secondary	Family observations critical
Mental status examination can be deferred	Mental status examination critical
Laboratory studies often critical for diagnosis	Laboratory studies are exclusionary, not diagnostic
Imaging studies may not be needed	Imaging studies critical

Another reason to divide the evaluation into separate visits is that time is necessary to build up a rapport with patients and families. When patients come to the clinic for an initial visit with laboratory studies and scans already completed and the diagnosis clear, it would seem logical to provide the diagnosis in that visit. However, we would not recommend doing this. It is our experience that many patients and families are simply not prepared to hear a diagnosis of Alzheimer's or another dementia from a clinician they have just met. Although it will still be emotionally difficult for patients and families, it is better to invite the patient back to the clinic to discuss the diagnosis and treatment plan on another day. In the initial visit, the patients quite correctly perceive that they are seeing "a new doctor." Upon returning to the clinic on a later day, many patients will now feel that they are seeing "one of their doctors."

In our memory clinics we have the opportunity to have the patient perform cognitive testing with a member of the clinic staff, and it is during this time that we talk with the family alone. On occasions when the patient would not have testing with a member of the clinic staff, we will simply ask the patient to sit in the waiting room for a few minutes while we speak with the family. There are, however, many other opportunities to speak with a family member alone. For example, in the busy internal medicine practice of one of our colleagues, when he is worried that a patient of his is having memory problems, he will talk with the family member for a few minutes in a spare examination room while the patient is changing into a gown. Calling the family member on the phone at a different time is of course another option, and a necessary one if the family member did not accompany the patient. If a patient does not have a close family member (or one that they want contacted), talking with a close friend is a good substitute. For those patients who are still working, talking with an employer can sometimes be helpful, particularly if difficulties at work are the main issue. One must be careful, however, to maintain patient confidentiality when talking with any of these individuals, but particularly when talking with friends and employers.

Setting the agenda

In all cases we believe it is important to begin by describing to the patient and the family what is going to happen in the appointment, and what the follow-up will be. Here is one example of a typical preamble that might be used by a clinician, in this case a neurologist:

> *Hi Mr. Jones, I hear there are some concerns about your memory. Let me begin by telling you how I like to do my memory evaluations. I want to start by talking with you, to find out what problems you have noticed, if any, with your thinking and memory. We will then go over your medical history, medications, family history, and other things like that. I am glad*

that you brought your family with you—I'm going to ask for their help when we go over your medical history, etc., so that I don't miss anything. We'll then do a physical and neurologic exam: listen to your heart and lungs, tap on your reflexes, that sort of thing. Next we'll decide what blood work and CT or MRI scans need to be performed. Then you're going to spend some time with my assistant, who will give you some paper and pencil tests of your thinking and memory. While you're doing that I'll spend a couple of minutes chatting with your family to get their perspective on your thinking and memory difficulties, if that is OK with you. That will be what we'll have time to do today, and then when I see you back in our next appointment we'll go over the results of all these tests, and make a plan of what to do to try to improve your memory. How does all that sound to you?

Here is another example, one that might better fit a busy internist's practice for an existing patient:

Hi Mr. Jones, your wife is worried that you are having a bit of difficulty with your memory. While it may be part of normal aging, I don't want to miss any treatable diseases. To find out if there is anything going on besides the fact that you're getting a bit older, I want to start by talking with you, to find out what problems you have noticed, if any, with your thinking and memory. We will then briefly review your medical history, medications, family history, and other things like that. We'll then do a physical exam. Next week I'd like you to come back to the office. At that visit I'll chat privately with your wife for a few minutes if that is OK with you, to get her perspective on things. We'll also do a few minutes' pencil and paper tests to see how your thinking and memory are doing. Finally we'll decide what blood work needs to be done, and we may get a CT or MRI scan to take a look at your brain. When I see you back next month we'll go over the results of all these tests, and see what we can do to improve your memory. How does all that sound to you?

AT THE BEDSIDE

Sometimes an evaluation of memory loss takes place in the inpatient setting of a hospital. Some things are much easier to accomplish in the hospital, and other things are more difficult. It is usually easier to find time to speak with a family member, and it may also be easier to have laboratory and imaging studies completed in the hospital. It is more difficult, however, to see patients at their cognitive best. Typically, the hospitalized setting will make a patient disoriented and confused, even aside from the illness or procedure that they are in the hospital for. Because of this, being in the hospital is a fine place to begin an evaluation of memory loss, but the evaluation must include an outpatient visit so that the clinician has the opportunity to see the patient at their cognitive best. Beware of diagnosing patients with memory loss or dementia having seen them only in the inpatient setting!

HISTORY
Location, location, location...

One of the keys to understanding the history of signs and symptoms in a patient with Alzheimer's disease is to understand the relative timing and distribution of Alzheimer's pathology in the brain. Alzheimer's pathology has a predilection for a number of particular regions of the brain (Fig. 2.1). These regions include the hippocampus and amygdala, and the parietal, temporal, and frontal lobes. Alzheimer's pathology also affects subcortical nuclei that project to the cortex, such as the basal forebrain cholinergic nuclei (which produce acetylcholine), the locus caeruleus (which produces norepinephrine), the raphe nuclei (which produce serotonin), and certain nuclei of the thalamus.

Memory Loss

The hippocampus and other medial temporal lobe structures are the earliest and most severely affected brain regions in Alzheimer's disease. The hippocampus is the brain structure that is most directly responsible for learning of new personal experiences, such as remembering a short story or what you had for dinner the previous night. This type of memory is usually referred to as *episodic memory* because it is memory for a specific episode of your life (see Appendix C: *Our current understanding of memory*). Thus, impairment of episodic memory is usually one of the earliest signs of Alzheimer's disease.

Common symptoms of this memory loss include asking the same questions repeatedly, repeating the same stories, forgetting important appointments, and leaving the stove on (Box 2.1). The memory disorder of Alzheimer's disease, like other disorders of episodic memory, follows a particular pattern that is known as Ribot's law (Ribot, 1881). Following Ribot's law, the patients show *anterograde amnesia* or difficulty learning new information. They also show *retrograde amnesia* or difficulty retrieving previously learned information. However, the patients typically demonstrate preserved memory for remote information. Thus, a patient may report, "I've got short-term memory problems—I cannot remember what I did yesterday but I can still remember things from thirty years ago." Not understanding that this pattern is suggestive of the memory impairment common in Alzheimer's disease, family members may report that they feel confident that whatever the patient's problem is, that "it isn't Alzheimer's disease," because the patient can still remember what happened many years ago. The memory deficits experienced by patients with Alzheimer's disease are often referred to as *rapid forgetting* of information they have recently learned.

Memory distortions

In addition to rapid forgetting, patients with Alzheimer's disease also experience distortions of memory and false memories. These distortions may include falsely remembering that they have already turned off the stove or taken their medications, leading patients to neglect performing these tasks. More dramatic distortions of memory may occur when patients substitute one person in a memory for another, combine two memories together, or think that an event that happened long ago occurred recently. Sometimes a false memory can be confused with a psychotic delusion or hallucination. For example, a patient may claim to have recently seen and spoken with a long-deceased family member. This patient is much more likely to be suffering from a memory distortion or a false memory than a true hallucination. The same is true for the patient who claims that people are breaking into the house, and moving things around. That these symptoms likely represent memory distortions rather than true hallucinations or delusions has implications when the time comes for treatment, as memory distortions are best treated with memory-enhancing medications (such as cholinesterase inhibitors) rather than antipsychotic medications. (A true hallucination, on the other hand, would suggest dementia with Lewy bodies rather than Alzheimer's disease; see Chapter 5: *Dementia with Lewy bodies (including Parkinson's disease dementia)*.)

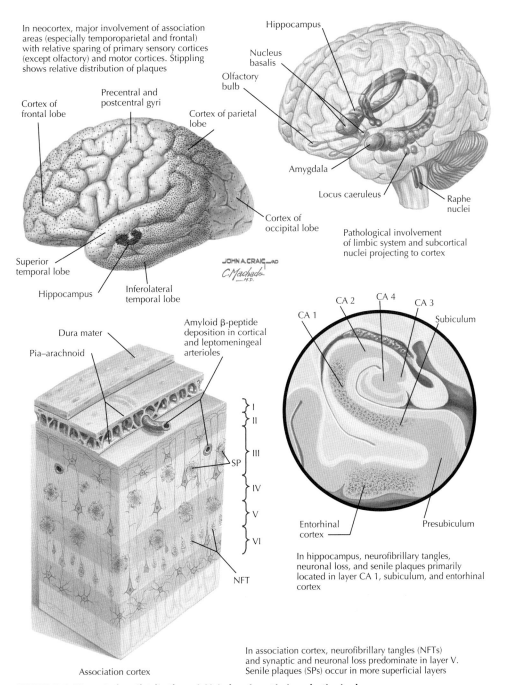

In neocortex, major involvement of association areas (especially temporoparietal and frontal) with relative sparing of primary sensory cortices (except olfactory) and motor cortices. Stippling shows relative distribution of plaques

Cortex of frontal lobe

Precentral and postcentral gyri

Cortex of parietal lobe

Cortex of occipital lobe

Superior temporal lobe

Hippocampus

Inferolateral temporal lobe

JOHN A. CRAIG—MD
C.Machado—M.D.

Hippocampus

Nucleus basalis

Olfactory bulb

Amygdala

Locus caeruleus

Raphe nuclei

Pathological involvement of limbic system and subcortical nuclei projecting to cortex

Dura mater

Pia–arachnoid

Amyloid β-peptide deposition in cortical and leptomeningeal arterioles

I
II
III
IV
V
VI

SP

NFT

Association cortex

CA 2   CA 4

CA 1   CA 3

Subiculum

Entorhinal cortex

Presubiculum

In hippocampus, neurofibrillary tangles, neuronal loss, and senile plaques primarily located in layer CA 1, subiculum, and entorhinal cortex

In association cortex, neurofibrillary tangles (NFTs) and synaptic and neuronal loss predominate in layer V. Senile plaques (SPs) occur in more superficial layers

FIGURE 2.1 The relative distribution of Alzheimer's pathology in the brain.

A color version of this figure is available online at http://www.expertconsult.com

---

BOX 2.1 COMMON SIGNS AND SYMPTOMS IN ALZHEIMER'S DISEASE

Memory
- Rapid forgetting
- Repeats questions and stories
- Loses items
- Puts items in wrong place
- Memory distortions

Language
- Word-finding difficulties
- Pauses in sentences
- Family members automatically filling in for missing words
- Word substitutions, either wrong word or a simpler word for a more complex one

Visuospatial
- Difficulty learning a new route
- Becomes confused or lost in familiar places

Reasoning and judgment (executive function)
- Makes poor decisions
- Difficulty planning and/or carrying out activities such as a simple repair or preparing a meal

Behavioral and psychiatric symptoms
- Apathy
- Depression
- Anxiety
- Irritability
- Delusions such as people are in the house or stealing money

---

Word-finding

After memory loss, difficulty finding words (often referred to as an anomia) is one of the most common symptoms of Alzheimer's disease. There are several areas of the brain that are critical for word-finding, the majority of which are affected by Alzheimer's disease. There is evidence to suggest that the lower, lateral portion of the temporal lobes is involved in the representations of words and their meanings (Damasio et al., 1996; Perani et al., 1999). This part of the brain is involved in our general store of conceptual and factual knowledge, such as the color of a lion or the first president of the United States, which is not related to any specific memory (see the section on Semantic memory in Appendix C: *Our current understanding of memory*). The frontal lobes, by contrast, are thought to be involved in the selection or choice of the particular word that is searched for (Balota et al., 1999). Both the inferolateral temporal lobes and the frontal lobes are affected by the pathology of Alzheimer's disease (Price & Morris, 1999) (Fig. 2.1).

Word-finding difficulties manifest in several different ways in patients with Alzheimer's disease. Frequently, patients will substitute a simpler word for a more complex one; later they may be unable to complete sentences. Sometimes there will be *circumlocutions*, in which patients will describe the word because they cannot retrieve it. For example, the patient may say, "He went to the place where they sell the food," referring to the grocery store. Some patients will refer to missing words by using generic terms, such as "Bring me the *whatchamacallit*" or "use the *thing* if you're going to do that." Family members become accustomed to filling in missing words. As the disease progresses, word substitutions (often referred to as paraphasic errors) occur. These word substitutions are typically not random, but instead are usually related to the word by meaning (often referred to as semantic paraphasic errors) or sound (often referred to as phonemic paraphasic errors). For example, the patient who meant to say "Are we going in the boat?" may instead say either "Are we going in the car?" or "Are we going in the coat?" Sometimes the speech is fluent, but is relatively uninformative (often called "empty speech"). For example, the patient may respond "I worked at my job," rather than mentioning a specific company or occupation, when asked what he or she did prior to retiring. As the disease progresses, speech may remain fluent, but almost devoid of content. For example, a patient attempting to describe what they did yesterday might say, "I went with my friend to the thing over there."

Getting lost

The parietal lobe is another region of the brain affected very early by Alzheimer's disease. The parietal lobe is involved in spatial function, and is particularly important for real-time spatial navigation, such as when walking or driving (Nitz, 2009). It is because of the parietal involvement in Alzheimer's disease that patients with the disorder often make wrong turns and become lost or confused. These difficulties occur even when traveling familiar routes, and patients with Alzheimer's disease have great difficulty planning new routes. Families often report that they suspected something was wrong when the patient became lost in an airport, couldn't find the way to a new place, or had to search the restaurant to find the right table after using the restroom. Later, the patient may become lost when going to a familiar location. For example, a patient we have cared for was trying to go to her doctor's office, a location that she had been to frequently for many years. Although it was only 20 minutes away in a neighboring town, she spent over 7 hours trying to find the office, driving through many towns which were far from the office. She ultimately gave up and went home.

Reasoning and judgment

Alzheimer's disease affects the frontal lobes, specifically the prefrontal cortex. This part of the frontal lobes is involved in many aspects of brain functioning, including problem solving, abstraction, reasoning, and judgment. These cognitive abilities are sometimes collectively referred to as *executive function*. The frontal lobes are also critical for attention, concentration, and working memory—the ability to temporarily maintain and manipulate information (see Appendix C: *Our current understanding of memory* for details).

Patients with Alzheimer's disease manifest difficulties in these areas in several different ways. Difficulties with complex tasks such as paying bills and balancing a checkbook occur frequently. They may be unable to perform tasks requiring even simple reasoning that would have been easy for them previously. For example, an electrical engineer may be unable to connect a DVD player to a television, and a gourmet cook may be unable to make anything but the simplest meals. They may also have difficulty planning and organizing a task such as a household repair or thanksgiving dinner.

Behavior issues

In addition to reasoning, judgment, and attention, the frontal lobes are involved in the control of behavior, as well as personality and affect. The amygdala, a small brain structure that is affected by Alzheimer's pathology early in the course of the disease, is also involved in regulation of behavior and affect. Over 80% of individuals diagnosed with Alzheimer's disease experience a change in behavior and affect at some point in the disease; these changes often occur early in the disease course and progress with the disease. Although how these changes manifest is somewhat variable, apathy is the most common behavioral change early in the disease, followed by irritability. As the disease progresses, many patients show an exacerbation of their previous personality characteristics. A person who was always competitive may become aggressive, whereas a person who was a wallflower may stop initiating conversation entirely. Sometimes patients exhibit more dramatic changes in personality, as when someone who was previously aggressive becomes passive, or vice versa. In general, however, the personality changes in Alzheimer's disease are relatively mild. Although the patient may be acting in a more aggressive or more passive manner than usual, family members still think of the patient as their "father" or "husband" acting differently, rather than as a completely different person (in contrast to many patients with frontotemporal dementia, see Chapter 7). Often these personality changes will not be apparent during the formal office evaluation or even in brief social settings. One good rule of thumb is that the patient with mild Alzheimer's disease can appear normal at a cocktail party for 5 minutes, and can "pull it together" in a doctor's office and behave normally during an evaluation. Because of this fact, it is important to discuss changes in behavior and personality during the interview with a family member or friend.

Several symptoms often result from the combination of frontal lobe dysfunction in conjunction with cognitive loss. Apathy and disinterest are two such symptoms. For example, an avid reader may not be able to remember enough of a book to enjoy it. A builder of model ships may no longer possess the attention, spatial, and problem-solving skills necessary to put together a model consisting of several hundred parts. Suspiciousness and paranoia are two other common symptoms that may result from frontal lobe dysfunction in conjunction with cognitive dysfunction. The usual scenario is that the patient puts his or her valuables away in a safe place so that they cannot be stolen, forgets where they were put, and then is certain that they were stolen—only to be found later.

Depression and anxiety

Depression and anxiety are extremely common in the earliest stages of Alzheimer's disease (Grut et al., 1993; Li et al., 2001; Zankd & Leipold, 2001). These symptoms are understandable, since there are few things as depressing and anxiety-provoking as realizing that one has memory loss or worrying that one has Alzheimer's disease. It has long been thought that depression is a common cause of memory problems. Although it is true that individuals with depression will often complain of memory problems, it has been our experience that it is more likely that patients with memory complaints in addition to depression or anxiety will have an underlying primary memory disorder such as Alzheimer's disease. We discuss the relationship between depression and Alzheimer's disease in Chapter 12: *Other disorders*.

Insight

An older rule of thumb that some clinicians have used is that if the patient complains of memory problems then he or she does not have a memory disorder; it is the patient who denies memory problems who has Alzheimer's disease or another dementia. This rule of thumb brings up the issue of insight. Commonly, patients in the very early stages of Alzheimer's disease—and those with the pre-Alzheimer's stage of mild cognitive impairment (MCI) (see Chapter 4: *Mild cognitive impairment* (MCI) for details)—show insight into their memory deficits (Grut et al., 1993). Occasionally, even patients with moderate Alzheimer's disease demonstrate preserved insight. In our experience younger patients, regardless of their disease stage, are more likely than older patients to demonstrate insight into their difficulties. Presumably this is attributable to younger patients having better preserved frontal lobe function than older patients. Thus, many patients in the very earliest stage of Alzheimer's disease are aware of and complain about their memory difficulties.

Function

Understanding the patient's ability to function is critical in any evaluation of memory loss. Part of the definition of dementia is that the patient has had a noticeable decline from their prior level of functioning. For mildly affected patients we often ask about their ability to organize and prepare meals (both simple and more involved for holiday gatherings), do volunteer or other work, pay bills, balance their checkbook, and go grocery shopping. For the more impaired patients we often ask about being able to take their medications independently, whether there is any wandering from the house, and whether there are any difficulties with bathing, dressing, and toileting. One good method of evaluating patients' level of function is to determine how they are doing in their basic and instrumental activities of daily living (Box 2.2).

BOX 2.2 ACTIVITIES OF DAILY LIVING AND INSTRUMENTAL ACTIVITIES OF DAILY LIVING

Knowing if a patient has difficulties with instrumental and/or basic activities of daily living is one way to quickly understand how much function the patient does and does not have. (See the section below in this chapter, *Evaluating function*, for additional information.)

Activities of daily living
- Bathing
- Dressing and undressing
- Eating
- Transferring from bed to chair and back
- Walking
- Control of bowel and bladder
- Using the toilet

Instrumental activities of daily living
- Light housework
- Preparing meals
- Taking medications
- Shopping for groceries and clothes
- Using the telephone
- Managing money and paying bills

REVIEW OF SYSTEMS

As with any disorder, it is important that the clinician conducts a review of systems that includes signs and symptoms of disorders in the differential diagnosis of memory loss. Ask about whether the following have ever occurred:

- a significant brain infection such as meningitis or encephalitis
- a significant head injury in which the patient lost consciousness
- a stroke or a transient ischemic attack
- a seizure
- fluctuating levels of alertness or periods of being relatively unresponsive
- visual hallucinations of people or animals
- a disturbance of gait
- falls
- a tremor
- rigidity and other signs of Parkinsonism
- a dramatic change in personality such that the patient seems like a different person
- any major psychiatric problems earlier in life, such as major depression or bipolar disease
- any weakness or numbness in the face or of an arm or a leg
- problems with fevers, chills, or night sweats
- problems with nausea, vomiting, or diarrhea
- problems with chest pain or shortness of breath
- any incontinence of bowel or bladder
- problems going to sleep (insomnia), staying asleep, or early morning awakening; any naps?
- acting out dreams during sleep or other abnormal movements while sleeping
- difficulty distinguishing dreams from reality when transitioning to and from sleep.

The significance of these signs and symptoms will be made clearer in Section II: *Differential Diagnosis of Memory Loss.*

MEDICAL HISTORY

In addition to obtaining a general medical history, it is worthwhile asking specifically about disorders that can predispose an individual to memory loss. These include the following, which are mainly related to cerebrovascular disease (note that disorders covered in the review of systems have not been repeated):

- hypertension
- hypercholesterolemia
- coronary artery disease
- atrial fibrillation and other cardiac arrhythmias
- obstructive sleep apnea.

ALLERGIES TO MEDICATIONS

When eliciting a history of allergies it is worthwhile to be attuned to two particular kinds of reactions to medications.

First, are there medications that caused significant confusion or agitation when administered? Susceptibility to confusion from medications may be present prior to the clinical onset of Alzheimer's disease or other dementia. Such medications may include narcotics such as Percocet or Darvocet, benzodiazepines such as diazepam and lorazepam, antihistamines such as Benadryl and Tylenol PM, and anticholinergic medications such as scopolamine and meclizine.

Second, are there reactions to medications used to treat Alzheimer's disease? If so, are these true allergic reactions to the medications, common side-effects, or rare and unusual problems? If side-effects to potential treatment medication are present (such as nausea to a cholinesterase inhibitor), these should be carefully noted. Discussions regarding how to best deal with side-effects to treatment medications are discussed in Section III: *Treatment of Memory Loss.*

SOCIAL HISTORY

Several elements of the social history are important when diagnosing memory loss.

Habits

Cigarette smoking, whether past or present, is of course a risk factor for cerebrovascular disease. Current smoking also poses a significant risk of fires, as the patient with memory loss may forget and leave their lit cigarette or cigar in a place where it may start a fire.

Alcohol use is important to ascertain for two reasons. First, when alcohol use is severe, it can cause memory loss from Wernicke–Korsakoff syndrome (see Chapter 12: *Other disorders*), and even more mild chronic alcohol use can cause frontal/executive dysfunction. Second, many patients with mild memory loss experience an exacerbation of their memory difficulties while drinking, and remember very little during the time that the alcohol is in their system. Some patients may become outright confused with as little as two glasses of wine. Patients may also not remember how many drinks they have had, and end up drinking too much. Lastly, patients with Alzheimer's disease may also be self-medicating for anxiety and/or depression.

Use or abuse of prescription medications and other drugs should also be elicited. Benzodiazepines and narcotics are all too commonly abused, and can explain an apparent dementia, particularly when fluctuations in mood, behavior, and cognition are present.

Education and occupation

When making a diagnosis of memory loss, particularly in a patient with very mild memory loss, it is critical to take into account the patient's education and previous occupation. We would, of course, expect that a college professor would score better on most standard cognitive tests than an individual with a lesser degree of education. Taking education and occupation into account is particularly important when interpreting standard cognitive tests. For example, scoring 28 out of 30 on the Mini-Mental State Examination (MMSE; Folstein et al., 1975) or making three errors out of 37 on the Blessed Dementia Scale (Blessed et al., 1968) may be normal for the 65-year-old factory worker with a 6th grade education, but would be very concerning for a retired physician of the same age with 20 years of education.

Does the patient have any longstanding prior problems with attention, memory, or other cognitive function, such as dyslexia, another learning disability, or attention-deficit hyperactivity disorder? Has she always had a poor memory for names? Did he always become lost when trying to find a new place? Understanding the patient's baseline memory and other cognitive abilities can help one interpret the current symptoms and the results of the cognitive tests appropriately.

Social supports

Patients with memory loss need the support of others. Support can be present in many forms, including emotional, financial, and assistance with daily function at many levels. Knowing what supports the patient has will help to guide treatment options such as whether prescribed medications can be complicated or need to be simple, and whether options such as day programs, moving in with a family member, or moving to an assisted living facility are available.

FAMILY HISTORY

Studies suggest that 25–40% of patients with Alzheimer's disease have a first-degree relative with the disorder (Jayadev et al., 2008). These statistics mean, of course, that there are more patients with Alzheimer's disease who do not have a first-degree relative with the disorder than those who do. This fact is probably attributable to a number of factors, including that the genetics of late-onset Alzheimer's disease are complex and that many times the parents of the patients died relatively young of other causes before they reached an age in which the disorder may have shown symptoms. Nonetheless, a family history of Alzheimer's disease can be a clue in a patient who presents with memory loss. Additionally, the family history may point to a disorder other than Alzheimer's disease, such as vascular disease, Parkinson's disease, or frontotemporal dementia.

We have found that it is best not to start by asking for a history of Alzheimer's disease, but instead to ask whether there is a history of memory loss late in life. Frequently the response will be something like, "yes, but they told me it was just 'senility,'" or "yes, but it was due to dementia, not Alzheimer's," or "yes, due to hardening of the arteries." Most of the time the correct diagnoses of these family members is Alzheimer's disease based upon what can be inferred from the history. Even a putative diagnosis of vascular or multi-infarct dementia in the era prior to the advent of CT and MRI was often Alzheimer's disease in reality. Similarly, the history of a parent or grandparent with a late-onset psychosis is much more likely to be a dementia (most commonly being due to Alzheimer's disease, frontotemporal dementia, or dementia with Lewy bodies) than a true primary psychotic disorder.

PHYSICAL EXAMINATION (see Box 2.3)
General physical examination

In evaluating memory loss, it is important to perform a thorough general physical examination. Many medical problems can contribute to memory difficulties, including congestive heart failure, pneumonia, and the like. Listening at the neck is useful because a carotid bruit, if found, may suggest cerebrovascular disease.

Neurological examination

There are three main types of abnormalities to look for on the neurological examination: signs of focal brain lesions, signs of other neurodegenerative disorders, and frontal release signs. Although an anatomical brain lesion should be detectable on an imaging study, it is still worthwhile to look for signs of brain pathology, such as focal weakness, brisk or asymmetric reflexes, and Babinski's sign. These focal signs may indicate a stroke, tumor, multiple sclerosis lesion, or other pathology.

BOX 2.3 RELEVANT ELEMENT OF THE NEUROLOGICAL EXAMINATION

Focal signs suggesting possible cerebrovascular disease or other cause of brain injury

- Neck auscultation (? carotid bruit)
- Focal weakness
- Asymmetric reflexes
- Extensor plantar (Babinski's sign)
- Focal sensory loss
- Visual field deficits
- Incoordination

Signs of possible extrapyramidal disease

- Tremor
- Rigidity
- Gait disorder

Signs of possible dementia

- Snout
- Grasp
- Palmomental reflex
- Apraxia (see Chapter 9: *Corticobasal degeneration*)

Unusual signs

- Alien limb (see Chapter 9: *Corticobasal degeneration*)
- Eye movement abnormalities (see Chapter 8: *Progressive supranuclear palsy*)

More important is to look for signs suggestive of other neurodegenerative diseases, since these will not typically show up on imaging or laboratory studies. For example, Parkinson's disease may present with a tremor, rigidity of the limbs, shuffling gait, a tendency to fall backwards, or all of these signs. Progressive supranuclear palsy, an atypical Parkinsonian syndrome, often presents with frequent falls, rigidity of the neck and spine, swallowing difficulty, and impaired voluntary gaze (i.e., difficulty moving the eyes to command, particularly up and down). We will discuss each of these disorders in greater detail in Section II: *Differential Diagnosis of Memory Loss*.

In our experience so-called frontal release signs are often more sensitive to the overall degree of bilateral brain pathology, and are not specific for frontal lobe dysfunction. These signs are discussed more below.

Tremor

One common etiology of tremor is "essential" tremor, a hereditary tremor, about 6–8 Hz, unrelated to other conditions (think of Katharine Hepburn in her later years). Another common cause is an enhanced physiological tremor. Everyone has a small amplitude, fast, physiological tremor, about 8–9 Hz, that can be noticeable when one is nervous or carrying something heavy. Physiological tremor can also be enhanced by medications, such as stimulants. A Parkinsonian tremor is slow, about 4–6 Hz, often present at rest (though can be with action), and is typically described as a "pill-rolling" tremor in the hands.

Rigidity

There are two main types of rigidity: one that primarily affects the limbs (appendicular rigidity) and one that primarily affects the neck and trunk (axial rigidity). Appendicular rigidity can often be brought out by using enhancement/distraction techniques such as drawing a circle in the air with the opposite hand. Parkinsonian rigidity is often described as "cogwheeling" when tremor is present and "lead pipe" when it is not. Axial rigidity is commonly tested by gently flexing the patient's neck.

Gait

Gait disorders are very common in the elderly, are often multifactorial, and are sometimes inscrutable. Two common gait disorders relevant for memory disorders are Parkinsonian gait disorders and frontal gait disorders. A Parkinsonian gait consists of slow, shuffling steps, which increase in speed after initiation. There is a tendency to retropulse and fall backwards. A frontal gait is sometimes described as a magnetic gait or (in French) a *marche à petits pas*, the walk of little steps. In a frontal gait disorder, the feet look like they are stuck to the floor, which is usually due to bilateral frontal subcortical white matter lobe pathology. The etiology of this bilateral frontal subcortical white matter pathology may in turn be due to small vessel ischemic vascular disease (as in a vascular dementia), normal pressure hydrocephalus, multiple sclerosis, traumatic brain injury, or other etiology.

Frontal release signs

Frontal release signs are so named because of the theory that these are reflexes present in infants that are inhibited once frontal lobes become myelinated; when the frontal lobes degenerate these infantile reflexes then become "released." In our experience these signs are more likely to be present with significant bilateral brain dysfunction, not necessarily confined to the frontal lobes. Frontal release signs are of little clinical importance in isolation, but can be helpful supportive evidence of a dementia when a patient presents with memory loss. Three of the more reliable frontal release signs are the snout, grasp, and palmomental reflexes.

Snout

The snout is commonly elicited by very gently tapping the broad aspect of the reflex hammer against the lips. It is a good idea to warn the patient that you are going to tap gently on their lips, and to make sure that the mouth is closed. If the lips protrude outward when they are tapped, this is an abnormal response. The snout is thought to be related to the rooting response observed in infants. Sometimes the lips and mouth open as the hammer approaches; this may indicate a visual suck response—another frontal release sign that is typically present in the more advanced dementia.

Grasp

A grasp response may be elicited in several different ways. One is to have the patient put their hands in a prone, palm down, relaxed position, and then to use your fingertips to stroke gently upwards as you move from palm to fingertips. The abnormal response is for the patient to close down and grasp your fingers. Sometimes the normal patient may not be clear what you are doing or what you want them to do and may grab your hand as well. For this reason, if the patient grasps your hands, repeat the action while instructing the patient not to hold your hand. If the grasp is strongly present, it will be apparent even when you tell the patient not to hold your hand, and also with different types of contact across the palm. The grasp is thought to be related to the reflex, common in infants, when they tightly hold your finger in their hand.

Palmomental reflex

When the palmomental reflex is present, the mentalis muscle of the chin below the lower lip contracts when the palm is stroked. The stroke in the palm may be performed by gently flicking the thumbnail from lower ulnar surface of the palm, up and across the palm to the base of the index finger. You must be watching the mentalis muscle as you do this, as it occurs quickly if present. The reflex often quickly habituates, so that it may only be present the first time it is performed in a several minute interval. There is one palmomental reflex on each side.

COGNITIVE TESTS AND QUESTIONNAIRES

Although the interview with the patient and informant(s) provides a wealth of information and may be in and of itself sufficient to make a preliminary diagnosis, supplementing the history with the results of cognitive tests and questionnaires is crucial. Our general approach is to both conduct an interview and perform cognitive tests. Cognitive tests can be performed by the clinician in the office, or as part of a formal neuropsychological evaluation by a neuropsychologist.

A neuropsychological evaluation for memory loss typically includes an interview with the patient and family member (or other caregiver), 4–6 hours of cognitive testing with the patient, and one or more functional activity questionnaires to be filled out by the family member or caregiver. Recommendations are made regarding further diagnostic tests and treatment.

Cognitive instruments can be used for a variety of purposes. First, they may be used to screen for subtle cognitive dysfunction. For example, some primary care practices are now using cognitive tests and questionnaires to screen for Alzheimer's disease. A second purpose is to determine the degree of cognitive impairment. For example, we might use a test to classify an Alzheimer's disease patient as mild, moderate or severe. A third purpose of cognitive testing is to help with diagnosis. Aiding diagnosis is possible because certain test result patterns are suggestive of different causes of dementing illness. For example, neuropsychological evaluation may be helpful in distinguishing between dementia caused by Alzheimer's disease and dementia caused by frontotemporal dementia. In general, using cognitive tests for differential diagnosis will not be carried out in primary care practices, but rather in the context of referral to specialists including behavioral neurologists and neuropsychologists.

There are numerous brief measures of cognition that can be helpful to the clinician. Several of these are discussed briefly below; see Appendix B: *Screening for memory loss* for more detail. One of the earliest, and still the most widely used, instruments is the Mini-Mental State Examination (Folstein et al., 1975; often referred to as the MMSE or the "Folstein" after its developer). The MMSE is often used for initial screening for cognitive dysfunction and is also for staging patients (mild, moderate, or severe dementia) based-upon the score. The Blessed Information, Memory, and Concentration (Blessed et al., 1968; BIMC) test is a similar test that is primarily used for screening in day-to-day practice. Both of these instruments briefly and quickly evaluate cognitive domains that can be affected by dementia including orientation, memory, attention, and concentration.

Since the development of these early instruments there have been many more contemporary instruments developed and validated. These contemporary instruments have the advantage of being based on recent developments in the neuropsychology of dementia and, as such, may be more accurate.

In this section we will briefly review these instruments. We begin with the two "standards," the MMSE and the Blessed Information-Memory-Concentration test. These tests are generally used to assess overall mental status and as noted can be used to screen for cognitive dysfunction. We also consider a newer version of an overall mental status test, the MoCA (the Montreal Cognitive Assessment; www.mocatest.org). We then discuss single neuropsychological tests that can be sensitive to Alzheimer's disease and other dementing illnesses. We conclude by considering a relatively new approach that appears to be highly accurate: combining multiple single cognitive tests into a very brief (5–10 minutes) screening battery. There are, of course, many brief tests of cognition which can also be used. Rather than advocating for a particular test, we believe it is most important that clinicians become comfortable with a test that is helpful for differentiating normal versus impaired cognition in their patient population. Please see Appendix A: *Cognitive test and questionnaire forms, instructions, and normative data* for samples of some of these tests and additional details on the use and administration of these and other cognitive tests.

Mental status screening tests
The Mini-Mental State Examination

Published by Folstein, Folstein, and McHugh in 1975, the MMSE is one of the most widely used tests in clinical medicine for assessing a patient's overall cognitive function (Folstein et al., 1975). A revised version is now available, published by Psychological Assessment Resources, Inc. (Lutz, Florida); more information about it is available online at www.minimental.com.

The MMSE evaluates orientation to time and place, recent memory, attention/concentration, praxis, and language. It is scored on a 30-point scale, with 30 as a perfect score. A rule of thumb is that patients with Alzheimer's disease who are untreated decline at a rate of about 2 or 3 points a year.

The advantages of the MMSE include that it is well known, it is easy to administer in about 5–10 minutes, it samples a number of cognitive functions, and it has test–retest and inter-rater reliability. A limitation is that only three words are to be remembered on the recall test, making the MMSE insensitive for patients with mild but clinically relevant memory problems. Another limitation is that the interval between registration and recall is not standard; instead, it is dependent upon the time it takes for the patient to perform the attention and calculation section. Thus, patients who take a long time to complete the attention and calculation section will end up with a more difficult memory test than those who complete the attention and calculation section more quickly. Lastly, the MMSE is not sensitive in detecting frontal/executive dysfunction.

Numerous studies have evaluated the MMSE in the last 30 years. When using the MMSE as a screening instrument for cognitive dysfunction, we favor flexible cut-offs with the understanding that a result below this number does not definitively indicate dementia or other cognitive impairment, but suggests that a more thorough evaluation is warranted. Scores which warrant concern are those below 29 for adults younger than 50 years old, below 28 for those aged 50–79 years, and below 26 for those aged 80–89 years (Bleecker et al., 1988). In addition to age, lower levels of education are also associated with lower scores in the absence of cognitive impairment.

When reporting the results of the MMSE, we encourage clinicians to report which items were missed in addition to the total score. The implications of scoring 26 out of 30 may be very different depending upon which items are missed. For example, a patient who misses all three of the recall items and the date shows evidence of episodic memory dysfunction, whereas the patient who misses only four points on the attention and calculation section does not.

The Blessed Dementia Scale

In 1968 Blessed, Tomlinson, and Roth published a study that correlated the number of senile plaques in several areas of the cortex of the brain in dementia patients with two quantitative measures of dementia severity (Blessed et al., 1968). One measure is a brief cognitive test given to patients, now known as the BIMC test. Another is a brief caregiver questionnaire now known as the Blessed Dementia Scale. These measures may be used together or separately.

The BIMC test is similar to the MMSE in that it measures orientation for time and place, recent memory, and attention and concentration. It also measures orientation for person, as well as personal information (autobiographical memory). It does not, however, measure praxis or language.

Note that the number of impaired responses (or errors) is commonly reported for the Blessed, rather than the number of unimpaired (or correct) responses. Thus, the most severely demented patient would score 28 on the caregiver scale and 37 on the BIMC test. For the caregiver scale, scoring less than 4 suggests that the patient is unimpaired; a score from 4 to 9 suggests mild impairment; scores higher that 10 suggest moderate to severe impairment (Eastwood et al., 1983). For the BIMC test, fewer than 4 errors suggests no impairment, 4–10 errors suggests mild impairment, 11–16 errors suggests moderate impairment, and more than 16 errors suggests severe impairment (Locascio et al., 1995). Untreated patients decline approximately 3 or 4 points per year.

As with the MMSE, when reporting the results of the Blessed, we encourage clinicians to report which items were missed in addition to the total score.

The Montreal Cognitive Assessment (MoCA)

This recently developed instrument (Nasreddine et al., 2005) evaluates orientation, memory, attention, language (naming), executive function, and visuospatial function. In head-to-head studies with the MMSE the MoCA appears more sensitive in detecting patients with MCI and Alzheimer's disease (Nasreddine et al., 2005).

The MoCA has a number of advantages as a screening test for memory loss and dementia. First, the test and instructions are freely available on a website, www.mocatest.org (see also Appendix A: *Cognitive test and questionnaire forms, instructions, and normative data*). Second, it has clear instructions and scoring. Third, it has been translated into 21 languages. Fourth, it covers a variety of cognitive domains. Its main limitations are that it is still quite new, normative data are limited, and it is not as well known as the older tests. The value of the MoCA will become clearer over time.

Single neuropsychological tests

Clock drawing test

The clock drawing test (CDT) is a rapidly administered test that is appropriate for primary care practices. Although there are multiple versions of this test, in general, they all ask the patient to draw the face of a clock and then to draw the hands to indicate a particular time. This single test may be sensitive to dementia because it involves many cognitive areas that can be affected by dementia, including executive function, visuospatial abilities, motor programming, and attention and concentration. Telling analogue time is a complex and demanding cognitive function. Many of our patients have difficulty with analogue watches in the early stages of a dementing illness (we often address this problem by suggesting they wear a digital watch). We would also note that children typically learn to read and write before they learn to tell analogue time.

There are many versions of the Clock Drawing Test, in terms of both administration procedures and scoring. We have used and validated a relatively straightforward system that is easy to administer and accurate (see Appendix A: *Cognitive test and questionnaire forms, instructions, and normative data* for details).

Category fluency

The category fluency test requires that the subject names as many members of a semantic category as possible in a fixed period of time – typically 1 minute. This type of test has been shown to be sensitive to Alzheimer's disease. One easily and quickly administered version of the category fluency test is animal naming. Patients are simply asked to name all the animals they can in 60 seconds. The total number of animals they name produces the score (Box 2.4) (see Appendix A: *Cognitive test and questionnaire forms, instructions, and normative data* for details).

Delayed word recall

This test was initially described by Knopman & Ryberg (1989) and takes advantage of the finding that healthy elderly individuals benefit from mnemonic strategies that facilitate the storage and retrieval of information whereas patients with dementia show substantially less benefit from some strategies. In an attempt to capture this as a brief memory test, Knopman and colleagues showed a list of 10 words to patients with Alzheimer's disease (and healthy elderly controls) and asked that they make up a sentence using each word. The rationale was that, by asking the subjects to make up a sentence, they were assuring that each individual was paying attention to the word and relating it to other words and concepts with which they were familiar. After a 5-minute delay, they asked the participants to recall as many of the 10 words as possible in any order. Patients with Alzheimer's disease typically recalled four or fewer words, while healthy elderly subjects typically recalled five or more.

Trailmaking A and B

These are two parts of a well-established neuropsychological test that was developed during World War II. "Trails" is generally sensitive to brain damage and is particularly sensitive to executive dysfunction. It consists of two parts (trails A and B) and takes 5 minutes to administer. In trails A the patient is given a single sheet of paper that contains 25 small circles consecutively numbered from 1 to 25. The circles are placed randomly on the page. The patient is asked to draw lines to join the consecutively numbered circles. In trails B, half the circles contain numbers and half letters, and the patient's job is to connect alternating consecutive numbers and letters (e.g., 1, A, 2, B, 3 etc. . . .). Scoring is simply the time it takes to complete the task. If a subject makes a mistake, the administrator points out the mistake and asks the subject to correct it before proceeding (imposing a time penalty).

BOX 2.4 INTERPRETING CATEGORY FLUENCY

A quick rule of thumb for determining performance on the category fluency test is that the individual should name approximately the number of animals that equals their number of years of education (e.g., a high school graduate has 12 years) plus 4.

Trails A requires attention, visual search, and psychomotor speed and trails B adds sequencing, working memory, and set shifting, which are all sensitive to executive/frontal lobe functioning. We have found this test particularly useful when we suspect frontal lobe dementias.

Screening instruments that combine single tests
The Mini-Cog
Developed in 2000, the Mini-Cog consists simply of three words which must be memorized (like the MMSE) and then recalled after the drawing of a clock with the hands at 10 minutes after 11 o'clock; the circle is provided (Borson et al., 2005). As a screening tool for dementia, the test is considered negative (i.e., no dementia) if either all three words are recalled or at least one word is recalled with a normal clock; the test is considered positive (i.e., suggestive of dementia) if no words are recalled or if fewer than three words are recalled with an abnormal clock.

The Mini-Cog has been shown to have good sensitivity and specificity. In a head-to-head comparison, it was equal to or better than the MMSE in detecting dementia in early-stage patients (Borson et al., 2005). Compared with the MMSE, the Mini-Cog is relatively insensitive to the level of education. It has also been shown to be accurate in multicultural settings, primarily because it relies minimally on language abilities. We agree that, when the Mini-Cog is positive (suggesting dementia), the patient likely has cognitive impairment. However, the criteria for a negative test are too insensitive to make the Mini-Cog a good instrument for screening. We would therefore be cautious in using the Mini-Cog.

The 7 Minute Screen
Like the Blessed, the 7 Minute Screen was also developed for use in dementia. In 1998 Solomon and colleagues published the first report of a screening assessment they developed consisting of four subtests: orientation (month, date, year, day, time), memory (16 items, four at a time, cued and uncued), clock drawing, and verbal fluency (naming animals in 1 minute) (Solomon et al., 1998). Unlike most tests, however, the interpretation is performed automatically by entering the results of the four subtests into a special calculator or website (http://www.memorydoc.org), leading to a high or low probability that the patient has Alzheimer's disease. (The calculated formula is based upon the results of a logistic regression comparing 60 patients with Alzheimer's disease and 60 healthy control subjects.) The 7 Minute Screen demonstrates sensitivity, specificity, test–retest reliability, and interrater reliability all greater than 90%. The test has been validated in the primary care setting as a screening tool for patients over the age of 60 (Solomon et al., 2000), and it has also been validated in other languages (Tsolaki et al., 2002; Meulen et al., 2004).

Advantages of this test include that it is sensitive, reliable, easy to administer, takes little time, and the interpretation is performed automatically. The main limitation is that a calculator is needed for interpretation, although now that most clinicians have ready Web access this issue is rarely a problem. If the result from the calculator reads "HI," the patient has a high probability of dementia characteristic of Alzheimer's disease, and it is suggested that the patient undergoes a full diagnostic evaluation. The test instructions caution (and we agree) that it is inappropriate to diagnose Alzheimer's disease based only on the results of the 7 Minute Screen. If the calculator reads "LO," the patient has a low probability of dementia characteristic of Alzheimer's disease; in this circumstance, the patient may or may not need further evaluation depending upon the history and clinical setting. In less than 5% of cases the calculator may also indicate that the data are insufficient to make a judgment; in this situation, either using other evaluation measures or rescreening the patient in 6–9 months would be appropriate.

Caregiver-completed questionnaires

Screening instruments generally fall into two categories: clinician-administered neuropsychological instruments or questionnaires that are completed by the patient and/or an informant. Informant-based questionnaires may be preferable to other methods because: (1) they require no time from medical professionals, (2) they do not require the cooperation of the patient, (3) they can potentially be completed via telephone, mail or Internet, and (4) they can be completed by the informant confidentially. It is for these reasons that the most recent trend in screening for cognitive dysfunction is a questionnaire completed by the caregiver. In general, these questionnaires ask someone who knows the patient well to answer a series of questions about the patient's memory and other cognitive functions. Because they are typically completed in the waiting room, the results can be made available to the clinician before he or she sees the patient. These caregiver-completed questionnaires are as accurate as the clinician-administered instruments. Examples of caregiver-completed questionnaires are the IQCODE, the Alzheimer's disease Caregiver Questionnaire, and the AD8 Dementia Screening Interview.

IQCODE

The IQCODE (the Informant Questionnaire on Cognitive Decline in the Elderly) is a 26-item questionnaire in which informants are asked to rate the degree of change in the patient's memory and intelligence over a 10-year period (Jorm & Jacomb, 1989). This rating is done on a five-point scale: much improved, a bit improved, not much change, a bit worse, much worse. Subsequent research has shown that a shortened 16-item version is just as accurate as the 26-item questionnaire (Jorm, 1994). Research has shown the IQCODE to be as sensitive as the MMSE in detecting patients with dementia (Jorm, 2004). The overall accuracy of the IQCODE ranged from 80% to 85% in detecting patients with dementia.

Alzheimer's Disease Caregiver Questionnaire

The Alzheimer's Disease Caregiver Questionnaire (ADCQ) is an 18-item yes/no questionnaire that can be completed by a caregiver in 5–10 minutes. It asks questions regarding multiple aspects of cognition, including memory, language, executive function, visuospatial abilities, and praxis. It also asks questions regarding functional abilities, mood, and behavior, as well as progression of symptoms. Validation studies have indicated that the instrument approaches 90% accuracy in determining which patients have symptoms of dementia suggestive of Alzheimer's disease (Solomon et al., 2003; Solomon & Murphy, 2008). The ADCQ can be completed either online (ADCQ.net) or in paper and pencil format (which can be later scored online). The online scoring program produces a caregiver report that contains a summary of the cognitive areas that appear problematic and the likelihood that the individual is experiencing symptoms of Alzheimer's disease. This report can then be discussed with the physician during the patient visit (see Appendix A: *Cognitive test and questionnaire forms, instructions, and normative data* for additional information.)

AD8 Dementia Screening Interview

The AD8 Dementia Screening Interview (AD8) is an eight-item questionnaire that can be completed by the caregiver. For each question the caregiver indicates "Yes" there has been a change in the patient's ability, "No" there has not been a change in the patient's ability or "N/A, don't know" they are unable to rate the item (Galvin et al., 2005, 2007). The score is simply the number of endorsed "Yes" items. The authors state that it is preferable for the questionnaire to be answered by the informant, but suggest that the patient can also complete it. They state that a score of 0 or 1 suggests normal cognition and a score of 2 or greater suggests that cognitive impairment is likely to be present. When administered to either the informant or the patient, the sensitivity is >84% and the specificity greater than 80% (see Appendix A: *Cognitive test and questionnaire forms, instructions, and normative data* for additional information).

SCREENING IN THE CLINIC (Box 2.5)

When and who to screen

As with any other disease, there is debate about whom to screen and how often to screen. Recently a set of guidelines has been suggested (Solomon & Murphy, 2005) and these have been adopted by several groups. These guidelines suggest that screening should be routine for people over 65 or those who have memory complaints, raised by either the patient or family, and that the frequency of screening be increased as individuals age and the probability of a dementing illness increases. Table 2.2 summarizes these guidelines.

How to interpret a screen (Table 2.3)

Positive screens

As is the case for screening instruments for all diseases, a positive memory screen should not be used to make a diagnosis of Alzheimer's disease or other dementia. Instead, a positive screen provides the opportunity to discuss the results with the patient and family and encourages patients to undergo a full diagnostic evaluation. We always emphasize that this

---

BOX 2.5 RECOMMENDATIONS FOR IN-OFFICE SCREENING

Clinicians often ask us if we have specific recommendations for in-office screening procedures. As we have discussed, there are many potentially useful screening instruments and what is most valuable is to routinely use one or two so that you gain comfort and familiarity with administering and interpreting the instrument. In terms of specific suggestions, we generally try to use both a clinician-administered instrument and a caregiver-completed instrument. Below are two recommended combinations that you may find helpful.

The 7 Minute Screen and the Alzheimer's Disease Caregiver Questionnaire (ADCQ)

We routinely use these two instruments that were developed in our centers. We find that input from both the patient and caregiver is useful. In some instances the patient comes alone and, of course, in these cases we use the 7 Minute Screen in the office and have a member of the clinic staff administer the ADCQ over the phone. Another advantage of the ADCQ is that this questionnaire can be filled out by one individual for multiple family members—only one of whom may be the identified patient—if there is concern about memory and/or other behavioral and functional issues for additional family members who may or may not be present at the visit.

The Montreal Cognitive Assessment (MoCA) and the AD8 Dementia Screening Interview (AD8)

A second combination of instruments that are being widely adopted are the MoCA, a clinician-administered instrument, and the AD8. Both are easily administered and accurate. Although these are relatively new and we do not have extensive experience with either, the published data from each and our experience to date indicate that they may be appropriate for in-office screening.

Table 2.2 Recommendations for screening for Alzheimer's disease in primary care practice

Age range	Prevalence	Recommendation
65–74	3%	Discretionary, based on risk factors including family history and cognitive complaints from either patients or family
75–84	19%	Every 2 years or if there are cognitive complaints from either patients or family
>85	47%	Annually

After Solomon, P.R., Murphy, C.A., 2005. Should we screen for Alzheimer's disease? A review of the evidence for and against screening Alzheimer's disease in primary care practice. Geriatrics, 60, 26–31.

Table 2.3 Summary of characteristics of various screening instruments

Instrument	Administration time	Level of clinical judgment/training to administer/score	Sensitivity	Specificity
Clinician-administered instruments				
Mini-Mental State Examination	5–10 minutes	Moderate	80–90%	<80%
Neurobehavioral Cognitive Status Examination	>10 minutes	Moderate	Not reported for dementia	Not reported for dementia
7 Minute Screen	5–10 minutes	Minimal (Web-based)	>90%	>90%
Time and Change Test	<5 minutes	Minimal	>90%	80–90% (dementia) >90% (Alzheimer's)
Clock drawing	Not reported	Moderate	80–90%	80–90%
The Mini-Cog	<5 minutes	Moderate	>90%	>90%
Informant-completed instruments				
Informant Questionnaire on Cognitive Decline in the Elderly	Not reported	Minimal	80–90%	80–90%
Alzheimer's Disease Caregiver Questionnaire	Not reported	Minimal (Web-based)	80–90%	80–90%
Symptoms of Dementia Screen	Not reported	Minimal	80–90%	80–90%

is only a screen and does not mean that the person has Alzheimer's disease. Rather it just means that we should carry out a more complete evaluation. We find that using the analogy of false positives for mammography for breast cancer often helps the patient and family understand the process. In our experience most patients and caregivers readily agree to an evaluation.

Negative screens

A negative screen provides the opportunity to reassure the patient and family that, although there are changes in memory that occur as people age, they are most likely a normal part of the aging process. Again, in most cases, the patients are accepting of this and indeed often relieved. Occasionally, a caregiver will tell us that, despite what the screen indicates, this is not the same person they knew a year ago and would like a more comprehensive evaluation. In these cases we almost always proceed with a full diagnostic evaluation.

Neuropsychological evaluation

In most cases, comprehensive neuropsychological evaluation is not necessary to make a diagnosis of Alzheimer's disease. A careful taking of history combined with office-based cognitive screening will usually provide the necessary information for making a diagnosis. In some cases, however, neuropsychological testing may be helpful. Neuropsychological evaluation consists of standardized tests which evaluate multiple cognitive areas, including: memory; executive function including reasoning, judgment, and problem-solving; language; visuospatial functioning; praxis; and attention. Additionally, the neuropsychologist will screen for mood, including anxiety and depression, and functional deficits (e.g., activities of daily living). He or she will also obtain a complete history of cognitive complaints. A typical neuropsychological evaluation takes 4–6 hours and is generally conducted in a single day.

In our experience, neuropsychological evaluation can be beneficial:

- when family members continue to be concerned, even in the presence of normal office-based cognitive screening
- when the patient has high premorbid intellectual functioning resulting in performing in the "normal" range on office-based screening instruments at the same time the family is reporting cognitive decline
- when a pre-existing cognitive problem is present such as mental retardation due to, for example, Down's syndrome or traumatic brain injury
- when a coexisting psychiatric condition is present
- to help with differential diagnosis, e.g. Lewy body disease vs. Alzheimer's disease or frontal lobe dementia vs. Alzheimer's disease.

Screening for depression

Depression is common in the elderly and even more common in patients with Alzheimer's disease. Major depressive disorder occurs in about 1–3% of community-dwelling elderly and in 10–15% of elderly patients in hospital and nursing home settings (Rinaldi et al., 2003). As many as 15–27% of the elderly have a subsyndromal depression that does not meet criteria for a specific depressive syndrome (Lebowitz et al., 1997). In Alzheimer's disease patients, the prevalence of depression is nearly 50%.

Because the symptoms of depression can overlap some of the symptoms of dementia, the two diseases can be confused. Further complicating the picture is recent evidence suggesting that the late-life onset of depression signals the onset of Alzheimer's disease. As such, clinicians should be suspicious of an emerging dementia in elderly patients who exhibit new-onset depression.

We will discuss in Chapter 12: *Other disorders*, some strategies for discriminating between cognitive deficits due to depression alone and those due to Alzheimer's disease, with or without comorbid depression. For now, we would just note that any evaluation for possible Alzheimer's disease should include a screen for depression. There are several instruments that may be helpful. We have found the Geriatric Depression Scale (GDS; either the 5-, 10-, 15-, or 30-item version) and the somewhat longer Neuropsychiatric Inventory (NPI) to be useful in detecting depression and other psychiatric symptoms in the elderly.

The Geriatric Depression Scale

The Geriatric Depression Scale (GDS) was designed specifically to screen for depression in geriatric populations. Therefore, it taps the affective and behavioral symptoms of depression and excludes most symptoms that may be confused with somatic disease (e.g., slowness, insomnia, sexuality) or dementia.

The original GDS is a 30-item yes/no self-report questionnaire completed by the patient that is widely used to screen for depression in the elderly. The instrument is most commonly used in primary care settings, geriatric clinics, and hospitals. The purpose of the scale is somewhat disguised to the patient by the title "Mood Assessment Scale." Shorter forms of the GDS have been developed and the 15-item and 10-item version are the most commonly used. The 15-item version takes about 5–7 minutes to complete. Less is known about the 5-item version (Table 2.4) but data suggest that accuracy can approach that of the 15-item version (Rinaldi et al., 2003).

Neuropsychiatric Inventory (NPI)

The Neuropsychiatric Inventory is a relatively brief interview with a family member or friend who knows the patient well and can evaluate 12 behavioral areas commonly affected in patients with dementia, including depression (Box 2.6). It is also routinely used to evaluate the effects of treatment on these symptoms. Evaluation in each of the 12 areas begins with a yes/no screening question. If the screening question is answered "Yes," the interviewer follows with additional questions.

Table 2.4 The 5-item Geriatric Depression Scale

Question: Over the past week…	Positive answer for depression screening
Are you basically satisfied with your life?	No
Do you often get bored?	Yes
Do you often feel helpless?	Yes
Do you prefer to stay home rather than going out and doing new things?	Yes
Do you feel pretty worthless the way you are now?	Yes
Depressed patients are likely to have >2 positive answers.	

BOX 2.6 NEUROPSYCHIATRIC INVENTORY (NPI)

Description of the NPI

The NPI consists of 12 behavioral areas:

1. Delusions
2. Hallucinations
3. Agitation
4. Depression
5. Anxiety
6. Euphoria
7. Apathy
8. Disinhibition
9. 9. Irritability
10. Aberrant motor behavior
11. Night-time behaviors
12. Appetite and eating disorders

Frequency is rated as:

1. Occasionally – less than once a week
2. Often – about once per week
3. Frequently – several times a week but less than every day
4. Very frequently – daily or essentially continuously present

Severity is rated as:

Mild – produces little distress in the patient
Moderate – more disturbing to the patient but can be redirected by the caregiver
Severe –very disturbing to the patient and difficult to redirect

Distress is scored as:

0 – no distress
1 – minimal
2 – mild
3 – moderate
4 – moderately severe
5 – very severe or extreme

For each domain there are four scores: frequency, severity, total (frequency x severity) and caregiver distress. The total possible score is 144 (i.e., a maximum of 4 in the frequency rating x 3 in the severity rating x 12 remaining domains)

A clinician generally administers the instrument in about 10 minutes. The scoring reflects not only the effect on the patient, but also the extent to which the symptom causes distress in the caregiver. There is also a brief version, the Neuropsychiatric Inventory Questionnaire (NPI-Q), that takes only 5 minutes to administer and may be more appropriate for primary care settings.

Evaluating function

Often one of the first signs of cognitive decline is difficulty performing day-to-day activities, often called activities of daily living (ADLs) (Fig. 2.2 and Box 2.2: *Activities of daily living and instrumental activities of daily living*). Validated scales that rate

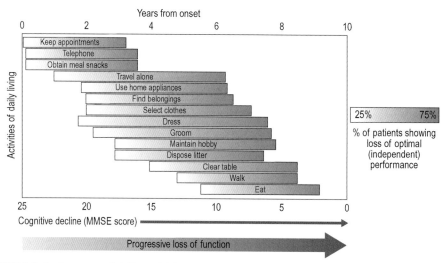

FIGURE 2.2 Performance of daily activities declines as Alzheimer's disease worsens.

From Galasko D. An integrated approach to the management of Alzheimer's disease: assessing cognition, function, and behaviour. Eur J Neurol. 1998;5:S9-S17.

activities of daily living are helpful in initial diagnosis as well as tracking progression and determining the effectiveness of treatment. Because these scales are completed by the caregiver, they are appropriate for primary care practices.

Functional Activities Questionnaire

The Functional Activities Questionnaire (FAQ) evaluates ADLs such as preparing meals, writing checks, and participating in hobbies (Pfeffer et al., 1982). The FAQ is completed by a family member or friend who routinely observes the patient in his or her day-to-day activities. The informant rates the patient in 10 areas (Box 2.7) as: dependent (on others to complete the task) (3 points), requires assistance (2 points), had difficulty, but performs independently (1 point), or performs independently with no difficulty (0 points). Scores range from 0 to 30, with higher scores indicating more functional difficulty. Scores higher than 10 suggest reduced functional ability.

BOX 2.7 ACTIVITIES OF DAILY LIVING RATED IN THE FUNCTIONAL ASSESSMENT QUESTIONNAIRE

1. Writing checks and maintaining other financial records
2. Assembling tax or business records
3. Shopping alone for clothes, household necessities, or groceries
4. Playing a game or skill or working on a hobby
5. Heating water for coffee or tea, turning off the stove
6. Preparing a balanced meal
7. Keeping track of current events
8. Paying attention to and understanding a TV show, book, or magazine
9. Remembering appointment, family occasions, holidays, or medications
10. Traveling out of the neighborhood (e.g., driving or arranging to take buses)

LABORATORY STUDIES
General laboratory studies

Although not causes of dementia, impairments in the function of almost any system of the body can impair cognition. Medical problems typically produce a delirium (also referred to as an encephalopathy), which impairs cognition by disrupting attention. We recommend obtaining general screening laboratory studies, including the electrolytes sodium (Na^+), potassium (K^+), chloride (Cl^-), and calcium (Ca^{++}); measures of renal function, including blood urea nitrogen (BUN) and creatinine (Cr), measures of liver function, including aspartate aminotransferase (AST), alanine aminotransferase (ALT), and bilirubin; measures of blood cells, including red blood cell count (RBC), possible signs of infection such as the white blood cell count (WBC), and general measures of inflammation including erythrocyte sedimentation rate (ESR).

Causes of reversible cognitive dysfunction

The two laboratory studies which are absolutely necessary to obtain are levels of vitamin B12 and thyroid-stimulating hormone (TSH), as abnormalities of both of these are common in the older adult and can impair cognition. There are several other laboratory studies which are worth carrying out if there is a clinical suspicion that they would be helpful.

Vitamin B12 deficiency is very common in older adults, owing primarily to a loss of intrinsic factor, a hormone released in the stomach that is necessary for B12 to be absorbed. Thus, B12 deficiency is typically not associated with diet, and oral vitamin supplementation will not correct the B12 loss. B12 is stored in the liver, and because of this the level can be normal for some months or more after the time when the patient can no longer absorb it. B12 deficiency can present in many different ways, including as a macrocytic anemia, as hyper-reflexia and loss of posterior column function (loss of joint position and vibration senses) when it is often called subacute combined degeneration, as a peripheral neuropathy, and—most relevant for this book—as a neuropsychiatric syndrome affecting mood and cognition. Fatigue, lethargy, sleepiness, and depression are the most prevalent symptoms, but loss of memory is also commonly reported. The treatment of B12 deficiency is either monthly parenteral injections of B12 (usually at a dose of 1000 micrograms), or nasal cyanocobalamin (Nascobal) taken weekly. Oral supplementation is not effective because of the inability to absorb B12. Once adequate stores have been built up in the liver, the frequency of injections can be reduced to every 2–4 months.

Thyroid disorders are also very common in older adults. In hypothyroidism, the usual cause of thyroid hormone deficiency is failure of the thyroid gland itself, and thus an elevation of the pituitary-derived TSH is the usual sign of hypothyroidism. Hypothyroidism may cause impaired memory, difficulty concentrating because of slowing of cognition, irritability, mood instability, and occasionally psychosis. Hyperthyroidism also presents with difficulty concentrating; here it is attributable to increased distractibility and restlessness. Hyperthyroidism may cause difficulty with memory as well as irritability, apathy, depression, and delirium.

Screening for *Lyme disease* should be considered in the appropriate clinical context by obtaining an enzyme immunoassay or immunofluorescent assay for IgG, with appropriate follow-up if positive with a western immunoblot for both IgG and IgM for confirmation. Lyme disease is common and even endemic in many areas of the country, and has replaced syphilis as the "great mimicker," often presenting as other diseases. Cognitively, Lyme disease presents with a primary impairment in attention. Patients can become disorganized, easily distracted, and somnolent. We have diagnosed a number of patients with Lyme disease who presented clinically with memory loss.

Although screening for **neurosyphilis** by obtaining an rapid plasma reagent is no longer routinely recommended, it is still worthwhile to consider it, particularly if the patient is immunocompromised. For example, neurosyphilis is now most common in patients with HIV infection. Neurosyphilis causing dementia (also known as "general paresis of the insane") is extremely rare, but can present with personality changes, memory loss, and poor judgment, and can progress to depression, mania, and psychosis.

Risk factors

Elevated levels of homocysteine have been associated with cerebrovascular disease (Khan et al., 2008) and with Alzheimer's disease (Miller et al., 2002; Seshadri et al., 2002). Homocysteine levels can be measured. There is also some evidence that levels of homocysteine can be lowered by treating with folate and its cofactors B6 and B12. Whether this lowering can reduce the risks of cerebrovascular and Alzheimer's disease is unknown (for review see Maron & Loscalzo, 2009). Because recommending supplementation of B12, B6, and folic acid in reasonable doses is not likely to be harmful, we typically recommend this vitamin supplementation to our patients who inquire about additional things that they can do to help slow decline.

Apolipoprotein E testing

We advise caution when considering apolipoprotein E testing. See Chapter 3: *Alzheimer's disease*, for further discussion of this issue.

Cerebrospinal fluid (CSF) Aβ and tau

Tests of cerebrospinal fluid measuring $A\beta_{42}$ and tau are being investigated. Although these tests are not part of routine clinical practice, they can be helpful in select circumstances. See Chapter 3: *Alzheimer's disease*, for the current status of these tests.

STRUCTURAL IMAGING STUDIES

A non-contrast, structural imaging study of the brain is essential in the work-up of memory loss. Strokes, tumors, hemorrhages, subdural hematomas and other fluid collections, normal pressure hydrocephalus, vascular dementia, and many other conditions may cause memory loss, and can only be accurately diagnosed with a structural imaging study. Additionally, most patients show some degree of small vessel ischemic strokes by the time they reach 70 years of age or older. It is our experience that, although this small vessel disease is unlikely to be the main cause of memory loss, it is often a contributing factor, making the underlying Alzheimer's disease present with more severe signs and symptoms than it otherwise would (Snowdon et al., 1997). Structural brain imaging allows a qualitative look at the contribution of this small vessel disease. Computed tomography (CT) and magnetic resonance imaging (MRI) are standard; each has advantages and disadvantages.

MRI versus CT

MRI scans have higher resolution than CT scans, and can use different sequences to highlight different tissues in the living brain (Figs 2.3 and 2.4). For this reason MRI scans provide an unparalleled view of the structure of the brain and almost any pathology. The one major exception is that MRI scans do not show an acute hemorrhage of almost any type as effectively as CT scans. Consequently, CT—and not MRI—is the modality of choice if an acute hemorrhage is suspected. Relative to CT, the MRI scan takes longer, is noisier, and involves going into a much narrower tube. If a patient is claustrophobic or agitated (as can often be the case in Alzheimer's disease after the early stages), a CT scan is easier to obtain than an MRI scan. Thus, CT scans are generally easier for the patient to tolerate than MRI scans. They are fast,

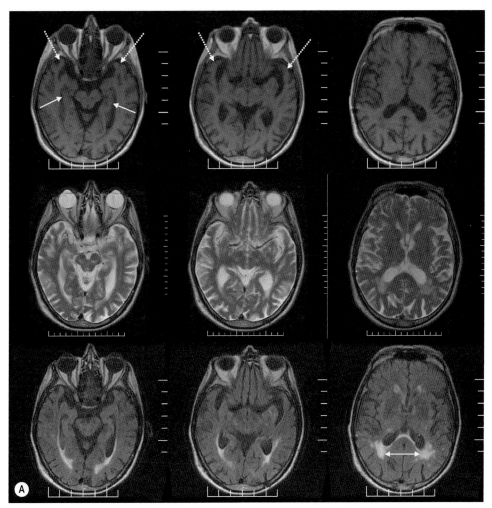

FIGURE 2.3 Selected slices of an MRI scan of a patient with mild Alzheimer's disease.

Panels (A) and (B) (below) show the same six axial slices of brain from T1 (top), T2 (middle), and FLAIR (bottom) sequences. Panel (C) (below) shows five T1 coronal slices and one T1 sagittal slice. The T1 images provide the best anatomical resolution, showing mild atrophy of hippocampus (thin solid arrows), anterior temporal lobe (thin dotted arrows), and parietal cortex (thick dotted arrows). FLAIR images (in combination with T2) show vascular disease best (double-headed arrow). Note that the small vessel ischemic cerebrovascular disease shown here is average for an older adult.

Continued

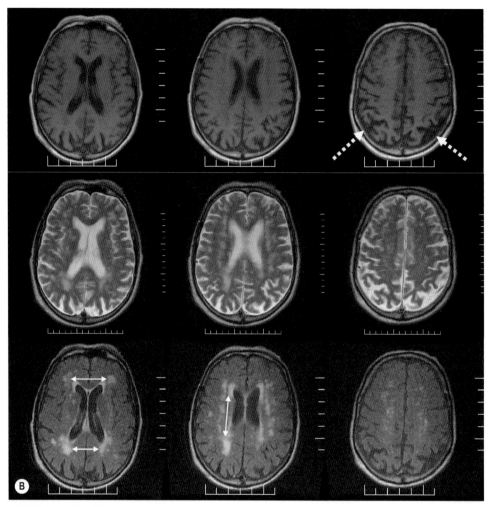

FIGURE 2.3—Cont'd

and provide a completely adequate look at the structure of the brain. Both studies allow a look at the extent of small vessel ischemic disease, and can also evaluate for strokes, tumors, subdural fluid collections, normal pressure hydrocephalus, and many other conditions. Note that some findings on a CT scan, such as a mass, will prompt a subsequent MRI for additional characterization.

Questions for structural imaging studies to answer

Three questions should be answered when examining an imaging study of the brain in a patient with memory loss.

First, what is the pattern of atrophy (shrinkage of the brain) that is present? Is the atrophy more than is expected for age? Is it bilateral temporal and parietal with relative sparing of other brain regions, consistent with Alzheimer's disease? Is it predominantly frontal consistent with a

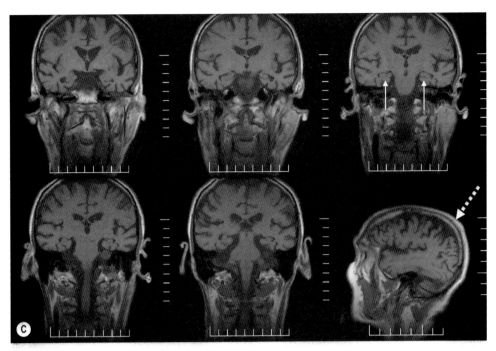

FIGURE 2.3—Cont'd

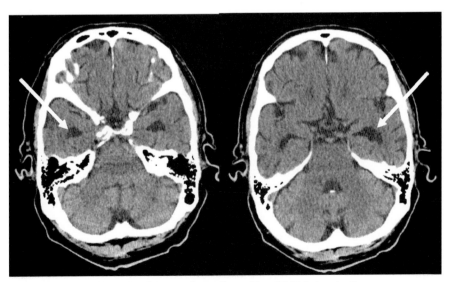

FIGURE 2.4 Selected slices of a CT scan of a patient with mild Alzheimer's disease.

Note the prominent dilatation of the temporal horns of the lateral ventricles bilaterally (arrows). This so-called "ex-vacuo" dilatation (or enlargement due to loss of tissue) of this part of the ventricles is due to underlying shrinkage of the hippocampi.

frontotemporal dementia? Is there hippocampal atrophy consistent with memory loss? Is there no significant atrophy? In our experience, atrophy is almost never "global," that is, atrophy is almost never evenly distributed throughout the brain. Note that, although atrophy on a structural imaging study can be consistent with a neurodegenerative disease, it is never diagnostic or exclusionary of such a disease. In Alzheimer's disease there is typically atrophy of bilateral hippocampi, anterior temporal lobes, and parietal lobes. Note that the atrophy is often asymmetric, for unknown reasons.

Second, how extensive is the small vessel ischemic disease? Is the amount of these tiny small vessel strokes average for the patient's age, less, or more? Has the small vessel disease affected critical areas of the brain such as the thalamus, where even a small stroke can cause memory loss? Note again that most patients aged 70 years or older have some small vessel ischemic disease. As mentioned above it is often a minor contributing factor, sometimes a major contributing factor, and only very rarely is it the sole cause of the patient's memory loss.

Third, is there any other pathology present? Is there an old cortical stroke in the right frontal cortex? Is there loss of brain tissue (encephalomalacia) due to an old head injury? Are there subdural or epidural fluid collections? Is there a tumor? In brief, are there any "surprises" evident on the imaging study that may be a primary or contributing factor to the patient's memory loss?

FUNCTIONAL IMAGING STUDIES

In a routine case of memory loss, one in which the history, physical examination, cognitive testing, and structural imaging studies are all consistent with Alzheimer's disease, vascular dementia, or another etiology, a functional imaging study is not necessary. In a situation, however, in which one or more of the elements of the evaluation suggests that the patient has an atypical neurodegenerative disease, a functional imaging study can be helpful. We would also strongly recommend a functional imaging study for a young person aged less than 66 years with dementia, even if the evaluation appears straightforward. The main reason to obtain a functional imaging study in a patient less than 66 years of age is simply that the prevalence of Alzheimer's disease causing memory loss relative to other etiologies is much less in the younger patient than in the older patient. For example, whereas the overall ratio of Alzheimer's disease to frontotemporal dementia may be 10:1 or even 100:1, this ratio drops to closer to 1:1 for individuals younger than 66 years (Brunnstrom et al., 2009). Note that the sensitivity and specificity of functional imaging studies is not terribly high, which is one reason why they should not be conducted routinely. For example, a false-positive test suggesting dementia in the case of someone with only mild cognitive issues can be devastating to the patient and family. Thus, these functional imaging studies are helpful in distinguishing between different types of dementia in a patient who clearly has a dementia. They are not helpful in distinguishing between, for example, normal aging and MCI, or between depression and mild Alzheimer's disease.

SPECT versus PET

There are two main functional imaging technologies used in clinical practice, SPECT (single photon emission computed tomography) and PET (positron emission tomography). In both cases a small amount of a radiolabeled dye (usually technetium-99 for SPECT and fluorodeoxyglucose for PET) is injected into the patient's bloodstream, and a collector outside the head records the amount of radioactivity detected in different areas of the brain. Areas that are more metabolically active show higher levels of radioactivity than areas that are less metabolically active. Before an area of the brain becomes atrophic, it is likely that it first becomes metabolically less active. Thus, functional imaging scans are typically more sensitive to early brain dysfunction than structural imaging scans. SPECT and PET imaging can vary widely from one institution to another, based upon the availability of the radiolabeled dye, quality of the SPECT and PET cameras detecting the radioactivity, and expertise of the radiologist interpreting the scans. Choosing between SPECT and PET imaging is thus dependent upon which technique is available in a given geographic area and, if both are available, which the radiologist feels is better for distinguishing between different neurodegenerative diseases. From a practical standpoint, both provide very similar information. The cost of these studies is covered by most insurance companies as well as Medicare.

Questions for functional imaging studies to answer

There is one question for a functional imaging study to answer. In a patient with cognitive impairment and a likely neurodegenerative disease, with which neurodegenerative disease is the pattern of impaired and preserved metabolism most consistent? In Alzheimer's disease the pattern is one of bilateral temporal and parietal hypometabolism (Fig. 2.5). As with structural imaging studies, for unknown reasons the hypometabolism is often asymmetric.

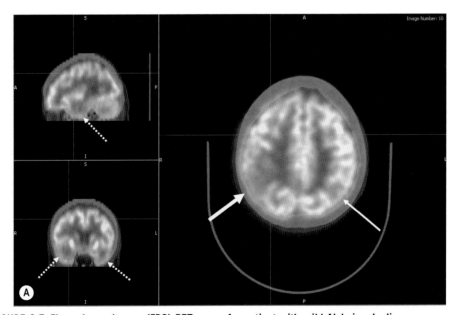

FIGURE 2.5 Fluorodeoxyglucose (FDG) PET scan of a patient with mild Alzheimer's disease.

Selected slices of a PET imaging study (A) of a patient with Alzheimer's disease demonstrating greatly reduced brain metabolism function in right parietal (thick solid arrow) and bilateral temporal (dotted arrows) regions, and more mild reduced metabolism in the left parietal (thin solid arrow) region. Note that both CT (B) and MRI (C) scans of this 67-year-old patient were essentially normal. A color version of this figure is available online at http://www.expertconsult.com.

Continued

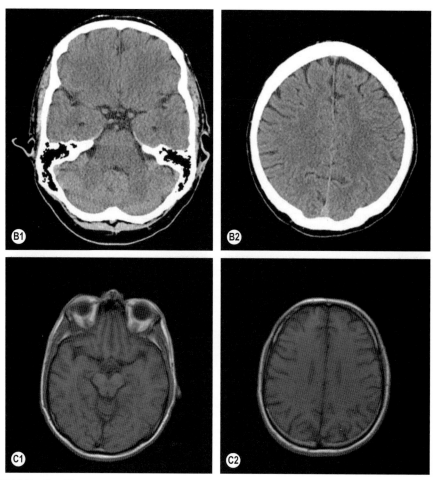

FIGURE 2.5—Cont'd

Note that these functional imaging studies are more likely than structural imaging studies to show significant changes over relatively brief periods of time, such as 6–12 months. Therefore, if an evaluation of a patient is inconclusive at one time-point and the patient continues to deteriorate, repeating the functional imaging study in 6–12 months is more likely to yield informative results than repeating the structural imaging study.

Functional imaging studies being developed

There are several novel functional imaging studies that are currently being developed and evaluated. Two of the more promising studies are the Pittsburgh compound B (PiB) PET and the dopamine transporter PET. As at the writing of this book, both imaging compounds are experimental and neither compound has been approved by the US Food

---

BOX 2.8 ESSENTIAL ELEMENTS IN THE WORK-UP OF MEMORY LOSS

- History from the patient
- History from the caregiver, including at least a few minutes in private
- History should include whether there are problems with:
  - Memory
  - Word-finding
  - Getting lost
  - Reasoning and judgment
  - Mood
  - Behavior
  - Delusions, hallucinations, memory distortions
  - Activities of daily living
  - Instrumental activities of daily living
- Review of systems and past medical history including:
  - A significant brain infection such as meningitis or encephalitis
  - A significant head injury in which the patient lost consciousness
  - A stroke or a transient ischemic attack
  - A seizure
  - Fluctuating levels of alertness or periods of being relatively unresponsive
  - Visual hallucinations of people or animals
  - A disturbance of gait
  - Falls
  - A tremor
  - Rigidity and other signs of Parkinsonism
  - A dramatic change in personality such that the patient seems like a different person
  - Any major psychiatric problems earlier in life, such as major depression or bipolar disease
  - Any incontinence of bowel or bladder
  - Problems going to sleep (insomnia), staying asleep, or early morning awakening. Any naps?
  - Acting out dreams during sleep or other abnormal movements while sleeping
  - Difficulty distinguishing dreams from reality when transitioning from sleep
- Habits including alcohol and smoking
- Previous education and occupation
- Family history of Alzheimer's disease, memory loss, or other neurological disorder
- Physical and neurological examination including:
  - Search for focal signs including weakness, abnormal reflexes, and Babinski's sign
  - Search for Parkinsonism including tremor, rigidity, and gait disorder
  - Careful evaluation of eye movements
- Cognitive testing with brief cognitive screening instrument such as Mini-Mental State Examination
- Laboratory studies including vitamin B12 and thyroid-stimulating hormone
- Structural imaging study, either MRI or CT (both non-contrast)

---

and Drug Administration for use in diagnosing patients. The PiB PET appears to be able to non-invasively identify β-amyloid in the brains of patients with Alzheimer's disease (Grimmer et al., 2009). This technology, therefore, has the potential to diagnose Alzheimer's pathology in a sensitive and specific manner, perhaps even before the onset of subtle cognitive symptoms. Similarly, the dopamine transporter PET study has the potential to aid in the diagnosis of both Parkinson's disease and dementia with Lewy bodies (Rinne et al., 1999).

BOX 2.9 ADDITIONAL ELEMENTS TO CONSIDER IN THE WORK-UP OF MEMORY LOSS

- Consultations
  - Neuropsychology
  - Psychiatry
- Laboratory studies
  - Rapid plasma reagent
  - Lyme titer
  - Erythrocyte sedimentation rate
  - Antibodies to detect limbic encephalitis and/or Hashimoto's thyroiditis
  - Cerebrospinal fluid evaluation for cells, Aβ42, total tau, and p-tau
  - Apolipoprotein E4 testing
  - Genetic testing for familial early-onset Alzheimer's disease
- Imaging studies
  - MRI with magnetic susceptibility (or other sequence looking for blood products)
  - SPECT
  - PET
  - Special SPECT and PET studies
- EEG
- Sleep study

SUMMARY

In summary, the key elements in an evaluation of memory loss include a history from both the patient and family to characterize the signs, symptoms, and current level of function, physical and neurological examinations, cognitive testing, and laboratory and brain imaging studies (Box 2.8), Additional elements of the evaluation can be included when required (Box 2.9).

References

Balota, D.A., Cortese, M.J., Duchek, J.M., et al., 1999. Veridical and false memories in healthy older adults and in dementia of the Alzheimer's type. Cogn. Neuropsychol. 16, 361–384.

Bleecker, M.L., Bolla-Wilson, K., Kawas, C., et al., 1988. Age-specific norms for the Mini-Mental State Exam. Neurology 38, 1565–1568.

Blessed, G., Tomlinson, B.E., Roth, M., 1968. The association between quantitative measures of dementia and of senile change in the cerebral grey matter of elderly subjects. Br. J. Psychiatry 114, 797–811.

Borson, S., Scanlan, J.M., Watanabe, J., et al., 2005. Simplifying detection of cognitive impairment: comparison of the Mini-Cog and Mini-Mental State Examination in a multiethnic sample. J. Am. Geriatr. Soc. 53, 871–874.

Brunnstrom, H., Gustafson, L., Passant, U., et al., 2009. Prevalence of dementia subtypes: a 30-year retrospective survey of neuropathological reports. Arch. Gerontol. Geriatr. 49, 146–149.

Damasio, H., Grabowski, T.J., Tranel, D., et al., 1996. A neural basis for lexical retrieval. Nature 380, 499–505.

Eastwood, M.R., Lautenschlaeger, E., Corbin, S., 1983. A comparison of clinical methods for assessing dementia. J. Am. Geriatr. Soc. 31, 342–347.

Folstein, M.F., Folstein, S.E., McHugh, P.R., 1975. A practical method for grading the cognitive state of patients for the clinician. J. Psychiatr. Res. 12, 189–198.

Galvin, J.E., Roe, C.M., Powlishta, K.K., et al., 2005. The AD8: a brief informant interview to detect dementia. Neurology 65, 559–564.

Galvin, J.E., Roe, C.M., Coats, M.A., et al., 2007. Patient's rating of cognitive ability: using the AD8, a brief informant interview, as a self-rating tool to detect dementia. Arch. Neurol. 64, 725–730.

Grimmer, T., Henriksen, G., Wester, H.J., et al., 2009. Clinical severity of Alzheimer's disease is associated with PIB uptake in PET. Neurobiol. Aging 30, 1902–1909.

Grut, M., Jorm, A.F., Fratiglioni, L., et al., 1993. Memory complaints of elderly people in a population survey: variation according to dementia stage and depression. J. Am. Geriatr. Soc. 41, 1295–1300.

Jayadev, S., Steinbart, E.J., Chi, Y.Y., et al., 2008. Conjugal Alzheimer disease: risk in children when both parents have Alzheimer disease. Arch. Neurol. 65, 373–378.

Jorm, A.F., 1994. A short form of the Informant Questionnaire on Cognitive Decline in the Elderly (IQCODE): development and cross-validation. Psychol. Med. 24, 145–153.

Jorm, A.F., 2004. The Informant Questionnaire on Cognitive Decline in the Elderly (IQCODE): a review. Int. Psychogeriatr. 16, 275–293.

Jorm, A.F., Jacomb, P.A., 1989. The Informant Questionnaire on Cognitive Decline in the Elderly (IQCODE): socio-demographic correlates, reliability, validity and some norms. Psychol. Med. 19, 1015–1022.

Khan, U., Crossley, C., Kalra, L., et al., 2008. Homocysteine and its relationship to stroke subtypes in a UK black population: the south London ethnicity and stroke study. Stroke 39, 2943–2949.

Knopman, D.S., Ryberg, S., 1989. A verbal memory test with high predictive accuracy for dementia of the Alzheimer type. Arch. Neurol. 46, 141–145.

Lebowitz, B.D., Pearson, J.L., Schneider, L.S., et al., 1997. Diagnosis and treatment of depression in late life. Consensus statement update. JAMA 278, 1186–1190.

Li, Y., Meyer, J.S., Thornby, J., 2001. Depressive symptoms among cognitive normal versus cognitive impaired elderly subjects. Int. J. Geriatr. Psychiatry 16, 455–461.

Locascio, J.J., Growdon, J.H., Corkin, S., 1995. Cognitive test performance in detecting, staging, and tracking Alzheimer's disease. Arch. Neurol. 52, 1087–1099.

Maron, B.A., Loscalzo, J., 2009. The treatment of hyperhomocysteinemia. Annu. Rev. Med. 60, 39–54.

Meulen, E.F., Schmand, B., van Campen, J.P., et al., 2004. The seven minute screen: a neurocognitive screening test highly sensitive to various types of dementia. J. Neurol. Neurosurg. Psychiatry 75, 700–705.

Miller, J.W., Green, R., Mungas, D.M., et al., 2002. Homocysteine, vitamin B6, and vascular disease in Alzheimer's disease patients. Neurology 58, 1471–1475.

Nasreddine, Z.S., Phillips, N.A., Bedirian, V., et al., 2005. The Montreal Cognitive Assessment, MoCA: a brief screening tool for mild cognitive impairment. J. Am. Geriatr. Soc. 53, 695–699.

Nitz, D., 2009. Parietal cortex, navigation, and the construction of arbitrary reference frames for spatial information. Neurobiol. Learn. Mem. 91, 179–185.

Perani, D., Cappa, S.F., Schnur, T., et al., 1999. The neural correlates of verb and noun processing. A PET study. Brain 122 (Pt 12), 2337–2344.

Pfeffer, R.I., Kurosaki, T.T., Harrah, C.H., Jr, et al., 1982. Measurement of functional activities in older adults in the community. J Gerontol. 37 (3), 323–329.

Price, J.L., Morris, J.C., 1999. Tangles and plaques in nondemented aging and "preclinical" Alzheimer's disease. Ann. Neurol. 45, 358–368.

Ribot, T., 1881. Les Maladies de la Mémoire. Félix Alcan, Paris.

Rinaldi, P., Mecocci, P., Benedetti, C., et al., 2003. Validation of the five-item geriatric depression scale in elderly subjects in three different settings. J. Am. Geriatr. Soc. 51, 694–698.

Rinne, J.O., Ruottinen, H., Bergman, J., et al., 1999. Usefulness of a dopamine transporter PET ligand [(18)F] beta-CFT in assessing disability in Parkinson's disease. J. Neurol. Neurosurg. Psychiatry 67, 737–741.

Seshadri, S., Beiser, A., Selhub, J., et al., 2002. Plasma homocysteine as a risk factor for dementia and Alzheimer's disease. N. Engl. J. Med. 346, 476–483.

Snowdon, D.A., Greiner, L.H., Mortimer, J.A., et al., 1997. Brain infarction and the clinical expression of Alzheimer disease. The Nun Study. JAMA 277, 813–817.

Solomon, P.R., Murphy, C.A., 2005. Should we screen for Alzheimer's disease? A review of the evidence for and against screening Alzheimer's disease in primary care practice. Geriatrics 60, 26–31.

Solomon, P.R., Murphy, C.A., 2008. Early diagnosis and treatment of Alzheimer's disease. Expert Rev. Neurother. 8, 769–780.

Solomon, P.R., Hirschoff, A., Kelly, B., et al., 1998. A 7 minute neurocognitive screening battery highly sensitive to Alzheimer's disease. Arch. Neurol. 55, 349–355.

Solomon, P.R., Brush, M., Calvo, V., et al., 2000. Identifying dementia in the primary care practice. Int. Psychogeriatr. 12, 483–493.

Solomon, P.R., Ruiz, M.A., Murphy, C.A., 2003. The Alzheimer's Disease Caregiver Questionnaire: initial validation of a screening instrument. Int. Psychogeriatr. 15 (Suppl. 2), 87.

Tsolaki, M., Iakovidou, V., Papadopoulou, E., et al., 2002. Greek validation of the seven-minute screening battery for Alzheimer's disease in the elderly. Am. J. Alzheimers Dis. Other Demen. 17, 139–148.

Zankd, S., Leipold, B., 2001. The relationship between severity of dementia and subjective well-being. Aging Ment. Health 5, 191–196.

Alzheimer's disease
(See Chapter 2 for additional information)

3

QUICK START 1: ALZHEIMER'S DISEASE

Definition	• Alzheimer's disease is a neurodegenerative disease of the brain characterized by a clinical dementia with prominent memory impairment and specific microscopic pathology including senile plaques and neurofibrillary tangles.
Prevalence	• Either alone or in combination with other disorders, Alzheimer's disease is the cause of approximately 75% of dementia cases. • Alzheimer's disease becomes more prevalent with age, although it is not part of normal aging.
Genetic risk	• Family history of Alzheimer's disease in a first-degree relative increases the risk approximately twofold.
Cognitive symptoms	• After memory loss, other symptoms develop including word-finding and visuospatial difficulties, and frontal/executive dysfunction including problems with reasoning and judgment.
Diagnostic criteria	• Two widely accepted sets of diagnostic criteria are from the NINCDS-ADRDA and the DSM-IV. • Both criteria require: (1) presence of dementia, (2) deficits in multiple cognitive areas, (3) gradual onset and progression, and (4) ruling out other causes of dementia.
Behavioral symptoms	• Behavioral and psychiatric symptoms may develop early, including apathy, irritability, agitation, anxiety, and exacerbation of premorbid personality traits.
Treatment	• Cholinesterase inhibitors are US Food and Drug Administration (FDA) approved for the treatment of mild, moderate, and severe Alzheimer's disease. • Memantine is FDA approved for the treatment of moderate and severe Alzheimer's disease. • The behavioral and psychiatric symptoms of Alzheimer's disease are often more distressing to caregivers than the cognitive ones, and should also be treated.
Top differential diagnoses	• Normal aging, mild cognitive impairment, dementia with Lewy bodies, vascular dementia, frontotemporal dementia.

PREVALENCE, PROGNOSIS, AND DEFINITION (Figs 3.1–3.4)

Alzheimer's disease is a neurodegenerative disease of the brain characterized by a clinical dementia with prominent memory impairment and specific pathology including senile plaques and neurofibrillary tangles (Box 3.1). Over time, Alzheimer's disease produces neurochemical deficits (Box 3.2) and prominent brain atrophy (Box 3.3). Alzheimer's disease is by far the most common form of dementia, being the cause of approximately 75% of dementia cases either by itself or in combination with other disorders. The overall prevalence of Alzheimer's disease in the community is estimated at about 10% in population-based studies. Alzheimer's disease becomes more prevalent with age, with most cases being diagnosed after the age of 65. In fact, the incidence roughly doubles every 5 years from ages 65 to 85, starting with an incidence of about 2.5% for 65- to

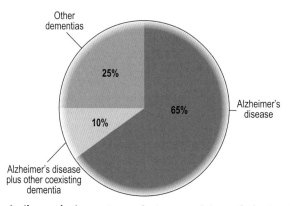

FIGURE 3.1 Alzheimer's disease is the most prevalent cause of dementia in the elderly.

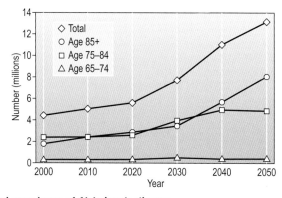

FIGURE 3.2 Projected prevalence of Alzheimer's disease.

The rapid growth of the oldest age groups in the US population will bring a significant increase in the prevalence of Alzheimer's disease. Projections show cases of Alzheimer's disease in the 85-plus age group will more than quadruple by 2050.

Reprinted with permission of Hebert LE et al., 2003. Alzheimer disease in the US population: prevalence estimates using the 2000 census. Arch. Neurol. 60,1119–1122.

BOX 3.1 ALZHEIMER'S PATHOLOGY

Microscopically, Alzheimer's pathology consists of two main features, senile plaques and neurofibrillary tangles (Figs 3.5 and 3.6). Additional microscopic features include selective loss of neurons and synapses, and an increase in the number and activation of astrocytes. Neuropil threads (short, often curly silver-stained fibers) also accumulate in the neocortex.

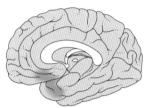 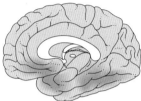 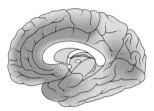

Preclinical Alzheimer's disease   Mild to moderate Alzheimer's disease   Severe Alzheimer's disease

FIGURE 3.5 Alzheimer's disease spreads through the brain.

Senile plaques contain a specific type of amyloid, often referred to as β-amyloid or as "Aβ." (Note that the amyloid in Alzheimer's disease has nothing to do with the amyloid in systemic amyloidoses; they both just happen to have similar properties under the polarized light microscope.) Aβ is a 40- or 42-amino acid peptide that is a fragment of a larger, membrane-spanning glycoprotein known as the amyloid precursor protein or APP. The normal function of Aβ is unclear at this time. Up to 50% of the Aβ found in plaques is Aβ42—despite the fact that Aβ42 constitutes only 5–20% of the total Aβ produced. Senile plaques are extracellular structures that are composed of Aβ, dystrophic neuritic processes (axons and dendrites), astrocytes and their processes, and microglial cells (Fig. 3.6). When axons and dendrites are disrupted the communication between neurons becomes impaired. When microglial cells attempt to remove amyloid and remnants of axons and dendrites, an inflammatory reaction can start causing more damage. Under light microscopy senile plaques appear to have a fluffy central core with surrounding thick irregular processes (Fig. 3.7). Various classifications of senile plaques have been proposed, including diffuse and neuritic types. Neuritic plaques are associated with the destruction of axons and dendrites of neurons. Diffuse plaques do not disrupt these neuronal processes, but are thought to be the precursor of neuritic plaques. The relationship between the amount of plaque and the degree of dementia is unclear at this time (Wilcock & Esiri, 1982; Josephs et al., 2008). Many researchers now consider that smaller fragments of Aβ, Aβ oligomers, may in fact cause the damage in Alzheimer's disease and that the plaques are important because they can serve as a reservoir for the oligomers. And some of the newest evidence could be interpreted as suggesting that, once the process of Alzheimer's disease has started and tangles have begun to form, one can remove all Aβ from the brain but the dementia will still progress (Holmes et al., 2008).

Neurofibrillary tangles are intraneuronal cytoplasmic structures that are composed of paired filaments with a regular helical periodicity (Fig. 3.6). Neurofibrillary tangles appear to be composed primarily of a hyperphosphorylated form of the microtubule-associated protein tau. Microtubules are one of the three major constituents of the neuronal cytoskeleton; neurofilaments and microfilaments being the other two. All of these can be thought of as infrastructural elements of neurons that participate in functions such as axonal transport and maintenance of the structural integrity of the cell. Among other roles, tau and other microtubule-associated proteins stabilize the microtubule assembly (think of tau as the support beams or rivets for this system). Although neurofibrillary tangles begin as intracytoplasmic structures, they may remain behind after the neuron dies, forming "ghost" or

BOX 3.1 ALZHEIMER'S PATHOLOGY—Cont'd

"tombstone" tangles in the neuropil. Under the microscope neurofibrillary tangles look like skeins of yarn (Fig. 3.7). Unlike plaques, the amount of tangles in the brain has been shown to correlate with dementia severity in Alzheimer's disease (Wilcock & Esiri, 1982).

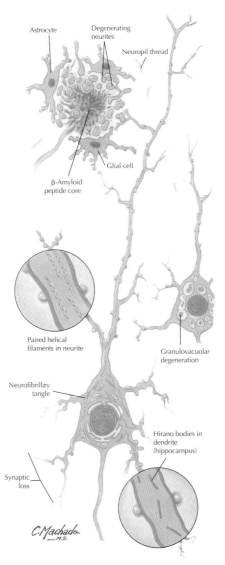

FIGURE 3.6 Some of the pathological features in Alzheimer's disease.

A color version of this figure is available online at http://www.expertconsult.com

Continued

BOX 3.1 ALZHEIMER'S PATHOLOGY—Cont'd

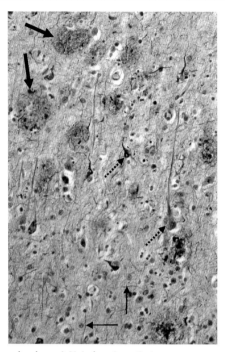

FIGURE 3.7 Light microscopic view of Alzheimer's pathology.

Plaques (thick arrows), tangles (dotted arrows), and neuropil threads (thin arrows) in Alzheimer's disease. A color version of this figure is available online at http://www.expertconsult.com.

BOX 3.2 NEUROCHEMISTRY

A deficit in acetylcholine is the most consistently found alteration of brain chemistry in Alzheimer's disease. Early in the disease there is a loss of choline acetyltransferase and reduced high-affinity choline uptake and acetylcholine synthesis (Mesulam et al., 2004). Studies have shown a correlation between the loss of choline acetyltransferase and impairment of cognition (Mesulam, 2004). These data have led to the cholinergic hypothesis of Alzheimer's disease that, in turn, has led to the development of acetylcholinesterase inhibitor therapies to treat this disorder (see Chapter 14: *Cholinesterase inhibitors*). Other studies have shown that, in addition to acetylcholine, many other neurotransmitters also become disrupted as the disease progresses, including norepinephrine, serotonin, glutamate, and dopamine (see Fig. 3.10).

BOX 3.3 GROSS PATHOLOGY (Figs 3.8 and 3.9)

Brain weight is typically reduced in Alzheimer's disease by 100–200 grams. Examination of the surface of the brain reveals cortical atrophy of the temporal, parietal, and frontal lobes, as well as the hippocampus. The ventricular system becomes enlarged. The occipital lobes, along with primary sensory and motor cortices, are usually preserved.

BOX 3.3 GROSS PATHOLOGY (Figs 3.8 and 3.9)—Cont'd

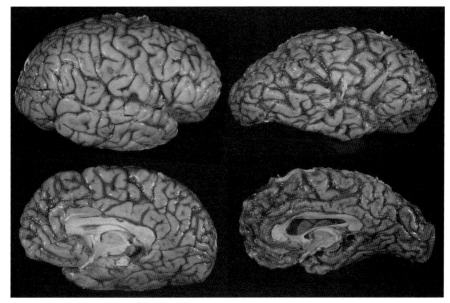

FIGURE 3.8 External view of gross pathology in Alzheimer's disease.

Comparison of a brain with Alzheimer's disease (right) with a healthy brain (left). Note that the meningeal vessels are more prominent in the brain with Alzheimer's disease because the brain gyri have shrunk, revealing the vessels. A color version of this figure is available online at http://www.expertconsult.com.

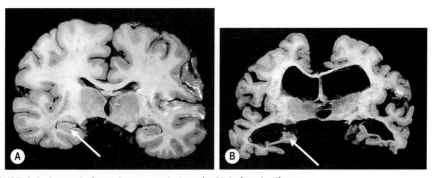

FIGURE 3.9 Coronal view of gross pathology in Alzheimer's disease.

Coronal view through a brain with Alzheimer's disease (B) compared with a healthy brain (A). Note the hippocampus (arrows), intact in the healthy brain and atrophic in the brain with Alzheimer's disease (note also the enlarged ventricles). A color version of this figure can be found online at http://www.expertconsult.com.

Continued

Alzheimer's is also a costly disease. Direct costs include paid home health aids, acute care, and nursing home costs. Indirect costs include unpaid care by family members and friends. Alzheimer's disease and related dementias are some of the most expensive health conditions in the USA with a total annual cost for 2010 estimated to be $172 billion for healthcare and long-term care (Alzheimer's Association, 2010).

DIAGNOSTIC CRITERIA

There are several different diagnostic criteria that are used for Alzheimer's disease. The two most common are from the Diagnostic and Statistical Manual of Mental Disorders (DSM; current edition IV-TR) and the National Institutes of Neurological and Communicative Disorders and Stroke–Alzheimer's Disease and Related Disorders Association (NINCDS-ADRDA) (McKhann et al., 1984) (Boxes 3.4–3.6). The key elements of each are:

- dementia—a progressive decline in cognition and function
- a progressive decline in:
  - memory and
  - at least one other major area of cognition, such as language or executive function
- no disturbance of consciousness, such as a delirium or acute confusional state, and
- the decline in function cannot be explained by another medical or brain disease.

BOX 3.4 DSM-IV-TR CRITERIA FOR DEMENTIA OF THE ALZHEIMER'S TYPE

A. The development of multiple cognitive deficits manifested by both: (1) memory impairment (impaired ability to learn new information or to recall previously learned information) and (2) one (or more) of the following cognitive disturbances:
  (a) aphasia (language disturbance)
  (b) apraxia (impaired ability to carry out motor activities despite intact motor function)
  (c) agnosia (failure to recognize or identify objects despite intact sensory function)
  (d) disturbance in executive functioning (i.e., planning, organizing, sequencing, abstracting).

B. The cognitive deficits in criteria A1 and A2 each cause significant impairment in social or occupational functioning and represent a significant decline from a previous level of functioning.

C. The course is characterized by gradual onset and continuing cognitive decline.

D. The cognitive deficits in criteria A1 and A2 are not due to any of the following:
  (1) other central nervous system conditions that cause progressive deficits in memory and cognition (e.g., cerebrovascular disease, Parkinson's disease, Huntington's disease, subdural hematoma, normal-pressure hydrocephalus, brain tumor)
  (2) systemic conditions that are known to cause dementia (e.g., hypothyroidism, vitamin B or folic acid deficiency, niacin deficiency, hypercalcemia, neurosyphilis, HIV infection)
  (3) substance-induced conditions.

E. The deficits do not occur exclusively during the course of a delirium.

F. The disturbance is not better accounted for by another axis I disorder (e.g., major depressive episode, schizophrenia).

Adapted from American Psychiatric Association, 2000. Diagnostic and Statistical Manual of Mental Disorders DSM-IV-TR, fourth ed. American Psychiatric Publishing, Inc., Arlington, VA.

BOX 3.5 NINCDS-ADRDA CRITERIA FOR CLINICAL DIAGNOSIS OF ALZHEIMER'S DISEASE

I. Clinical diagnosis of <u>probable</u> Alzheimer's disease:
   a. Dementia established by clinical examination and documented by the Mini-Mental State Examination, Blessed Dementia Scale, or some similar examination, and confirmed by neuropsychological tests.
   b. Deficits in two or more areas of cognition.
   c. Progressive worsening of memory and other cognitive functions.
   d. No disturbance of consciousness.
   e. Onset between ages 40 and 90, most often after age 65.
   f. Absence of systemic disorders or other brain diseases that could account for progressive deficits in memory and cognition.

II. Diagnosis of <u>probable</u> Alzheimer's disease is supported by:
   a. Progressive deterioration of specific cognitive function such as language (aphasia), motor skills (apraxia), and perception (agnosia).
   b. Impaired activities of daily living, and altered patterns of behavior.
   c. Family history of similar disorders, particularly if confirmed neuropathologically.
   d. Laboratory results of
      i. Normal lumbar puncture
      ii. Normal pattern or non-specific changes in EEG, such as increased slow-wave activity
      iii. Evidence of cerebral atrophy on CT with progression documented by serial observation.

III. Other clinical features consistent with the diagnosis of <u>probable</u> Alzheimer's disease, after exclusion of causes of dementia other than Alzheimer's disease, include:
   a. Plateaus in the course of the progression of the illness.
   b. Associated symptoms of depression, insomnia, incontinence, delusions, illusions, hallucinations, catastrophic verbal, emotional, or physical outbursts, sexual disorders, and weight loss.
   c. Other neurological abnormalities in some patients, especially with more advanced disease, including:
      i. Motor signs (such as increased muscle tone)
      ii. Myoclonus
      iii. Gait disorder.
   d. Seizures in advanced disease.
   e. CT normal for age.

IV. Features that make the diagnosis of <u>probable</u> Alzheimer's disease uncertain or unlikely include:
   a. Sudden, apoplectic onset.
   b. Focal neurological findings such as hemiparesis, sensory loss, visual field deficits, and incoordination early in the course of the illness.
   c. Seizures or gait disturbances at the onset or very early in the course of the illness.

V. Clinical diagnosis of <u>possible</u> Alzheimer's disease
   a. May be made on the basis of the dementia syndrome, in the absence of other neurological, psychiatric, or systemic disorders sufficient to cause dementia, and in the presence of variations in the onset, presentation, or clinical course.
   b. May be made in the presence of a second systemic or brain disorder sufficient to produce dementia, but which is not considered to be the cause of the dementia.
   c. Should be used in research studies when a single, gradually progressive severe cognitive deficit is identified in the absence of other identifiable cause.

VI. Criteria for the diagnosis of <u>definite</u> Alzheimer's disease
   a. The clinical criteria for probable Alzheimer's disease and
   b. Histopathological evidence obtained from biopsy or autopsy.

VII. Classification of Alzheimer's disease for research purposes should specify features that may differentiate subtypes of the disorder, such as
   a. Familial occurrence.
   b. Onset before age 65.
   c. Presence of trisomy 21.
   d. Coexistence of other relevant conditions such as Parkinson's disease.

Adapted from McKhann, G. et al., 1984. Clinical diagnosis of Alzheimer's disease: report of the NINCDS/ADRDA Work Group, Dept. of HHS Task Force on Alzheimer's Disease. Neurology 34,939.

BOX 3.6 SIMILARITIES AND DIFFERENCES BETWEEN DSM-IV AND NINCDS-ADRDA CRITERIA

Similarities

- Presence of dementia
- Progression of cognitive deficits
- Deficits are not caused by other systemic or CNS conditions

Differences

- DSM requires deficits in memory plus one other cognitive area, NINCDS-ADRDA requires deficits in any two cognitive areas.
- Only DSM requires a significant loss of social or occupational functioning
- Only NINCDS-ADRDA distinguishes between probable, possible and definite Alzheimer's disease
- Only NINCDS-ADRDA specifies an age range (40–90)

RISK FACTORS, PATHOLOGY, AND PATHOPHYSIOLOGY

Age is the primary risk factor for Alzheimer's disease. Other risk factors include family history of Alzheimer's disease, female gender, few years of education, head injury, strokes, elevated plasma homocysteine levels and other risk factors for cerebrovascular disease, late-onset depression, and inheritance of certain allelic forms of the gene coding for apolipoprotein E (APOE) (Table 3.1). In addition, as many as 90% of individuals with trisomy 21 (Down's syndrome) who die over the age of 30 show Alzheimer's disease pathology in their brains, suggesting that it may be found in all older individuals with Down's syndrome. Several studies have suggested that having high premorbid intelligence (often correlated with many years of education) may be protective, as are other forms of the APOE gene. Some possible disease-modulating factors have shown mixed results: some studies show a beneficial effect whereas other studies show either no effect or a detrimental effect. The factors with mixed results include estrogen supplementation, certain non-steroidal anti-inflammatory drugs (NSAIDs), certain statin-based lipid-lowering agents, and smoking. Note that intervention trials with NSAIDs and statins have been negative to date. One reason that NSAIDs have been suspected as possibly being protective is that inflammation has been postulated as playing an important role in the pathophysiology of Alzheimer's disease (Box 3.7).

Alzheimer's disease is not part of normal aging

Given that age is the primary risk factor for Alzheimer's disease and that such a high percentage of older adults develop Alzheimer's disease, it is reasonable to wonder whether Alzheimer's disease is simply part of the normal aging process. We do not believe that this idea is correct. Alzheimer's disease is simply more common in aging, as are hypertension, type 2 diabetes, and cancer. At least three lines of evidence support the idea that Alzheimer's is a distinct age-related, but not age-determined, disease. First, many individuals live into their 80s and 90s without evidence of significant cognitive impairment, as do roughly half of centenarians. Second, patients with the accelerated aging disorder progeria do not develop dementia. Third, although autopsies may show some Alzheimer's pathology in the brains of normal older adults without cognitive impairment, the density of these neurofibrillary tangles and senile plaques is markedly lower in these individuals than in those with clinically diagnosed Alzheimer's disease.

Table 3.1 Risk factors for Alzheimer's disease

Fairly definite	Putative
Advanced age	Inverse association with smoking
Female sex	Alcohol or other drug abuse
Family history of dementia in first-degree relatives	Exposure to metals such as aluminum, zinc, mercury
Down's syndrome	Exposure to industrial solvents and pesticides
Presenilin mutations and the abnormal amyloid precursor protein gene	Electromagnetic fields
Apolipoprotein E-ε4 allele	Advance maternal age
Head trauma, particularly in the preceding 10 years	Maternal inheritance
Low educational attainment	Family history of Down's syndrome
Low life-long occupational attainment	Infectious processes
Small head size and brain volume	Cerebrovascular disease
	Cardiovascular disease
	Thyroid disease

Adapted with permission from Mendez, M.F., Cummings, J.L., 2003. Dementia: A Clinical Approach, third ed. Butterworth-Heinemann, Philadelphia, PA.

BOX 3.7 INFLAMMATION

The role of inflammation in Alzheimer's disease is both controversial and under continued investigation. One hypothesis is that inflammation may play a key role in Alzheimer's disease, by transforming benign, diffuse plaques into destructive mature plaques (Fig. 3.10), although studies to date have been mixed. Supporting the clinical importance of the role of inflammation in Alzheimer's disease, several correlational and retrospective studies have found that chronic use of non-steroidal anti-inflammatory drugs (NSAIDs) was associated with a lower risk of Alzheimer's disease but not other types of dementia. However, the results of randomized controlled trials of NSAIDs for the prevention or treatment of Alzheimer's disease have thus far been negative. Similar studies evaluating trials of prednisone have also been negative. These negative studies cast doubt on the clinical relevance of inflammation in this disease. However, it is certainly possible that the use of anti-inflammatories must be initiated much earlier in the disease process. Furthermore, certain NSAIDs have direct effects on the cleavage of the amyloid precursor protein by γ-secretase, independent of their inhibition of cyclooxygenase and other inflammatory mediators. It therefore remains unclear whether treatment with certain NSAIDs may be able to prevent or slow down the progression of Alzheimer's disease, and, if so, by what mechanism.

Genetic predisposition

Specific mutations on chromosomes 21, 14, and 1 have been associated with early-onset familial Alzheimer's disease. These patients with autosomal dominant early-onset disease are incredibly rare, and are typically easy to diagnose by family history. Patients with early-onset disease present clinically in their 40s and 50s, and usually family members can detect subtle changes years before clinical onset. The genetics of late-onset Alzheimer's disease has been harder to elucidate. The strongest genetic risk factor for late-onset Alzheimer's disease is the APOE allele. Relative to having an APOE ε3 allele, patients having an APOE ε4 allele are at increased risk of developing Alzheimer's disease (Boxes 3.8 and 3.9).

BOX 3.8 GENETICS AND PATHOPHYSIOLOGY OF β-AMYLOID (Aβ)

Chromosome 21 and the amyloid hypothesis

(See Figs 3.10 and 3.11.) Abnormal forms of Aβ are the cause of senile plaques in Alzheimer's disease. The gene coding for Aβ has been localized to the long arm of chromosome 21. Aβ is formed by the cleavage of the amyloid precursor protein, a normal constituent protein in humans whose function is unknown. The amyloid precursor protein can be cleaved into proteins of different lengths. Two of the more common products of this protein are Aβ of 40 and 42 amino acids. Mutations of the amyloid precursor protein that cause either an increase in the total production of Aβ or an increase in the relative production of $Aβ_{42}$ can lead to Alzheimer's disease. Although both $Aβ_{42}$ and $Aβ_{40}$ can cause Alzheimer's disease, $Aβ_{42}$ is more toxic—presumably because the two additional amino acids cause it to be more hydrophobic and more likely to self-aggregate and form oligomers. Although $Aβ_{42}$ totals only 5–20% of all Aβ produced, $Aβ_{42}$ constitutes close to 50% of the Aβ found in plaques.

When there is an increase in either the total amount of Aβ or the relative amount of $Aβ_{42}$, Aβ forms soluble oligomers, which further transform into insoluble fibrils, which deposit as diffuse plaques. These diffuse plaques may induce an inflammatory reaction with microglial and astrocytic activation, which then leads to a mature or neuritic plaque. It is these neuritic plaques that likely cause synaptic and neural injury, disrupt neuronal homeostasis, and cause oxidative injury. These disruptions alter kinase and phosphatase activity in the cell, which ultimately produces neurofibrillary tangles. Neurofibrillary tangles, in turn, cause neuronal death and dysfunction. In addition to this directly mediated neuronal damage and dysfunction, indirect brain dysfunction occurs when neurons producing neurotransmitters are affected by plaque and tangle pathology. Acetylcholine is affected first, primarily due to damage to the nucleus basalis of Meynert. In addition to the damage produced by plaques, there is also evidence that soluble oligomers of Aβ, acting extra- and/or intracellularly, may be directly responsible for cellular and synaptic dysfunction.

Chromosomes 14 and 1 and the secretases

In addition to the amyloid precursor protein on chromosome 21, two other genes, presenilin 1 on chromosome 14 and presenilin 2 on chromosome 1, have also been associated with early-onset familial Alzheimer's disease. Patients with mutations of these genes develop Alzheimer's disease in their 40s and 50s. These genes code for proteins of a critical part of the enzyme complex γ-secretase, which is involved in cleaving the amyloid precursor protein and forming Aβ.

Cleavage of the amyloid precursor protein may or may not result in Aβ formation, depending upon which proteolytic enzymes are initially active. The amyloid precursor protein is first cleaved by either α-secretase (the default pathway) or β-secretase (also known as the aspartyl protease BACE) (the alternative pathway), which releases α and β fragments of the amyloid precursor protein. After this initial cleavage, γ-secretase then splits the part of the amyloid precursor protein that remains on the cell membrane. When α-secretase performs the initial cleavage, the Aβ domain is split, precluding toxic Aβ formation. Thus, only when the amyloid precursor protein is first cleaved by β-secretase followed by γ-secretase can toxic Aβ fragments be released into the extracellular fluids. Understanding this pathophysiology is important because many of the medications currently in clinical trials are targeting these secretase enzymes.

Chromosome 10 and the clearance of Aβ

Because the concentration of Aβ is critical to its self-aggregation and subsequent cascade toward Alzheimer's pathology, the rate at which Aβ is cleared is as important as its formation in the pathophysiology of Alzheimer's disease. Two enzymes, insulin-degrading enzyme and neprilysin, have been shown to degrade Aβ. Levels of Aβ rise by 20–60% without insulin-degrading enzyme, and by 60–100% without neprilysin. The gene for insulin-degrading enzyme is on chromosome 10, and there is a genetic linkage between Alzheimer's disease and that gene locus.

Family history

A family history of Alzheimer's disease in a first-degree relative increases the risk of developing Alzheimer's disease approximately twofold (Lautenschlager et al., 1996). Knowledge of this increase in risk causes many middle-aged children of patients with

BOX 3.8 GENETICS AND PATHOPHYSIOLOGY OF β-AMYLOID (Aβ)—Cont'd

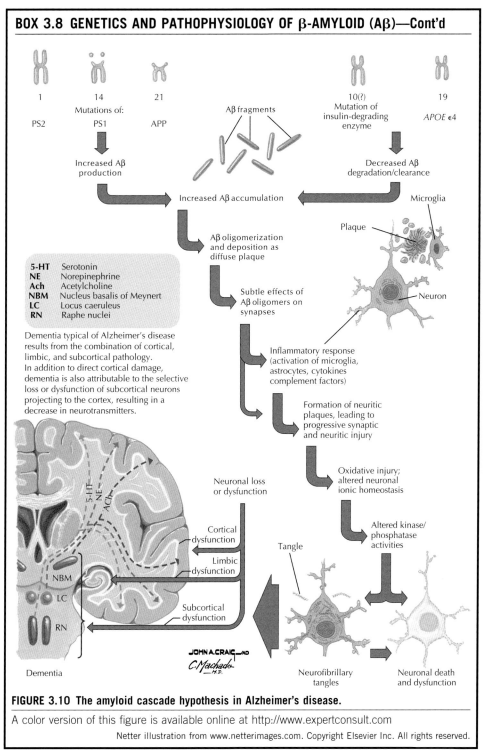

FIGURE 3.10 The amyloid cascade hypothesis in Alzheimer's disease.

A color version of this figure is available online at http://www.expertconsult.com

Continued

BOX 3.8 GENETICS AND PATHOPHYSIOLOGY OF β-AMYLOID (Aβ)—Cont'd

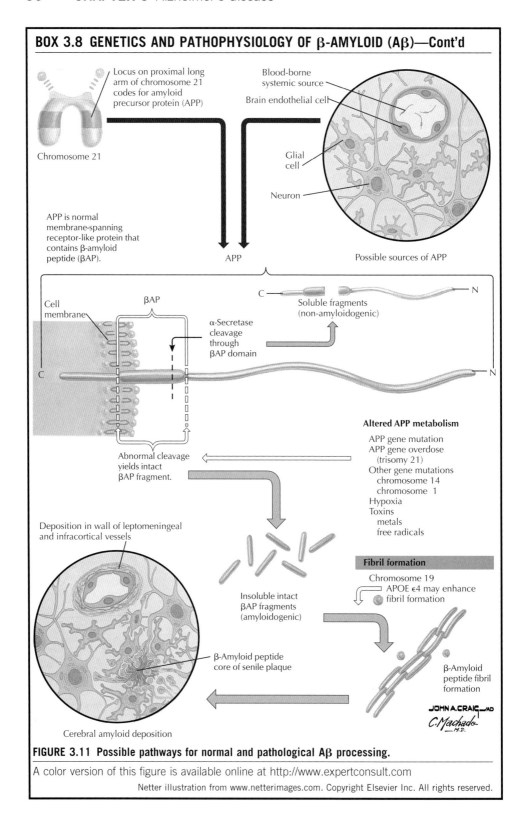

FIGURE 3.11 Possible pathways for normal and pathological Aβ processing.

A color version of this figure is available online at http://www.expertconsult.com

---

BOX 3.9 CHROMOSOME 19 AND APOLIPOPROTEIN E (APOE)

APOE is a major component of lipoproteins and has many normal functions, including lipid transport. The gene coding for APOE is on chromosome 19. The brain contains the second highest concentration of APOE, after the liver. In the brain, APOE is found primarily in macrophages and astrocytes. The three common isoforms of APOE are APOE-2, APOE-3, and APOE-4, coded for by alleles ε2, ε3, and ε4, respectively. APOE ε3 is the most common allele in the population, with a frequency of about 80%. Patients with familial and sporadic late-onset Alzheimer's disease (onset after age 55) have an approximately threefold increased likelihood of having an APOE ε4 allele. Conversely, the likelihood of having an APOE ε2 allele is lower than expected by allelic frequencies alone. Numerous studies have confirmed these findings, which suggest that APOE ε4 is a risk factor for developing Alzheimer's disease, whereas APOE ε2 is a protective factor.

In addition to conferring increased risk of developing Alzheimer's disease, having an APOE ε4 allele also lowers the age of onset of the disease compared with those without an ε4 allele who develop it. The majority of studies suggest that the course of Alzheimer's disease is not affected by the presence of an ε4 allele, although a few studies have disagreed with this finding. Neuropathologically, in patients with Alzheimer's disease there is more Aβ deposition in the brains of those with an ε4 allele than in those who have only ε3 alleles.

Evidence suggests that, as with insulin-degrading enzyme and neprilysin, APOE may be involved in Aβ clearance. APOE is thought to bind Aβ through the low-density lipoprotein receptor-related protein. In vitro experiments have demonstrated that APOE-3 binds Aβ with higher avidity than does APOE-4, which may suggest that APOE-3 is better able to clear Aβ than APOE-4. Other functions of APOE have been reported, which may also be clinically relevant. Binding of APOE to Aβ can promote the polymerization of Aβ into toxic oligomers and fibrils. Also consistent with the clinical data, this catalytic effect occurred fastest with APOE-4, slowest with APOE-2, and intermediate with APOE-3.

Should APOE genotyping be ordered routinely? Given the wealth of clinical and basic science data on the relationship between APOE and Alzheimer's disease, the question arises as to whether APOE genotyping should be performed routinely. We would argue that, in general, it is not clinically useful. Although carrying an APOE ε4 allele is a significant risk factor, it is neither necessary nor sufficient to cause Alzheimer's disease. First, approximately half of patients with Alzheimer's disease do not carry an APOE ε4 allele. Second, up to one-quarter of patients with non-Alzheimer's dementias carry an ε4 allele. Third, 10–19% of healthy older adults carry one or two ε4 alleles. Fourth, since APOE alleles are present from birth, APOE genotyping cannot be used to distinguish mild Alzheimer's disease from normal aging. Thus, using the APOE ε4 allele as a marker of Alzheimer's disease would result in huge numbers of both false positives and false negatives. Although it can be helpful in research, we do not recommend APOE genotyping in clinical practice.

Alzheimer's disease to become apprehensive that they, too, will develop this disorder. We generally point out to these family members that, although the risk of Alzheimer's disease is increased with a family history of the disorder, Alzheimer's disease is unfortunately extremely common as we age, such that everyone is at risk for the disorder, with or without a family history. More importantly, if the overall risk of Alzheimer's disease is about 2.5% between ages 65 and 70, the risk without a family history is probably around 1.5% and the risk with a family history is probably around 3%. Thus, although the relative risk may be doubled, the overall risk is still quite small. See Chapter 25: *Special issues* for more on this important topic.

Gender

In many studies women have been found to be at greater risk for Alzheimer's disease than men. This finding is not related to the longer life expectancy of women nor to the larger number of women consequently living to old age. Factors that have been suggested to explain this phenomenon include hormonal differences between men and women, different lifelong environmental exposures, and differences in years of education.

Education

It has been suggested that an increased number of years of education may reduce the risk of Alzheimer's disease, possibly by creating a "cognitive reserve" or a higher mental threshold that delays the onset of clinical symptoms. High educational attainment may also allow patients to compensate for some memory loss (by using memorization strategies, for example), disguising their symptoms and making diagnosis more challenging. Several studies suggest that low educational attainment is a risk factor for Alzheimer's disease: one study found that an uneducated person over the age of 75 is twice as likely to suffer dementia as is a person who has completed the 8th grade or higher. In another study, low linguistic ability early in life predicted poor cognitive function and Alzheimer's disease in late life (Snowdon et al., 1996, 2000). In the Framingham Heart Disease Study, however, low educational attainment was not found to be a significant risk factor for Alzheimer's disease (although it was for vascular dementia) (Cobb et al., 1995). Overall we do consider education to be an important factor when considering a patient's risk of Alzheimer's disease.

Trauma

Traumatic head injury associated with loss of consciousness or post-traumatic amnesia has been shown to be a risk factor for Alzheimer's disease, with some studies showing a relative risk greater than 2 (Fleminger et al., 2003). Several studies have suggested that the risk of Alzheimer's disease related to head injury is mediated through a specific genetic predisposition. One study found a 10-fold increase in Alzheimer's disease in individuals with traumatic head injury and an APOE ε4 allele, whereas no increase in the disease was seen in individuals without an APOE ε4 allele (Mayeux et al., 1995). Chronic traumatic encephalopathy, also known as dementia pugilistica, is found in boxers and other individuals with a history of repeated head injury (e.g., football players with multiple concussions); its relationship to Alzheimer's disease is still being determined (McKee et al., 2009) (see also Chapter 12: *Other disorders*).

Strokes

Strokes do not cause Alzheimer's pathology, but may contribute to cognitive dysfunction in patients who already have Alzheimer's pathology. Patients who have Alzheimer's pathology as well as small vessel ischemic strokes in the white matter and deep gray structures in the brain (basal ganglia, thalamus) are thus likely to have more cognitive dysfunction and dementia than those without these strokes (Snowdon et al., 1997). Cerebrovascular disease can thereby turn an individual with asymptomatic Alzheimer's pathology into a patient with Alzheimer's disease. It is for this reason that reducing cerebrovascular risk factors can help prevent Alzheimer's disease. Elevated plasma homocysteine levels—a known risk factor for strokes—is also a risk factor for the development of clinical

Alzheimer's disease (Seshadri et al., 2002). This effect of homocysteine is likely present because strokes may hasten a clinical diagnosis of dementia in a patient who already has Alzheimer's pathology (Miller et al., 2002; Luchsinger et al., 2004).

COMMON SIGNS, SYMPTOMS, AND STAGES

Alzheimer's disease typically first presents with memory loss for recent information, followed by word-finding difficulties, visuospatial difficulties, and frontal/executive dysfunction. As the disorder progresses, behavioral problems often develop such as irritability, exacerbation of premorbid personality traits, and sometimes aggression. Patients continue to lose function until they require round-the-clock care, usually in a long-term care facility.

Although there are no universally accepted definitions for the staging of patients with Alzheimer's disease, most clinicians agree that there are at least four stages of the disease—very mild, mild, moderate, and severe—each with its own cognitive, functional, and behavioral issues (Tables 3.2 and 3.3).

Very mild

Patients with very mild Alzheimer's disease show a slight but definite decline in memory, and sometimes in word-finding as well. They tend to be fully oriented, except perhaps for knowing the date. They show slight impairments in judgment and problem-solving,

Table 3.2 Clinical Dementia Rating (CDR) scale for Alzheimer's disease

CDR rating	0 (Normal)	0.5 (Very mild)	1 (Mild)	2 (Moderate)
MMSE Mean (range)	29 (27–30)	25.7 (24–27)	20.0 (16–26)	13.6 (6–17)
Memory (major category)	No memory loss or slight inconsistent forgetfulness	Consistent slight forgetfulness, partial recollection of events, "benign" forgetfulness	Moderate memory loss; more marked for recent events; defect interferes with everyday activities	Severe memory loss; only highly learned material retained; new material rapidly lost
Secondary categories				
Orientation	Fully oriented	Fully oriented except for slight difficulty with time relationships	Moderate difficulty with time relationships; oriented for place at examination; may have geographic disorientation elsewhere	Severe difficulty with time relationships; usually disoriented to time, often to place

Continued

Table 3.2 Clinical Dementia Rating (CDR) scale for Alzheimer's disease—cont'd				
CDR rating	**0 (Normal)**	**0.5 (Very mild)**	**1 (Mild)**	**2 (Moderate)**
MMSE Mean (range)	*29 (27–30)*	*25.7 (24–27)*	*20.0 (16–26)*	*13.6 (6–17)*
Judgment and problem-solving	Solves everyday problems and handles business and financial affairs well; judgment good in relation to past performance	Slight impairment in solving problems, and understanding similarities and differences	Moderate difficulties in handling problems, understanding similarities and differences; social judgment usually maintained	Severely impaired in handling problems, understanding similarities and differences; social judgment usually impaired
Community affairs	Independent function at usual level in job, shopping, and volunteer and social groups	Slight impairment in these activities	Unable to function independently at these activities although may still be engaged in some; appears normal to casual inspection	No pretense of independent function outside home. Appears well enough to be taken to function outside a family home
Home and hobbies	Life at home, hobbies, and intellectual interests are well maintained	Life at home, hobbies, and intellectual interests slightly impaired	Mild but definite impairment of function at home, more difficult chores abandoned, more complicated hobbies and interests abandoned	Only simple chores preserved; very restricted interests, poorly maintained
Personal care	Fully capable of self-care	Fully capable of self-care	Needs prompting	Requires assistance in dressing, hygiene, keeping of personal effects

Adapted from Morris, J.C., 1993. The Clinical Dementia Rating (CDR): current version and scoring rules. Neurology 43, 2412–2414.

community affairs, and home life and hobbies. For example, balancing the checkbook and keeping track of bills may become more difficult, and they may buy the same grocery items a number of times. They can usually manage their medications with a pill-box or other system of organization. These patients are typically able to prepare simple meals, and can usually be on their own for a few days at a time without getting into trouble. Most patients with very mild Alzheimer's disease are safe to drive, although they may become

Table 3.3 Alzheimer's disease (Alzheimer's disease) staging and clinical signs

Prodromal, MCI	Mild Alzheimer's disease	Moderate Alzheimer's disease	Severe/late-stage Alzheimer's disease
Very mild cognitive decline	Memory loss	Increasing memory loss	Inability to recognize family or to communicate
Memory lapses	Confusion about location or familiar places	Confusion	Lost sense of self
Poor word-finding	Taking longer to accomplish normal daily tasks	Problems recognizing friends and family	Weight loss
Decline in ability to plan and organize	Trouble handling money and paying bills	Poor judgment leading to bad decisions	Groaning, moaning, grunting
	Poor judgment leading to bad decisions	Difficulty organizing thoughts and thinking logically	Increased sleeping
	Loss of spontaneity and sense of initiative	Inability to learn new things or to cope with new or unexpected situations	Lack of bladder and bowel control
	Mood and personality changes, increased anxiety	Restlessness, agitation, anxiety, tearfulness, wandering	Seizures, skin infections, difficulty swallowing
		Repetitive statements or movement	Aspiration pneumonia
		Hallucinations, delusions, suspiciousness, paranoia	Death

lost on occasion, particularly when driving at night or to a new location (for more on driving see Chapter 23: *Life adjustments*). (See Chapter 4: *Mild cognitive impairment* for differences between very mild Alzheimer's disease and mild cognitive impairment.)

Mild

Patients with mild Alzheimer's disease show noticeable declines in memory and often word-finding, and these declines interfere with everyday activities. They usually show some disorientation to time and place. Judgment and problem-solving are moderately impaired. They are unable to function independently in community affairs. They cannot perform complicated hobbies and household tasks, but may still be able to perform simple ones. They are able to perform personal care tasks such as brushing teeth, changing clothes, and bathing, although they may need reminding to do these activities. These patients are usually safe to be on their own for a few hours, but may forget to eat, take medications, bathe, and change their clothes if left alone for a few days. Most patients with mild Alzheimer's disease should not drive, as their judgment, processing speed, and executive and visuospatial function all begin to be impaired.

Moderate

In moderate Alzheimer's disease, memory loss is severe; only remote and/or very prominent memories are retained, and almost all new material is rapidly lost. Disorientation to time and place are common. Judgment and problem-solving show severe impairment. Although the patient appears well enough to be taken to activities outside the home, there is no pretense of independent function. Only simple hobbies and household tasks can be maintained. Assistance is needed in personal care activities such as dressing and hygiene, and urinary incontinence often develops. Patients with moderate Alzheimer's disease should not be left alone due to potential issues of wandering, incontinence, and safety.

Severe

In the severe stage of Alzheimer's disease, memory is severely impaired and only fragments of memory remain. The patient is typically only oriented to self. Judgment and problem-solving are not possible. The patient appears too ill to be taken to activities outside the home, and the patient is not capable of pursuing hobbies or performing household tasks. The patient requires help with all aspects of personal care and is frequently incontinent of both urine and feces. Patients with severe Alzheimer's disease are usually managed in a long-term care facility.

THINGS TO LOOK FOR IN THE HISTORY

Alzheimer's disease typically starts insidiously with either memory loss or word-finding difficulties. Different family members often date the onset of symptoms to different months or years; such disagreement is common and suggests an insidious onset. Usually symptoms are noticeable for 6 months to several years prior to coming to the attention of a healthcare professional.

In addition to memory loss and word-finding difficulties, other common signs and symptoms to look for in the history include geographical disorientation (getting lost) and impairments in reasoning, problem-solving, and judgments. Apathy, depression, and anxiety are common in very mild and mild Alzheimer's disease, and impairment in controlling one's behavior increases as the disease progresses. See Chapter 2: *Evaluating the patient with memory loss* for an in-depth discussion of these and other elements of the history in Alzheimer's disease.

THINGS TO LOOK FOR ON THE PHYSICAL AND NEUROLOGICAL EXAMINATION

In very mild Alzheimer's disease, the physical and neurological examination is typically normal, except for trouble with praxis. As the disease progresses into the mild, moderate, and severe stages, a number of neurological signs often develop, including brisk deep tendon reflexes and frontal release signs such as the snout, grasp, and palmomental reflexes. See Chapter 2: *Evaluating the patient with memory loss* for a discussion of these frontal release signs. Although none of these signs are sensitive or specific for Alzheimer's disease, they do suggest that something is wrong in the central nervous system, and thus support the diagnosis of a brain disease of some type (as opposed to, for example, depression or normal aging).

PATTERN OF IMPAIRMENT ON COGNITIVE TESTS

Memory, language, reasoning and judgment, visuospatial function, and attention may all be impaired in Alzheimer's disease. However, in the very mild and mild stages there are common patterns that may be observed on cognitive tests that may aid in diagnosis. In addition to the discussions below, please also see Chapter 2: *Evaluating the patient with memory loss* for additional information on the pattern of cognitive impairment in Alzheimer's disease.

Memory

Although Alzheimer's disease may affect episodic memory in several different ways, one hallmark of the disease is that memory is impaired even when the learning or encoding of information is maximized by multiple rehearsals, and after retrieval demands have been minimized with the use of a multiple choice recognition test. In other words, even when patients appear to have successfully learned new information by repeating it back over several learning trials, they are typically unable to recall the information and often even to recognize this information on a multiple choice test. This type of memory loss is often referred to as a "rapid rate of forgetting," although whether the information has been truly learned or not in the first place has been a matter of debate (e.g., Budson et al., 2007).

From a practical standpoint, this means that in very mild and mild Alzheimer's disease on the MMSE and the Blessed Dementia Scale (BDS), for example, the registration or learning of the items is usually intact, but recall is usually impaired (and, although it is not part of these tests, patients are also unable to choose the registered words from a list). Similarly, on more comprehensive tests that include both recall and recognition components (such as the CERAD word list memory test (Welsh et al., 1992)), there will be a number of words successfully learned in the encoding trials that are not recognized on the multiple choice recognition test.

Language

The problems with language in Alzheimer's disease are usually attributable to the combination of an anomia plus an impairment of semantic memory. From a cognitive testing standpoint, two aspects of this impairment are typically found. First, there is an anomia, or impairment in naming uncommon objects. In very mild and mild Alzheimer's disease this impairment may be observed in tests such as the Boston Naming Test (Balthazar et al., 2008). In this test, line drawings of items are presented, with very common items shown at the beginning of the test (e.g., comb) and less common items shown toward the end of the test (e.g., trellis). Although the official Boston Naming Test consists of 60 items, 30- and 15-item versions have been successfully used. Note that only when patients reach the moderate stage of Alzheimer's disease do they typically show difficulty in naming the two items on the MMSE.

The second aspect of language that is typically impaired in Alzheimer's disease is the ability to generate an adequate number of words in 1 minute in certain semantic categories, such as "animals," "fruits," and "vegetables." In fact, many patients with very mild and mild disease show impairment on these tests of word generation to categories, but perform normally on tests of word generation to letters. See Appendix A: *Cognitive test and questionnaire forms, instructions, and normative data* for additional discussion of these tests.

Reasoning and judgment

Patients with Alzheimer's at almost all stages of disease are impaired in their reasoning, judgment, problem-solving, abstraction, and insight. Although an idea of impairment in these abilities is typically best obtained from the history, they may be evaluated in several other ways as well. First, there are a number of standard neuropsychological tests to evaluate this aspect of cognition. Second, impairment in these abilities may also be observed in the clinic by asking patients:

- what they would do in certain situations (e.g., "What would you do if you found an envelope on the street with an address and a stamp on it?"),
- to interpret proverbs (e.g., "What does it mean to say: a rolling stone gathers no moss?"), or
- to make abstractions (e.g., "How are a table and chair alike?").

Visuospatial function

Visuospatial function is impaired in Alzheimer's disease, and it becomes progressively worse as the disease worsens. In the very mild or mild stage of disease, difficulty with somewhat complex tasks such as clock drawing and copying intersecting pentagons may be impaired. In later stages even less demanding tasks such as copying familiar shapes (such as a triangle) becomes difficult.

Attention

It is important to differentiate simple versus complex attention. Simple attention, such as counting from one to 20, reciting the months of the year forwards, spelling a common word, or performing simple addition (e.g., 2 plus 5) is typically intact in very mild and mild Alzheimer's disease. More complex attention requiring the use of working memory (the ability to maintain information in memory while at the same time manipulating this information), however, is often impaired at this stage of the disease. Complex attention includes tasks such as counting from 20 back down to one, reciting the months of the year backwards, spelling a common word backwards, and performing more complex arithmetic (e.g., subtracting 7s serially from 100).

Examples

On the MMSE, the patient with very mild Alzheimer's disease may show difficulty with the date, recall of one to three of the items, and intersecting pentagons. In addition to those items, patients with mild Alzheimer's disease may also show difficulty with the year, month, day, county, city, name of place, floor, serial 7s/WORLD backwards, the three-step command, and writing a sentence. In the moderate and severe stages of Alzheimer's disease, as language becomes more impaired, patients may show difficulty with the remaining items as well.

On the Blessed Dementia Scale patients with very mild Alzheimer's disease may show difficulty with the date, street address, one to five of the items of the 5-minute recall, dates of WWI, and the Vice-President of the USA. Patients with mild Alzheimer's disease may also show difficulty with the year, month, day, specific time of day, city, name of place, dates of WWII, President of the USA, months of the year backwards, and counting from 20 back to one. Patients with moderate Alzheimer's disease may show additional difficulties with age, general time of day, type of place, recognition of persons, school attended, occupation, town where patient worked, name of employer, and counting from one to 20. Finally, patients with severe Alzheimer's disease may show difficulty with the few remaining items, including their date and place of birth, and ultimately their own name.

LABORATORY STUDIES

There are no routine laboratory studies that support the diagnosis of Alzheimer's disease. It is, of course, important to obtain a number of screening laboratory studies to search for readily treatable causes of cognitive dysfunction. At a minimum these should include vitamin B12 and thyroid-stimulating hormone, and this list should be expanded to include a rapid plasma reagent test, Lyme titer, complete blood count, or measurement of electrolyte levels, depending upon the patient's exposure and previous studies. Tests of cerebrospinal fluid measuring $A\beta42$ and tau are being investigated but are not part of routine clinical practice (Box 3.10). Please see Chapter 2: *Evaluating the patient with memory loss* for additional tests that may be important to consider in the evaluation.

BOX 3.10 CEREBROSPINAL FLUID STUDIES

There are three biomarkers that can be measured in the cerebral spinal fluid that may be helpful in the diagnosis of Alzheimer's disease in the future: $A\beta_{42}$, total tau, and a new biomarker, hyperphosphorylated tau. Initial studies using the ratio of low $A\beta_{42}$ and high total tau were able to differentiate between patients with Alzheimer's disease and controls with high sensitivity (85%) and specificity (86%), but were unable to separate patients with Alzheimer's disease from those with other forms of dementia (specificity 58%). Tau protein can by phosphorylated at several amino acids, forming different types of hyperphosphorylated tau or "p-tau." Types of hyperphosphorylated tau that have been studied include $p\text{-tau}_{231P}$, $p\text{-tau}_{181P}$, and $p\text{-tau}_{199P}$. Recent investigations have found that, when the biomarkers $A\beta_{42}$, total tau, and p-tau are combined, Alzheimer's disease could be distinguished from other forms of dementia with sensitivity and specificity of 85–90%, and a 6-year study found that it was also possible to predict which patients with mild cognitive impairment would develop Alzheimer's disease with a sensitivity of 95% and specificity of 85% (Hansson et al., 2006). We view this research as highly promising but not yet ready for routine clinical practice; see Hampel et al. (2008), for review.

STRUCTURAL IMAGING STUDIES

It should first be clearly stated that Alzheimer's disease cannot be either ruled in or ruled out by the pattern of atrophy observable on a structural imaging scan, or the lack of such atrophy. The primary purpose in obtaining a structural imaging study is to identify or rule out other etiologies which may cause dementia. Thus, a structural imaging study is ordered to evaluate for the presence of large strokes, tumors, hemorrhages, hydrocephalus, the extent of small vessel ischemic disease, and other such pathology.

Having stated that structural imaging studies cannot be used to diagnose Alzheimer's disease or to refute it, as mentioned in Chapter 2 it is worthwhile looking to determine whether there is atrophy bilaterally in hippocampi, anterior temporal lobes, and parietal lobes (see Fig. 3.12). If this pattern of atrophy is present in combination with the appropriate clinical context it may suggest Alzheimer's disease. Structural imaging studies are also invaluable for showing the extent of small vessel ischemic disease that a patient has. Because almost every patient aged 70 years or older has some small vessel ischemic

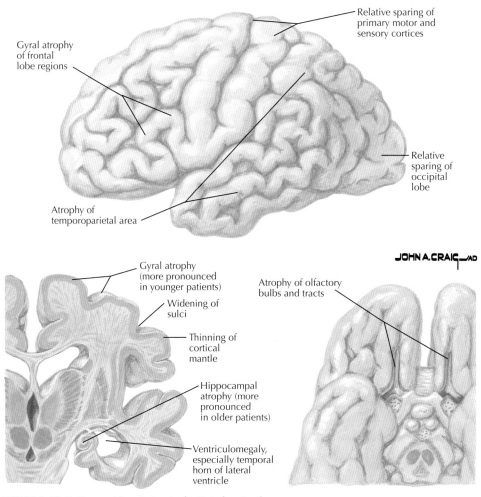

FIGURE 3.12 Patterns of focal atrophy in Alzheimer's disease.

A color version of this figure is available online at http://www.expertconsult.com

disease, the question for the clinician is whether the extent of the small vessel ischemic disease is the minor, major, or (rarely) sole factor in the patient's memory loss. See Figure 2.3 for an example of an MRI scan of a patient with mild Alzheimer's disease and an average amount of small vessel ischemic cerebrovascular disease. See Figure 2.4 for a CT scan of a patient with mild Alzheimer's disease showing hippocampal atrophy.

FUNCTIONAL IMAGING STUDIES

A functional imaging study (an FDG-PET or a ^{99}Tc SPECT) is not necessary in the evaluation of the vast majority of patients in whom Alzheimer's disease is suspected. If the history and cognitive examination suggest a case of straightforward Alzheimer's disease in a patient older than age 65, the history, physical and neurological examination, cognitive testing, and laboratory and structural imaging studies are sufficient to make an accurate diagnosis given the high prevalence of Alzheimer's disease in older adults. Furthermore, although functional imaging studies can be helpful in differentiating different types of dementia, they are not helpful in distinguishing between mild Alzheimer's disease and normal aging or depression—some of the more common diagnostic possibilities.

Functional imaging studies are helpful, however, in two circumstances when considering a diagnosis of Alzheimer's disease, as discussed in Chapter 2. First, when the patient is 65 years old or less, we recommend supporting the diagnosis with a SPECT or PET scan even if the rest of the work-up strongly suggests a case of Alzheimer's disease. The prevalence of Alzheimer's is much less likely in someone so young; for this reason the differential diagnosis is broad, and it becomes as important to "rule in" Alzheimer's disease as it is to "rule out" all other causes of memory loss and dementia. Second, in addition to Alzheimer's disease, when other forms of dementia are being strongly considered, such as frontotemporal dementia, the SPECT or PET scan can help distinguish between Alzheimer's disease and these other forms of dementia. For additional information see Chapter 2: *Evaluating the patient with memory loss* and Figure 2.5.

DIFFERENTIAL DIAGNOSIS

In our experience, the most common disorders to be confused with Alzheimer's disease are other degenerative dementias. If the patient showed behavioral problems and/or personality changes first and foremost, then a frontotemporal dementia should be considered. A frontotemporal dementia should also be considered if problems with language or judgment and reasoning predominate. See Chapter 7 for more information on frontotemporal dementia.

If there is any evidence of visual hallucinations or visual misperceptions, perhaps around the time of sleep, dementia with Lewy bodies should be considered (see Chapter 5). Dementia with Lewy bodies should also be considered if there is Parkinsonism. Parkinsonism should also of course lead one to consider Parkinson's disease, and Parkinsonian syndromes which affect cognition such as progressive supranuclear palsy (see Chapter 8) and corticobasal degeneration (see Chapter 9).

Vascular dementia should be considered if there are many large or small ischemic strokes on the structural imaging scan (CT or MRI) (see Chapter 6). However, if the history and cognitive examination suggest Alzheimer's disease, then we would argue that the patient most likely has Alzheimer's disease, the symptoms of which may be exacerbated to some extent by the amount of small vessel ischemic disease. Whether the patient can be said to have a mixed dementia of Alzheimer's disease plus small vessel ischemic disease depends upon the amount of small vessel ischemic disease present on the structural imaging study, and whether a number of the symptoms are consistent with vascular dementia (see Chapter 6: *Vascular dementia and vascular cognitive impairment*).

TREATMENTS

As discussed in detail in Section III: *Treatment of Memory Loss*, current pharmacological therapies to treat Alzheimer's disease include medications approved by the US Food and Drug Administration (FDA) to enhance cognition in Alzheimer's disease (cholinesterase inhibitors and memantine), medications to treat mood, anxiety, agitation, and other behavioral problems, as well as vitamins, herbs, and supplements.

For patients with Alzheimer's disease, we would recommend treatment with a cholinesterase inhibitor: donepezil (Aricept, now available as generic), sustained release galantamine (Razadyne SR, now available as generic), or the rivastigmine (Exelon) patch; oral rivastigmine is not well tolerated. Donepezil (Aricept) has been approved by the FDA for use in mild (including very mild), moderate, and severe Alzheimer's disease, and galantamine (Razadyne) and rivastigmine (Exelon) have been approved for use in patients with mild and moderate disease. (We would note, however, that we have used galantamine (Razadyne) and rivastigmine (Exelon) in patients with severe Alzheimer's disease to good effect as well.) These cholinesterase inhibitors improve memory and other aspects of cognition, improve function, and reduce behavioral and neuropsychiatric symptoms. Cholinesterase inhibitors should be initiated as soon as the diagnosis is established, and continued until the goal of treatment is only hospice, that is, until the goal of treatment is to help the patient die with care, comfort, and dignity. See Chapter 14: *Cholinesterase inhibitors*, for more on this class of medications.

In addition to treatment with cholinesterase inhibitors, we also recommend treatment with memantine (Namenda) in patients with moderate and severe Alzheimer's disease, as well as in patients with milder forms, who we believe would benefit. As discussed in Chapter 15, memantine (Namenda) tends to improve functional and neuropsychiatric symptoms in patients with Alzheimer's disease more than it improves memory. Although impairment in functional status and neuropsychiatric symptoms are most prominent in patients with moderate and severe Alzheimer's disease, these problems are also present in many patients with more mild disease, and it is therefore worthwhile trying memantine (Namenda) in these patients, especially when it is used in combination with a cholinesterase inhibitor.

Although many patients with Alzheimer's disease lack insight into their condition, those few patients who retain even a small amount of insight are understandably quite depressed and anxious about their memory loss and the fact that they have Alzheimer's disease. Sometimes patients articulate this, and sometimes they feel anxious because they know at some level things are wrong even if they cannot say just what it is. And in some patients with Alzheimer's disease in the moderate stage, anxiety can manifest itself as agitation. It is therefore not surprising that approximately one-half to two-thirds of patients with Alzheimer's disease benefit from selective serotonin reuptake inhibitor medication. In our experience, sertraline (Zoloft) or escitalopram (Lexapro) work best because they work well to treat both depression and anxiety, and because they are well tolerated with few side-effects in the patient with dementia.

As patients with Alzheimer's disease progress to moderate and severe stages, additional medications to control behavior are often necessary, including atypical antipsychotics and trazodone (Desyrel). Please see Section IV: *Behavioral and Psychological Symptoms of Dementia* for additional information on pharmacological and non-pharmacological treatment of these symptoms.

QUICK START 2: MEDICAL TREATMENT FOR ALZHEIMER'S DISEASE

Medication class	FDA approved?	Summary of benefits	Common side-effects
Cholinesterase inhibitors (see Chapter 14 for comparison of cholinesterase inhibitors)	Yes	Multiple studies demonstrating cognitive, behavioral, and functional benefit	Gastrointestinal (nausea, diarrhea), vivid dreams

---

QUICK START 2: MEDICAL TREATMENT FOR ALZHEIMER'S DISEASE—Cont'd

Memantine (Namenda) (see Chapter 15)	Yes	Multiple studies demonstrating cognitive, behavioral, and functional benefit	Drowsiness and confusion, dose-related, sometimes transient, worse in milder patients
Selective serotonin reuptake inhibitors – particularly those that treat both anxiety and depression (Lexapro, Zoloft) (see Chapter 22)	No – off-label use	Treatment if depression that often accompanies MCI (clinical experience, but no published studies)	Gastrointestinal upset; sexual dysfunction
Atypical antipsychotics (see Chapter 22)	No – off-label use	Treatment of hallucinations, delusions, and agitation	Sedation at higher doses, increased risk of stroke

---

References

Alzheimer's Association, 2010. 2010 Alzheimer's disease facts and figures. Alzheimers Dement. 6, 158–194.

American Psychiatric Association, 2000. Diagnostic and Statistical Manual of Mental Disorders DSM-IV-TR, fourth Ed. American Psychiatric Publishing, Inc, Arlington, VA.

Balthazar, M.L., Cendes, F., Damasceno, B.P., 2008. Semantic error patterns on the Boston Naming Test in normal aging, amnesic mild cognitive impairment, and mild Alzheimer's disease: is there semantic disruption? Neuropsychology 22, 703–709.

Budson, A.E., Simons, J.S., Waring, J.D., et al., 2007. Memory for the September 11, 2001, terrorist attacks one year later in patients with Alzheimer's disease, patients with mild cognitive impairment, and healthy older adults. Cortex 43, 875–888.

Cobb, J.L., Wolf, P.A., Au, R., et al., 1995. The effect of education on the incidence of dementia and Alzheimer's disease in the Framingham Study. Neurology 45, 1707–1712.

Fleminger, S., Oliver, D.L., Lovestone, S., et al., 2003. Head injury as a risk factor for Alzheimer's disease: the evidence 10 years on; a partial replication. J. Neurol. Neurosurg. Psychiatry 74, 857–862.

Hampel, H., Burger, K., Teipel, S.J., et al., 2008. Core candidate neurochemical and imaging biomarkers of Alzheimer's disease. Alzheimers Dement. 4, 38–48.

Hansson, O., Zetterberg, H., Buchhave, P., et al., 2006. Association between CSF biomarkers and incipient Alzheimer's disease in patients with mild cognitive impairment: a follow-up study. Lancet Neurol. 5, 228–234.

Holmes, C., Boche, D., Wilkinson, D., et al., 2008. Long-term effects of Abeta42 immunisation in Alzheimer's disease: follow-up of a randomised, placebo-controlled phase I trial. Lancet 372, 216–223.

Josephs, K.A., Whitwell, J.L., Ahmed, Z., et al., 2008. Beta-amyloid burden is not associated with rates of brain atrophy. Ann. Neurol. 63, 204–212.

Lautenschlager, N.T., Cupples, L.A., Rao, V.S., et al., 1996. Risk of dementia among relatives of Alzheimer's disease patients in the MIRAGE study: What is in store for the oldest old? Neurology 46, 641–650.

Luchsinger, J.A., Tang, M.X., Shea, S., et al., 2004. Plasma homocysteine levels and risk of Alzheimer disease. Neurology 62, 1972–1976.

Mayeux, R., Ottman, R., Maestre, G., et al., 1995. Synergistic effects of traumatic head injury and apolipoprotein-epsilon 4 in patients with Alzheimer's disease. Neurology 45, 555–557.

McKee, A.C., Cantu, R.C., Nowinski, C.J., et al., 2009. Chronic traumatic encephalopathy in athletes: progressive tauopathy after repetitive head injury. J. Neuropathol. Exp. Neurol. 68, 709–735.

McKhann, G., Drachman, D., Folstein, M., et al., 1984. Clinical diagnosis of Alzheimer's disease: report of the NINCDS-ADRDA Work Group under the auspices of Department of Health and Human Services Task Force on Alzheimer's Disease. Neurology 34, 939–944.

Mesulam, M., 2004. The cholinergic lesion of Alzheimer's disease: pivotal factor or side show? Learn. Mem. 11, 43–49.

Mesulam, M., Shaw, P., Mash, D., et al., 2004. Cholinergic nucleus basalis tauopathy emerges early in the aging-MCI-Alzheimer's disease continuum. Ann. Neurol. 55, 815–828.

Miller, J.W., Green, R., Mungas, D.M., et al., 2002. Homocysteine, vitamin B6, and vascular disease in Alzheimer's disease patients. Neurology 58, 1471–1475.

Seshadri, S., Beiser, A., Selhub, J., et al., 2002. Plasma homocysteine as a risk factor for dementia and Alzheimer's disease. N. Engl. J. Med. 346, 476–483.

Snowdon, D.A., Kemper, S.J., Mortimer, J.A., et al., 1996. Linguistic ability in early life and cognitive function and Alzheimer's disease in late life. Findings from the Nun Study. JAMA 275, 528–532.

Snowdon, D.A., Greiner, L.H., Mortimer, J.A., et al., 1997. Brain infarction and the clinical expression of Alzheimer disease. The Nun Study. JAMA 277, 813–817.

Snowdon, D.A., Greiner, L.H., Markesbery, W.R., 2000. Linguistic ability in early life and the neuropathology of Alzheimer's disease and cerebrovascular disease. Findings from the Nun Study. Ann. N. Y. Acad. Sci. 903, 34–38.

Welsh, K.A., Butters, N., Hughes, J.P., et al., 1992. Detection and staging of dementia in Alzheimer's disease. Use of the neuropsychological measures developed for the Consortium to Establish a Registry for Alzheimer's Disease. Arch. Neurol. 49, 448–452.

Wilcock, G.K., Esiri, M.M., 1982. Plaques, tangles and dementia. A quantitative study. J. Neurol. Sci. 56, 343–356.

Mild cognitive impairment

4

QUICK START: MILD COGNITIVE IMPAIRMENT

Definition	• Mild cognitive impairment is a term used to indicate patients who may be in the prodromal stage of Alzheimer's disease or another dementia. • Patients with mild cognitive impairment are not functionally impaired enough to meet the criteria for dementia, but still show cognitive problems.
Prevalence	• Estimates vary widely from 3–22% with higher percentages associated with increasing age. • Approximately 70% of patients with mild cognitive impairment ultimately develop Alzheimer's disease or another dementia at the rate of about 7–15% per year.
Genetic risk	• Little is currently known about the genetic risk. • For patients with amnestic mild cognitive impairment, the genetic risk is similar to that of Alzheimer's disease.
Cognitive symptoms	• Patients with mild cognitive impairment who have primarily memory problems are termed as having "amnestic" mild cognitive impairment and typically develop Alzheimer's disease. • Patients with mild cognitive impairment who have impairment in domains other than memory (such as executive function and language) are termed as having "non-amnestic" mild cognitive impairment and often progress to a non-Alzheimer's dementia.
Diagnostic criteria	• The most widely accepted set of criteria are the "Petersen criteria." • The Petersen criteria essentially require: (1) complaints of cognitive dysfunction (2) presence of cognitive impairment in one or more domains (typically memory) (3) the cognitive impairment does not affect functioning (4) dementia is not present.
Behavioral symptoms	• Changes in behavior have not been reported in published research. • Depression and other mood changes are often noted by clinicians.
Treatment	• There is no FDA approved treatment for mild cognitive impairment. However, studies suggest that patients with amnestic mild cognitive impairment can be successfully treated with cholinesterase inhibitors, improving memory and delaying Alzheimer's disease by a year or more, resulting in cholinesterase inhibitors being prescribed for these patients at most major memory centers in the USA.
Top differential diagnoses	• Normal aging, early Alzheimer's disease, depression, cerebrovascular disease.

PREVALENCE, PROGNOSIS, AND DEFINITION

Mild cognitive impairment (often referred to by its abbreviation, MCI) is not a specific disease entity or even a clinical syndrome; it is a conceptual entity. Nevertheless, the concept of MCI has proved to be extremely useful (Jicha & Petersen, 2007). There are many patients whose evaluation demonstrates that their cognition is not normal, but they do not meet criteria for any type of dementia. MCI is used as a label for these patients. Because degenerative diseases such as Alzheimer's disease (AD) and frontotemporal dementia progress slowly over years, patients with these dementias must have gone through a prodromal stage prior to obvious clinical manifestations of their disorder (Fig. 4.1). In fact, studies have found that about 70% of patients with a diagnostic label of MCI "convert" to Alzheimer's disease or another dementia at a rate of about 7–15% per year (Fig. 4.2). This conversion rate is much higher than that of individuals older than 65 in the general population, whose conversion rates are approximately 1–2%. That 70% of patients with MCI develop dementia indicates that 30% of patients with this diagnostic label do not. This 30% either remain stable over time, or improve back toward normal cognition. Depending upon the study, the incidence of MCI has been reported as being from 1–6% per year, with the prevalence ranging from 3% to 22% in individuals older than 65 years, and rising with increasing age. MCI is usually divided into amnestic versus non-amnestic, and single versus multiple cognitive domains of impairment, leading to four common types (Table 4.1).

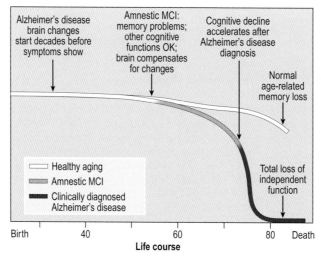

FIGURE 4.1 Charting the course from healthy aging to Alzheimer's disease (AD). MCI, mild cognitive impairment.

From NIA/NIH Alzheimer's Disease, 2008. Unraveling the Mystery, NIH Publication 08-3782, September.

http://www.nia.nih.gov/Alzheimers/Publications/Unraveling/

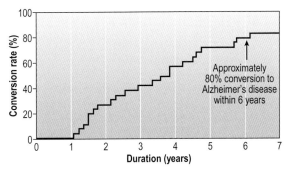

FIGURE 4.2 Between 70% and 80% of patients with mild cognitive impairment eventually develop dementia.

From Petersen, R.C., Stevens, J.C., Ganguili, M., et al., 2001. Practice parameter: early detection of dementia: mild cognitive impairment (an evidence-based review): report of the Quality Standards Subcommittee of the American Academy of Neurology. Neurology 56,1133–1142.

Table 4.1 Common types of mild cognitive impairment

	Amnestic	**Non-amnestic**
Single domain	Amnestic single domain	Non-amnestic single domain
Multiple domain	Amnestic multiple domain	Non-amnestic multiple domain
Likely etiology	Alzheimer's disease	Other (cerebrovascular disease, non-Alzheimer's neurodegenerative diseases)

DIAGNOSTIC CRITERIA

The clinical criteria for the diagnosis of MCI are listed in Box 4.1.

These clinical criteria are purposefully vague so that they can be implemented in a wide variety of settings and populations. It is important for each clinician to formally or informally "operationalize" these criteria. That is, each clinician must decide what is normal and abnormal for the tests that they use for an individual with a given education in their own population. These criteria have been operationalized in several different ways in the context of research. A common example can be found in Box 4.2, which shows criteria that were developed for a clinical trial of amnestic MCI.

BOX 4.1 CLINICAL CRITERIA FOR MILD COGNITIVE IMPAIRMENT

1. Memory or other cognitive complaint by patient and/or informant.
2. Memory or other cognitive impairment for age and education.
3. General cognitive function essentially normal.
4. Activities of daily living largely preserved.
5. Not demented.

Adapted from Jicha, G.A., Petersen, R.C., 2007. Mild cognitive impairment. In: Growdon, J., Rossor, M. (Eds.), The Dementias 2. Butterworth Heinemann, Philadelphia, PA.

BOX 4.2 EXAMPLE OF RESEARCH CRITERIA FOR AMNESTIC MILD COGNITIVE IMPAIRMENT

---

1. Memory complaint corroborated by an informant.
2. Abnormal memory function:
    A. Impaired delayed recall on one paragraph from the Wechsler Memory Scale-Revised Logical Memory II
        i. Cut-off scores:
            a. < or = to 8 for 16 or more years of education
            b. < or = to 4 for 8 to 15 years of education
            c. < or = to 2 for less than 8 years of education.
3. Overall function and cognition sufficiently preserved such that the patient does not meet criteria for Alzheimer's disease.
4. Not demented by the National Institute of Neurological and Communicative Disorders and Stroke—Alzheimer's disease and Related Disorders Association criteria (McKhann et al., 1984), which rely upon clinical judgment.
5. Selected additional criteria included for this study:
    A. Mini-Mental State Examination 24–30.
    B. Normal vitamin B12 levels, thyroid function studies, and non-reactive rapid plasma reagent test.
    C. No significant cerebrovascular disease, infarcts, or focal lesions.
    D. No significant depression or other psychiatric disorders.

Adapted from Petersen, R.C., Thomas, R.G., Grundman, M., et al., 2005. Vitamin E and donepezil for the treatment of mild cognitive impairment. N. Engl. J. Med. 352, 2379–2388.

COMMON MILD COGNITIVE IMPAIRMENT SCENARIOS

There are several scenarios in which we commonly diagnose a patient with MCI in our clinical practice. One such scenario occurs when we see a patient who has experienced a clear decline over time in their memory or other cognitive function, but at the same time can easily live independently. For example, the 85-year-old former college professor who, because of increasingly impaired memory, can no longer perform research, write books, or teach a class, but is fully capable of getting his groceries, making his meals, and paying his bills, in addition to performing all of his activities of daily living. In this case our best guess is that the patient has underlying Alzheimer's pathology but he is not clinically demented and therefore does not meet clinical criteria for Alzheimer's disease or other dementia at this time. This patient is at high risk for developing Alzheimer's disease in the future.

Another scenario in which we commonly make a diagnosis of MCI is in the patient who has again had a clear decline in his or her memory or other cognitive function, but at the same time has generally preserved function including activities of daily living, and the cause of the cognitive impairment is not clear. An example is the 69-year-old patient with a long-standing psychiatric disorder, on multiple psychoactive medications, who is having increasing trouble living independently; her psychiatric disorder has also been worsening and her psychoactive medications have increased in both number and dosage. Another example is the 72-year-old man with memory problems that his family believes began at the time of his cardiac surgery and have not worsened since then. In these cases it is difficult to determine whether the patient has the beginnings of a neurodegenerative disease (such as Alzheimer's) or not. Neurodegenerative diseases can certainly exacerbate or (particularly in the case of frontotemporal dementia) cause psychiatric symptoms. Although cardiac surgery can sometimes lead to significant memory and other cognitive impairment, it is more often that the physical stress of the surgery and hospitalization unmasks an incipient neurodegenerative disease. In each of these cases the prudent clinician will see the patient back in 6–12 months to determine whether the patient shows any signs of additional decline prior to making the diagnosis of a neurodegenerative disease.

RISK FACTORS, PATHOLOGY, AND PATHOPHYSIOLOGY

Because mild cognitive impairment is not a specific disease, the predominant risk factors, pathology, and pathophysiology, which are important in any individual patient with mild cognitive impairment will, of course, depend upon the particular etiology of the cognitive impairment (see Box 4.3). Although in theory this could include a myriad of possibilities (including virtually every disease entity mentioned in this book), the two most common etiologies of mild cognitive impairment in clinical practice are Alzheimer's disease and cerebrovascular disease. Studies have shown that most cases of amnestic mild cognitive impairment, whether single or multiple domain, convert to Alzheimer's disease. Many cases of non-amnestic mild cognitive impairment are attributable to cerebrovascular disease, particularly when executive function is impaired. Some clinicians and researchers have begun to use the term "vascular cognitive impairment" or "VCI" to indicate patients with mild cognitive impairment attributable to cerebrovascular disease (see Chapter 6: *Vascular dementia and vascular cognitive impairment*). Mimicking their relative prevalence, other common etiologies of mild cognitive impairment include dementia with Lewy bodies (and other Parkinsonian syndromes) and frontotemporal dementia. Depression can also be a cause of mild cognitive impairment. Although we believe that in the vast majority of cases there should be little confusion regarding whether a patient's cognitive problems are attributable to depression or attributable to Alzheimer's disease (because the history and cognitive profile are so different), differentiating mild cognitive impairment due to depression and that due to cerebrovascular disease or an early neurodegenerative disease can sometimes be difficult.

BOX 4.3 COMMON DISORDERS WHICH CAN CAUSE MILD COGNITIVE IMPAIRMENT

- Alzheimer's disease
- Cerebrovascular disease
- Other dementias
- Hippocampal sclerosis
- Normal aging
- Depression and other psychiatric disorders
- Disorders which cause a static encephalopathy:
  - Encephalitis
  - Head injury
  - Subdural fluid collection
  - Stroke
- Medical disorders

COMMON SIGNS, SYMPTOMS, AND STAGES

Again, because mild cognitive impairment is not a specific disease, the signs and symptoms will be different depending upon the type of mild cognitive impairment and of course upon the underlying etiology. In the common case of amnestic mild cognitive impairment, a decline in memory would, by definition, be present. Although in the amnestic single domain type, only memory difficulties would be present, word-finding difficulties and/or executive dysfunction, either prominent or subtle, are common in amnestic multiple domain mild cognitive impairment.

THINGS TO LOOK FOR IN THE HISTORY

One particular difference between patients with amnestic mild cognitive impairment and those with more severe impairment, such as Alzheimer's disease, is that insight is often preserved in patients with amnestic mild cognitive impairment. This insight, although often helpful in using compensatory strategies when dealing with memory difficulties, also often leads to depression. This very common secondary depression is certainly one of the reasons that it is easy to confuse amnestic mild cognitive impairment due to underlying Alzheimer's pathology with a primary depression causing secondary memory problems. (See the section on Depression and anxiety in Chapter 12: *Other disorders*, for more on how to distinguish depression from other etiologies of memory loss.)

THINGS TO LOOK FOR ON THE PHYSICAL AND NEUROLOGICAL EXAMINATION

Since mild cognitive impairment may have a number of different etiologies, it will be important to examine the patient carefully for all elements of the neurological examination described in Chapter 2, including eye movements, focal weakness or numbness, brisk or asymmetric reflexes, Babinski's sign, tremor, rigidity, gait, and frontal release signs.

PATTERN OF IMPAIRMENT ON COGNITIVE TESTS

In general, the impairment on cognitive tests should, of course, be mild. In the amnestic single domain type, only memory will be affected, and memory plus one or more additional domains will be affected in amnestic multiple domain mild cognitive impairment. For non-amnestic mild cognitive impairment domains other than memory will be affected. To detect these mild deficits, tests more sensitive than the MMSE or Blessed Dementia Scale are often needed. (See the section on Cognitive tests and questionnaires in Chapter 2: *Evaluating the patient with memory loss* for descriptions of some of these more sensitive tests.)

Examples

The score on the MMSE in the patient with amnestic mild cognitive impairment will typically range from 25 to 30, with points lost recalling the three items, and perhaps the date. Similarly on the Blessed Dementia Scale these patients will typically make between zero to seven errors, often missing some of the five recall items, the date, and perhaps the name of the Vice-President. Although scoring similarly to those with amnestic mild cognitive impairment, those patients with non-amnestic mild cognitive impairment will often have trouble with attention and executive function on the MMSE and the Blessed Dementia Scale, such as calculations, spelling WORLD backwards, and reciting the months of the year in backwards order.

LABORATORY STUDIES

Although there are no laboratory studies which support the diagnosis of mild cognitive impairment, it is particularly important to obtain a number of screening laboratory studies to search for readily treatable causes of cognitive dysfunction, as described in Chapter 2: *Evaluating the patient with memory loss.* At a minimum these should include vitamin B12 and TSH, and this list should be expanded to include a RPR, Lyme titer, CBC, or electrolytes depending upon the patient's exposure and previous studies.

STRUCTURAL IMAGING STUDIES

As in Alzheimer's disease, structural imaging studies are necessary to evaluate for the presence of large strokes, tumors, hemorrhages, hydrocephalus, the extent of small vessel ischemic disease, and other such pathology. Mild cognitive impairment itself cannot be "ruled-in" or "ruled-out" by a structural imaging scan. In patients with amnestic mild cognitive impairment, atrophy may be found in the hippocampi, anterior temporal lobes, and parietal lobes. In patients with mild cognitive impairment attributable to cerebrovascular disease (i.e.,vascular cognitive impairment, VCI), small vessel ischemic disease and/or other types of cerebrovascular disease will of course be present, typically of moderate to severe extent (see Chapter 6: *Vascular dementia and vascular cognitive impairment*).

FUNCTIONAL IMAGING STUDIES

Functional imaging studies such as FDG-PET and ^{99}Tc SPECT are neither sensitive nor specific enough to detect and/or determine the underlying etiology in a patient with mild cognitive impairment. Thus, we do not recommend routinely obtaining functional imaging studies in patients with mild cognitive impairment.

DIFFERENTIAL DIAGNOSIS

To a large extent, the diagnosis of mild cognitive impairment is a shorthand way of saying that we do not know exactly what the diagnosis is at this time. The "differential diagnosis" of mild cognitive impairment is not what other diagnosis the patient could have, but, instead, what underlying pathology or pathophysiology the patient does have that may evolve into a definitive diagnosis. Therefore, the "differential diagnosis" of mild cognitive impairment is quite broad, and includes normal aging, in addition to mild forms of almost every disease entity discussed in this book. Disorders which should always be considered are listed in Box 4.3.

Table 4.2 Comparison between mild Alzheimer's disease (AD) and amnestic mild cognitive impairment

	Mild Alzheimer's disease	Amnestic mild cognitive impairment
Cognitive complaints by patient or family	Present	Present
Cognitive deficits	Present, mild deficits	Present, very mild deficits
Functional impairment	Present	Absent
Dementia	Present	Absent
Deterioration over time	Always occurs	May occur, but may also remain stable or improve
FDA-approved treatment	Cholinesterase inhibitors	None
Recommended treatment	Cholinesterase inhibitors, SSRI if depression or anxiety	Cholinesterase inhibitors, SSRI if depression or anxiety

TREATMENTS

Although there are no FDA approved treatments for patients with mild cognitive impairment, several studies have shown that patients with amnestic mild cognitive impairment are improved by donepezil (Aricept), at least for 1 year if not longer (Petersen et al., 2005) (Table 4.2). We therefore recommend treatment with donepezil or another cholinesterase inhibitor for patients with amnestic MCI. Treatment of patients with amnestic mild cognitive impairment with cholinesterase inhibitors has become the standard of care in most specialized memory centers in the USA.

Other treatments may also be helpful. As in patients with mild Alzheimer's disease, most patients with mild cognitive impairment are anxious and depressed because of their awareness of their cognitive deficits, and benefit from an SSRI medication such as sertraline (Zoloft). Memantine (Namenda) can occasionally be worth considering in those patients with mild cognitive impairment who present with problems in functional and/or neuropsychiatric domains, although there are no published studies supporting its use in this population (see Chapter 15: *Memantine (Namenda)*).

References

Jicha, G.A., Petersen, R.C., 2007. Mild cognitive impairment. In: Growdon, J., Rossor, M. (Eds.), The Dementias 2. Butterworth Heinemann, Philadelphia, PA.

Petersen, R.C., Thomas, R.G., Grundman, M., et al., 2005. Vitamin E and donepezil for the treatment of mild cognitive impairment. N. Engl. J. Med. 352, 2379–2388.

McKhann, G., Drachman, D., Folstein, M., et al., 1984. Clinical diagnosis of Alzheimer's disease: report of the NINCDS-ADRDA Work Group under the auspices of Department of Health and Human Services Task Force on Alzheimer's Disease. Neurology 34, 939–944.

Dementia with Lewy bodies (including Parkinson's disease dementia)

QUICK START 1: DEMENTIA WITH LEWY BODIES (INCLUDING PARKINSON'S DISEASE DEMENTIA)

Definition	• Dementia with Lewy bodies is a neurodegenerative disease of the brain characterized clinically by dementia, visual hallucinations, and Parkinsonism, and characterized pathologically by Lewy body formation and abnormal alpha-synuclein metabolism. • Parkinson's disease dementia is an older term used for dementia with Lewy bodies when extrapyramidal motor features are present for more than a year prior to the onset of dementia.
Prevalence	• Autopsy studies have suggested that dementia with Lewy bodies accounts for up to 20% of cases of dementia, either by itself or in combination with other disorders.
Genetic risk	• There are familial cases of dementia with Lewy bodies related to mutations or repeats of the alpha-synuclein gene located on chromosome 4. Most patients with dementia with Lewy bodies, however, do not show abnormalities of this gene.
Cognitive and other symptoms	• Impairment in attention, executive function, and visuospatial ability are often prominent. Memory impairment may or may not be prominent initially. • In patients who also have Alzheimer's pathology, memory and word-finding deficits are prominent as well. • Sleep disturbances are common in dementia with Lewy bodies, leading to disrupted circadian rhythm, fluctuating levels of attention and alertness, and rapid eye movement sleep behavior disorder.
Diagnostic criteria	• Dementia with Lewy bodies should be suspected in any patient with dementia who has well-formed visual hallucinations of people and animals and/or Parkinsonism. • Criteria: essential for a diagnosis is dementia. • Core features (two are sufficient) include: **(1)** fluctuating cognition (pronounced variations in attention and alertness) **(2)** visual hallucinations (recurrent, well formed, detailed, of people and/or animals, often initially present around transitions between sleep and wake) **(3)** spontaneous features of Parkinsonism (i.e., Parkinsonism not related to medications).

Continued

Memory Loss: A Practical Guide for Clinicians.

QUICK START 1: DEMENTIA WITH LEWY BODIES (INCLUDING PARKINSON'S DISEASE DEMENTIA)—Cont'd

Behavioral symptoms	• Changes in behavior include visual hallucinations (which may or may not be frightening) and fluctuations in attention and alertness.
Treatment	• Cholinesterase inhibitors have been found to be beneficial; one has been approved by the US Food and Drug Administration.
	• Other medications, including levodopa/carbidopa (Sinemet), memantine, selective serotonin reuptake inhibitors, and atypical antipsychotics, may be used with caution
Top differential diagnoses	• Most common: Alzheimer's disease and mixed dementia (dementia with Lewy bodies plus Alzheimer's disease).
	• Less common: vascular dementia and atypical Parkinsonian syndromes (e.g., corticobasal degeneration, progressive supranuclear palsy).

PREVALENCE, PROGNOSIS, AND DEFINITION

Dementia with Lewy bodies is a neurodegenerative disease of the brain characterized clinically by dementia, visual hallucinations, and/or Parkinsonism, and characterized pathologically by Lewy body formation and abnormal alpha-synuclein metabolism. Parkinson's disease dementia (PDD), which used to be diagnosed when extrapyramidal motor features are present for more than a year prior to the onset of dementia, is now recognized to be a different point on the spectrum of dementia with Lewy bodies. In this book, we will refer to such cases of Parkinson's disease dementia by the more inclusive term "dementia with Lewy bodies," regardless of whether motor symptoms preceded cognitive symptoms. Older, infrequently used terms for dementia with Lewy bodies include diffuse Lewy body disease, dementia associated with cortical Lewy bodies, the Lewy body variant of Alzheimer's disease, senile dementia of the Lewy body type, and Lewy body dementia.

It used to be regarded as uncommon, several autopsy studies have suggested that dementia with Lewy bodies accounts for up to 20% of cases of dementia (Perry et al., 1989). Further, many clinical studies have found that dementia with Lewy bodies is the second most common cause of dementia in the older adult after Alzheimer's disease, with one study finding a rate of dementia with Lewy bodies of 22% of all patients with dementia over the age of 84 (Rahkonen et al., 2003). Although some studies have suggested that the prognosis of patients with dementia with Lewy bodies is similar to those with Alzheimer's disease, other studies suggest that patients with dementia with Lewy bodies show a more rapid decline in function, leading to earlier nursing home placement and death. Our clinical experience is that most patients with dementia with Lewy bodies do progress more rapidly than those with Alzheimer's disease. The combination of Parkinsonism, dementia, and visual hallucinations typically leads to nursing home placement in 2–6 years, and death in 3–8 years. (There are, however, exceptions of patients who show a much slower disease progression.)

It is important to note that a subset of patients with dementia with Lewy bodies also meet clinical and pathological criteria for Alzheimer's disease, with some studies suggesting an overlap of greater than 90% (Merdes et al., 2003). Not surprisingly, these patients' dementias often present more like Alzheimer's disease. Although some clinicians would label these patients as having the "Lewy body variant of Alzheimer's disease," we think a simpler and more accurate description is to simply state that these patients have a mixed dementia of Alzheimer's disease and dementia with Lewy bodies.

CRITERIA AND DIAGNOSIS

The most important features of dementia with Lewy body are dementia (which must of course always be present), fluctuating cognition, visual hallucinations, and Parkinsonism (Fig. 5.1). Additional features which are suggestive of the disorder include rapid eye movement (REM) sleep behavior disorder and neuroleptic sensitivity (that is, even small doses of neuroleptics may cause Parkinsonism). See Box 5.1 for a summary of the current clinical diagnostic criteria. Regarding the Parkinsonism, it is important to note that up to 25% of patients with autopsy-proven dementia with Lewy bodies showed no signs of Parkinsonism during life, perhaps attributable to having mainly cortical and little brainstem pathology. See the section on the neurological examination below for more details on the Parkinsonism observed in this disorder.

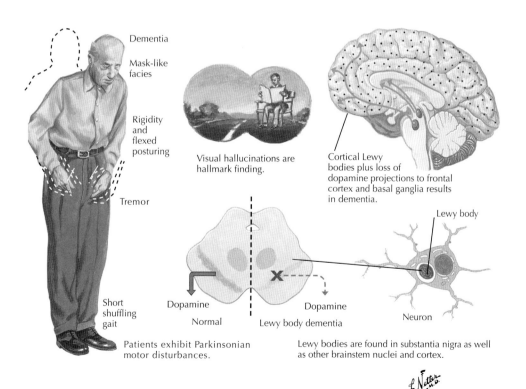

FIGURE 5.1 Major clinical and pathological abnormalities in dementia with Lewy bodies.

A color version of this figure is available online at http://www.expertconsult.com

---

BOX 5.1 SELECTED REVISED CRITERIA FOR CLINICAL DIAGNOSIS OF DEMENTIA WITH LEWY BODIES

I. Essential for a diagnosis:
  A. Dementia defined as progressive cognitive decline sufficient to interfere with normal social or occupational function. Impairment in attention, executive function, and visuospatial ability are often prominent. Memory impairment may or may not be prominent initially.
II. Core features (two are sufficient for a diagnosis of probable dementia with Lewy bodies; one for a possible diagnosis):
  A. Fluctuating cognition (pronounced variations in attention and alertness).
  B. Visual hallucinations (recurrent, well formed, detailed, of people and/or animals, often initially present around transitions between sleep and wake).
  C. Spontaneous features of Parkinsonism.
III. Suggestive features (one or more plus one core feature allows a probable diagnosis; one or more without any core features allows a possible diagnosis):
  A. Rapid eye movement sleep behavior disorder.
  B. Severe neuroleptic sensitivity.
  C. Low dopamine transporter uptake in basal ganglia demonstrated by SPECT or PET imaging.
IV. Supportive features (commonly present but have not been proven to have diagnostic specificity):
  A. Repeated falls.
  B. Transient unexplained loss of consciousness.
  C. Orthostatic hypotension.
  D. Reduced occipital activity and generalized low uptake on SPECT/PET perfusion scan.
V. A diagnosis of dementia with Lewy bodies is less likely:
  A. In the presence of clinically significant cerebrovascular disease noted on examination or radiology study.
  B. If Parkinsonism only appears for the first time at a stage of severe dementia.
  C. In the presence of any other disorder sufficient to account for some or all of the clinical picture.

Adapted from McKeith, I.G., Dickson, D.W., Lowe, J., et al., 2005. Diagnosis and management of dementia with Lewy bodies: third report of the DLB Consortium. Neurology 65, 1863–1872.

Regarding the characteristics of the dementia, it may appear identical to Alzheimer's disease, with memory problems being prominent, or memory may be relatively normal with major difficulties present in attention, executive function, and visuospatial ability. If the dementia appears quite similar to that of Alzheimer's disease, it is reasonable to presume that (as is common in patients with dementia with Lewy bodies) Alzheimer's pathology of senile plaques and neurofibrillary tangles is likely present along with Lewy bodies and abnormal alpha-synuclein metabolism.

Determining whether "fluctuating cognition" is present is quite difficult for most clinicians, for the simple reason that all dementing illnesses produce waxing and waning, with some days and times of day better than others. In our experience, the key aspect of fluctuating cognition to look for is relative dramatic fluctuations of alertness. In one patient we cared for, this manifested rather dramatically: the patient literally fell asleep during dinner and could not be awakened. Quite reasonably, the family was concerned that he had suffered a stroke or other catastrophic medical illness, and he was taken by ambulance to the hospital. By the time he reached the hospital he had awakened, and was back to baseline (the work-up, including MRI, EEG, and laboratory studies, was unrevealing). Other patients who we have cared for have had similar, though less dramatic, alterations in alertness.

BOX 5.2 TRUE HALLUCINATIONS?

Many times families of patients who are suffering from dementias other than that due to Lewy bodies inform us that the patient is having hallucinations. A common example is the patient with Alzheimer's disease who reports that she was talking with her mother last night, even though her mother died many years ago. Another example is the patient who reports that people were up having a party in her house all night long. Typically these symptoms are not true hallucinations but are instead memory distortions (thinking that a real memory from long ago happened recently), confabulations, or delusions. Memory distortions and delusions can usually be easily distinguished from true hallucinations because in the former case the patient is never observed to be actively hallucinating. Interestingly, all of these symptoms—true hallucinations, memory distortions, confabulations, and delusions—will often improve, at least partly, with cholinesterase inhibitors. Thus, cholinesterase inhibitors should always be used prior to atypical antipsychotics to treat these symptoms.

Visual hallucinations are perhaps the most definitive criteria for dementia with Lewy bodies. In our experience actual well-formed hallucinations of people or animals are simply not present in other disorders (see Box 5.2 for discussion). The hallucinations are always visual, and are almost always of people or animals. These hallucinations are remarkable in several ways. First, patients with mild dementia may be fully or partially aware that they are having hallucinations. We have had many patients who can both describe in detail their hallucinations and also know, at least some of the time, that they are not real (that is, they do not always have a delusional component). During a consultation, one patient said that he could see a man curled up under the desk, but knew that this could not be real. In other cases, the hallucinations can be incredibly realistic, and typically as the dementia progresses there is usually no ability of the patient to separate them from reality. One patient asked his wife why she was not serving dinner to the other people sitting at the table. Another patient thought she was petting an imaginary dog in the waiting room. And another patient used to see little children playing in the corner of the room. This last patient was thought initially to be suffering from a psychotic depression (she had lost a child) until the correct diagnosis was made. Unfortunately she had already received several courses of electroconvulsive therapy that may have exacerbated her hallucinations or her dementia. The cause of visual hallucinations in Lewy body dementia is unknown. One study found an association between the concentration of Lewy bodies in the temporal lobe and well-formed visual hallucinations (Harding et al., 2002). However, the hallucinations may also relate to sleep disturbances, as discussed in Box 5.2.

Although we are all normally paralyzed during rapid-eye movement (REM) sleep, those with REM sleep behavior disorder are not, and these individuals act out their dreams while sleeping. These actions can be disturbing and even frightening or life-threatening to their sleeping partners. It has been noted for a number of years that REM sleep behavior disorder can be one of the earliest signs of dementia with Lewy bodies (Ferman et al., 2002) (Box 5.3). One clue as to the reason for this association comes from a patient with dementia with Lewy bodies whose brain at autopsy showed a marked loss of brainstem monoaminergic nuclei (including locus caeruleus and substantia nigra) that inhibit cholinergic neurons in the pedunculopontine nucleus, which usually cause paralysis during REM sleep (Turner et al., 2000). When suspecting that a patient may have dementia with Lewy bodies, it is therefore important to ask whether the patient ever acts out his or her dreams while sleeping, or simply moves around a lot in their sleep. Probably the most common sign of this disorder is that the

---

BOX 5.3 IS DEMENTIA WITH LEWY BODIES ASSOCIATED WITH A PRIMARY SLEEP DISORDER?

The association of dementia with Lewy bodies and disturbances in alertness, visual hallucinations, and REM sleep behavior disorder has led researchers to investigate whether many of the symptoms of dementia with Lewy bodies are related to a sleep disorder. Harper et al. (2004) have found that, although both patients with Alzheimer's disease and those with dementia with Lewy bodies have disrupted circadian rhythms, the disruption was greatest in those with dementia with Lewy bodies (Harper et al., 2004). It may be that in dementia with Lewy bodies disruption of circadian rhythm causes loss of alertness owing to drowsiness or actual sleep, and REM phenomena breaking into wakeful consciousness cause the well-formed visual hallucinations.

---

sleeping partner complains that the patient has begun kicking them at night, and frequently by the time the history is taken the spouse has sought refuge by sleeping in another bed! For patients who sleep alone, a telltale sign is often covers and pillows on the floor in the morning.

RISK FACTORS, PATHOLOGY, AND PATHOPHYSIOLOGY

Other than age (mean of approximately 75 years) and male sex there are no known risk factors for dementia with Lewy bodies. Its pathology involves neurodegeneration associated with abnormal alpha-synuclein metabolism and formation of Lewy bodies and Lewy neurites in various brain regions including brainstem, basal forebrain, limbic regions, and neocortical regions (Fig. 5.2). The pathophysiology is attributable not only to the direct loss of neurons but also to neuronal loss in brainstem centers that produce

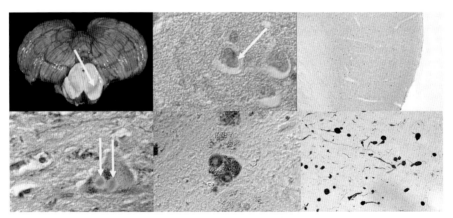

FIGURE 5.2 Pathological changes that occur in dementia with Lewy bodies.

Clockwise from top left: gross view of the brain through the midbrain to show the pallor of the substantia nigra (should be black, see arrow); high-power view showing the eosinophilic (pink in color) Lewy body (arrow) in a cortical neuron; low-power view of Lewy bodies in the cortex; alpha-synuclein stain technique to visualize only Lewy bodies and Lewy neurites; two Lewy bodies (rings) stare up at us via a ubiquitin stain; and high-power view of Lewy bodies in the substantia nigra—note the two Lewy bodies in a single large neuron. A color version of this figure is avaliable online at http://www.expertconsult.com.

neurotransmitters, including the substantia nigra (producing dopamine) and the nucleus basalis of Meynert (producing acetylcholine). Thus, patients with dementia with Lewy bodies have reduced levels of cortical dopamine and acetylcholine, which has important treatment implications (see below).

There are familial cases of dementia with Lewy bodies related to mutations or repeats of the alpha-synuclein gene located on chromosome 4. Most patients with dementia with Lewy bodies, however, do not show abnormalities of this gene.

COMMON SIGNS, SYMPTOMS, AND STAGES

As described in more detail in the section Criteria and diagnosis, the most important features of dementia with Lewy body are dementia, fluctuating cognition, visual hallucinations, Parkinsonism, rapid-eye movement (REM), sleep behavior disorder, and neuroleptic sensitivity.

When considering the stages of dementia with Lewy bodies, there are at least two axes to consider. The first axis is that of distribution of Lewy bodies in the brain. Those patients who initially have more Lewy bodies in their brainstem will present with the motor symptoms of Parkinson's disease. Those patients who present with Lewy bodies more evenly distributed throughout the brainstem, basal forebrain, limbic regions, and neocortical regions usually present with both cognitive impairment and Parkinsonism. And those patients who present with mainly cortical Lewy bodies present with cognitive impairment. The second axis to consider is that of disease severity, since each of these patients can demonstrate mild, moderate, or severe magnitude of motor and cognitive symptoms.

THINGS TO LOOK FOR IN THE HISTORY

It is generally not difficult to make the diagnosis of dementia with Lewy bodies in patients who began with idiopathic Parkinson's disease and develop prominent visual hallucinations. For those patients who do not have early or prominent Parkinsonism, the diagnosis can be more difficult—and as mentioned above 20–25% of autopsy-proven patients with dementia with Lewy bodies never develop Parkinsonism.

A number of signs and symptoms may often be harbingers of the disorder. REM sleep behavior disorder may be present for years preceding the clinical onset of cognitive impairment. Other sleep disturbances, such as nightmares, difficulty distinguishing dreams from being awake, and daytime drowsiness, are common. Brief episodes of poor attention and/or being poorly responsive may also be present early on. In addition to visual hallucinations, visual perceptual difficulties and misperceptions may be prominent early on. (One example is of a patient we cared for who could not see well enough to distinguish different types of paper money; he was referred to us by his ophthalmologist, who found nothing wrong with his eyes.) Autonomic dysfunction may also occur early in the course, leading to orthostatic hypotension, cardiovascular instability, urinary incontinence, constipation, impotence, eating and swallowing difficulties, falls, and syncope. Lastly, depression and apathy may precede the clinical onset of dementia with Lewy bodies, but these symptoms are common in most dementias.

Because dementia with Lewy bodies is a common cause of dementia, as discussed above, we recommend that clinicians simply incorporate many of the important signs and symptoms of this disorder into their history of present illness, review of systems, and physical examination. These include:

- fluctuating levels of alertness or periods of being relatively unresponsive
- visual hallucinations of people or animals
- a disturbance of gait
- falls
- a tremor
- rigidity and other signs of Parkinsonism
- acting out dreams during sleep or other abnormal movements while sleeping
- difficulty distinguishing dreams from reality when transitioning from sleep.

THINGS TO LOOK FOR ON THE PHYSICAL AND NEUROLOGICAL EXAMINATION

Parkinsonism is the main feature of dementia with Lewy bodies that can be identified in the physical and neurological examination (although signs of autonomic dysfunction can also sometimes be observed). The Parkinsonism is generally similar to age-matched, non-demented patients with Parkinson's disease in overall severity, but shows greater symmetry, axial involvement, postural instability, and facial impassivity, and less tremor. It is important to keep in mind that a lack of Parkinsonism does not exclude the disorder, as up to 25% of autopsy-proven patients with dementia with Lewy bodies showed no clinical signs of Parkinsonism. (Consistent with this finding is that the diagnostic guidelines do not require that Parkinsonism is present.)

PATTERN OF IMPAIRMENT ON COGNITIVE TESTS

In patients with pure dementia with Lewy bodies, cognitive impairment is prominent on measures of attention and visuospatial and executive function with relative sparing of memory. However, in the common scenario in which there is an underlying mixed dementia with Alzheimer's pathology as well as cortical Lewy bodies, the cognitive deficits may be similar to those of Alzheimer's disease.

LABORATORY STUDIES

There are no laboratory, genetic, or cerebrospinal fluid studies that are helpful in either confirming or ruling out dementia with Lewy bodies.

STRUCTURAL IMAGING STUDIES

There are no features of dementia with Lewy bodies that can be observed on structural imaging, although finding the hippocampal/medial temporal atrophy associated with Alzheimer's disease makes pure dementia with Lewy bodies less likely, but does not lessen the possibility of a mixed dementia of Alzheimer's disease plus dementia with Lewy bodies.

FUNCTIONAL IMAGING STUDIES

There are two types of functional imaging studies which can be helpful in confirming the diagnosis of dementia with Lewy bodies. Standard SPECT (^{99m}Tc-HMPAO) or PET (FDG) imaging, available in many institutions, has often (but not invariably) shown occipital hypoperfusion on SPECT imaging (Fig. 5.3) and occipital hypometabolism on PET imaging. Functional imaging of the dopamine transporter by either SPECT or PET using specialized tracers is typically available only in the research setting, but is relatively sensitive and specific.

When the diagnosis of dementia with Lewy bodies is relatively straightforward there is no reason to obtain a functional imaging study. In the complicated case, however, obtaining such a study can be helpful. Which you choose depends mainly upon what is available in your institution. We have had experience with standard ^{99m}Tc-HMPAO SPECT and FDG-PET studies which have been helpful in making difficult diagnoses.

DIFFERENTIAL DIAGNOSIS

The first issue that we bear in mind when considering a diagnosis of dementia with Lewy bodies is whether the patient's dementia would be best characterized by that diagnosis alone, Alzheimer's disease alone, or both (Table 5.1). If the patient meets criteria for both dementias, then the patient has a mixed dementia: dementia with Lewy bodies plus Alzheimer's disease. After Alzheimer's disease, the main differential diagnosis of dementia with Lewy bodies is vascular dementia and atypical Parkinsonian syndromes including progressive supranuclear palsy, multiple system atrophy, and corticobasal degeneration. Creutzfeldt–Jakob disease (CJD) should also be considered, although the pace of the dementia will usually distinguish between these disorders.

Vascular dementia should be considered if there are many large or small ischemic strokes on the structural imaging scan (CT or MRI). Strokes in the basal ganglia can produce

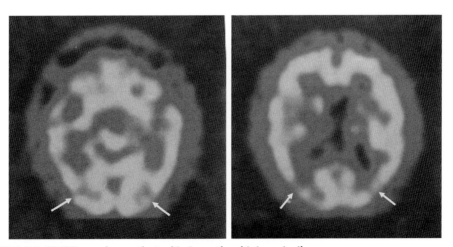

FIGURE 5.3 SPECT scan in a patient with dementia with Lewy bodies

Note decreased occipital function (arrows). A color version of this figure is avaliable online at http://www.expertconsult.com.

Table 5.1 Comparison between Alzheimer's disease and dementia with Lewy bodies

	Alzheimer's disease	**Dementia with Lewy bodies**
Cognitive deficits	Multiple cognitive areas, with memory deficits most prominent	More prominent deficits in visuospatial, attentional, and executive function with memory deficits less prominent
Behavioral symptoms	Visual hallucinations and sleep disturbances may occur late in the disease	Visual hallucinations and sleep disturbances often present early in the disease
Motor symptoms	None until the late stages	Parkinsonian symptoms often present early in the disease

Parkinsonism. However, if the history and cognitive examination strongly suggest dementia with Lewy bodies, then we would argue that the patient most likely has dementia with Lewy bodies, although the dementia may be exacerbated to some extent by small vessel ischemic disease. If the small vessel disease is moderate to severe, yet the patient has clear signs of dementia with Lewy bodies such as visual hallucinations or REM sleep behavior disorder, then diagnosis of a mixed dementia of dementia with Lewy bodies plus vascular dementia is most appropriate.

Progressive supranuclear palsy should be considered if there is an abnormality of vertical gaze (particularly downgaze), axial rigidity (rigidity of the neck and trunk), difficulty swallowing, and frequent falls. Corticobasal degeneration should be considered if there are strong asymmetric findings, such as focal or asymmetric rigidity or dystonia, inability to control a limb or apraxia of the limb, visual or sensory hemineglect, and focal or asymmetric myoclonus. See Chapters 8 and 9 for a more detailed description of these disorders.

Lastly, there are several non-dementia conditions that could be confused with dementia with Lewy bodies in that they may cause cognitive impairment, fluctuating cognition, repeated falls, and transient unexplained loss of consciousness. These conditions include complex partial seizures (including temporal lobe epilepsy), multiple sclerosis, and cardiac dysfunction (particularly arrhythmias).

TREATMENTS

Anticholinergic medications should be avoided, as medications with this property may impair cognition, cause confusion, aggravate or cause visual hallucinations, and often exacerbate behavioral disturbances. Regarding treatment, the FDA has approved the rivastigmine (Exelon) patch to treat Parkinson's disease dementia, which, as discussed above, is the same pathological entity as dementia with Lewy bodies.

Cholinesterase inhibitors have been shown in a number of studies to improve both cognition and neuropsychiatric/behavioral symptoms in patients with dementia with Lewy bodies. The most careful of these studies are two rivastigmine (Exelon) studies, one in patients labeled "dementia with Lewy bodies" (McKeith et al., 2000) and the other in patients labeled "Parkinson's disease dementia" (Emre et al., 2004). Smaller and less controlled studies have found similar results with donepezil (Aricept) (Ravina et al., 2005) and galantamine (Razadyne) (Bhasin et al., 2007). Our clinical experience confirms that cholinesterase inhibitors can improve cognitive, neuropsychiatric, and behavioral symptoms in patients with dementia with Lewy bodies.

The motor symptoms of Parkinsonism are generally best treated with levodopa (along with carbidopa, usually referred to as Sinemet) in low dose. Side-effects, however, in patients with dementia with Lewy bodies can include confusion and worsening of (or causing) visual hallucinations. Thus, as a general rule of thumb, levodopa is initiated only when the patient has significant functional impairment, such as difficulty getting out of a car or off a toilet.

Memantine (Namenda), as discussed in Chapter 15, enhances dopamine in addition to any effects on glutamate at the *N*-methyl-D-aspartic acid receptor. Thus, like levodopa, memantine has the potential to be useful but it could also make things worse. This view is supported by the literature: some reports are of patients benefiting and some are of patients worsening. We do not recommend routine use of memantine, but do recommend giving memantine a try when neuropsychiatric symptoms, particularly apathy, are not responsive to cholinesterase inhibitors.

Successfully treating hallucinations is difficult, and pharmacological treatment should be initiated when hallucinations become threatening or otherwise problematic. Only atypical antipsychotics should be used, such as quetiapine (Seroquel) at bedtime, since traditional neuroleptics like haloperidol (Haldol) are highly likely to cause worsening Parkinsonism. Even atypical antipsychotics may worsen Parkinsonism. REM sleep behavior disorder may also be treated with atypical antipsychotics such as quetiapine (Seroquel). (Please carefully review Chapter 21 prior treating with an atypical antipsychotic.)

The quandary for the clinician treating patients with Lewy body disease is often referred to as the "motion–emotion" dilemma. Treating the "emotion" deficit of hallucinations with antipsychotics which are dopaminergic antagonists can exacerbate the Parkinsonian symptoms such as rigidity, and treating the "motion" component with dopaminergic agonists can exacerbate the hallucinations.

Lastly, as in Alzheimer's disease and mild cognitive impairment, depression and anxiety are common in patients with mild disease and preserved insight. If these symptoms are present, we again recommend a selective serotonin reuptake inhibitor such as sertraline (Zoloft).

QUICK START 2: MEDICAL TREATMENT FOR DEMENTIA WITH LEWY BODIES

Medication class	Medication and FDA approval?	Summary of benefits
Cholinesterase inhibitors	Rivastigmine (Exelon patch) is FDA approved to treat Parkinson's disease dementia (dementia with Lewy bodies) Donepezil (Aricept), galantamine (Razadyne) can be used "off-label"	Our experience and a number of studies have found improved cognition as well as neuropsychiatric and behavioral symptoms
Memantine (Namenda)	Memantine (Namenda) "off-label"	Small study suggests improvement in clinical status
Selective serotonin reuptake inhibitors	Sertraline (Zoloft) and, escitalopram (Lexapro) "off-label"	Treatment if depression and/or anxiety is present
Dopaminergic agents	Levodopa/carbidopa (Sinemet) "off-label"	Use with caution to improve movement; can worsen hallucinations
Atypical antipsychotics	Quetiapine (Seroquel) "off-label"	Use with caution to improve frightening hallucinations; can worsen Parkinsonism

References

Bhasin, M., Rowan, E., Edwards, K., et al., 2007. Cholinesterase inhibitors in dementia with Lewy bodies: a comparative analysis. Int. J. Geriatr. Psychiatry 22, 890–895.

Emre, M., Aarsland, D., Albanese, A., et al., 2004. Rivastigmine for dementia associated with Parkinson's disease. N. Engl. J. Med. 351, 2509–2518.

Ferman, T.J., Boeve, B.F., Smith, G.E., et al., 2002. Dementia with Lewy bodies may present as dementia and REM sleep behavior disorder without parkinsonism or hallucinations. J. Int. Neuropsychol. Soc. 8, 907–914.

Harding, A.J., Broe, G.A., Halliday, G.M., 2002. Visual hallucinations in Lewy body disease relate to Lewy bodies in the temporal lobe. Brain 125, 391–403.

Harper, D.G., Stopa, E.G., McKee, A.C., et al., 2004. Dementia severity and Lewy bodies affect circadian rhythms in Alzheimer disease. Neurobiol. Aging 25, 771–781.

McKeith, I., Del Ser, T., Spano, P., et al., 2000. Efficacy of rivastigmine in dementia with Lewy bodies: a randomised, double-blind, placebo-controlled international study. Lancet 356, 2031–2036.

McKeith, I.G., Dickson, D.W., Lowe, J., et al., 2005. Diagnosis and management of dementia with Lewy bodies: third report of the DLB Consortium. Neurology 65, 1863–1872.

Merdes, A.R., Hansen, L.A., Jeste, D.V., et al., 2003. Influence of Alzheimer pathology on clinical diagnostic accuracy in dementia with Lewy bodies. Neurology 60, 1586–1590.

Perry, R.H., Irving, D., Blessed, G., et al., 1989. Senile dementia of Lewy body type and spectrum of Lewy body disease. Lancet 1, 1088.

Rahkonen, T., Eloniemi-Sulkava, U., Rissanen, S., et al., 2003. Dementia with Lewy bodies according to the consensus criteria in a general population aged 75 years or older. J. Neurol. Neurosurg. Psychiatry 74, 720–724.

Ravina, B., Putt, M., Siderowf, A., et al., 2005. Donepezil for dementia in Parkinson's disease: a randomised, double blind, placebo controlled, crossover study. J. Neurol. Neurosurg. Psychiatry 76, 934–939.

Turner, R.S., D'Amato, C.J., Chervin, R.D., et al., 2000. The pathology of REM sleep behavior disorder with comorbid Lewy body dementia. Neurology 55, 1730–1732.

Vascular dementia and vascular cognitive impairment

6

QUICK START: VASCULAR DEMENTIA AND VASCULAR COGNITIVE IMPAIRMENT

Definition	• Vascular cognitive impairment occurs when cognitive dysfunction is due to cerebrovascular disease (i.e., strokes).
	• Vascular dementia occurs when cerebrovascular disease causes both cognitive dysfunction and impairment in daily functioning.
	• The exact cerebrovascular disease that can cause cognitive and functional impairment may be varied, and can include:
	• Small vessel ischemic disease
	• Multiple cortical strokes
	• Strategic infarcts
	• Cerebral amyloid angiopathy.
Prevalence	• Approximately 5–10% of patients with dementia have a pure vascular dementia, that is, dementia entirely attributable to cerebrovascular disease.
	• Another 10–15% of patients with dementia suffer from a mixed dementia of cerebrovascular disease plus a neurodegenerative disease.
Genetic risk	• The genetic risk is related to the varied underlying cerebrovascular pathology.
	• One disorder, CADASIL (cerebral autosomal dominant arteriopathy with subcortical infarcts and leukoencephalopathy), is due to mutation of the Notch3 gene at the chromosome locus 19p13.
Cognitive symptoms	• Neuropsychological testing typically shows impairment in multiple domains, including attention, frontal/executive function, and speed of processing. Memory impairments are typically secondary to attention and frontal/executive dysfunction.
Diagnostic criteria	• The history shows the signs and symptoms of strokes and often reveals a stepwise decline.
	• The neurological examination shows evidence of strokes including focal signs and extensor plantar reflexes.
	• Neuropsychological testing typically shows impairment in multiple domains, including attention, frontal/executive function, and speed of processing. Memory impairments are typically secondary to attention and frontal/executive dysfunction.
	• To make a diagnosis of vascular dementia or vascular cognitive impairment, the CT or MRI scan shows sufficient cerebrovascular disease to explain the cognitive dysfunction.
	• The existing formal diagnostic criteria are for research purposes and are not necessarily helpful in clinical situations.

Continued

QUICK START: VASCULAR DEMENTIA AND VASCULAR COGNITIVE IMPAIRMENT—Cont'd

Behavioral symptoms	• Depression is often present.
Treatment	• There are no FDA approved medications to treat vascular dementia and vascular cognitive impairment. However, clinical trials have found both cholinesterase inhibitors and memantine to be helpful. For memory problems we recommend a trial of cholinesterase inhibitors, and for apathy we recommend a trial of memantine.
	• The underlying cause of the cerebrovascular disease must also be evaluated and treated.
Top differential diagnoses	• Mixed dementia (vascular dementia or vascular cognitive impairment plus another neurodegenerative disease such as Alzheimer's disease or Lewy body disease), Alzheimer's disease, depression.

PREVALENCE, PROGNOSIS, AND DEFINITION

Vascular dementia is dementia due to cerebrovascular disease (i.e., strokes; Box 6.1 and Fig. 6.1). When cerebrovascular disease causes cognitive dysfunction but not severe enough to lead to functional impairment, the term *vascular cognitive impairment* is used. Vascular cognitive impairment is analogous to the concept of mild cognitive impairment: cognitive impairment is present in each but the impairment is not great enough to cause functional decline. In vascular dementia, as in Alzheimer's disease, the cognitive impairment is sufficient to cause functional decline (Table 6.1).

The prevalence of vascular dementia and vascular cognitive impairment depends on how they are defined. If vascular dementia is defined such that patients with Alzheimer's disease and other neurodegenerative diseases are excluded, then vascular dementia is a relatively small cause of memory loss and dementia, of the order of 5–10% of all dementias, depending upon the particular population (closer to 10% in US veterans, for example). We would describe such patients as having a "pure vascular dementia." Like most older adults, the majority of patients with Alzheimer's disease and other degenerative diseases (such as dementia with Lewy bodies) have some cerebrovascular disease, usually in the

---

BOX 6.1 SO WHAT'S A STROKE?

Terminology can be confusing. In this chapter we discuss three different pathologies—small vessel ischemic vascular disease, multiple cortical strokes, and strategic infarcts—each using different words to describe the same underlying process. Although the etiology of these pathologies may be very different (as described in detail below), they all come under the rubric of cerebrovascular disease, which is also known as vascular disease, or strokes, or infarcts. In each of these disorders there is a lack of blood flow to a part of the brain, which dies, causing the injury. Because there is a lack of blood flow, they could also each be called "ischemic": ischemic vascular disease, ischemic stroke, an ischemic infarct. The fourth pathology discussed in this chapter, cerebral amyloid angiopathy, can cause a part of the brain to die as a result of bleeding rather than lack of blood flow (see below). But when bleeding occurs, damaging the brain tissue, the terms cerebrovascular disease, vascular disease, stroke, and infarct all apply to the resulting injury.

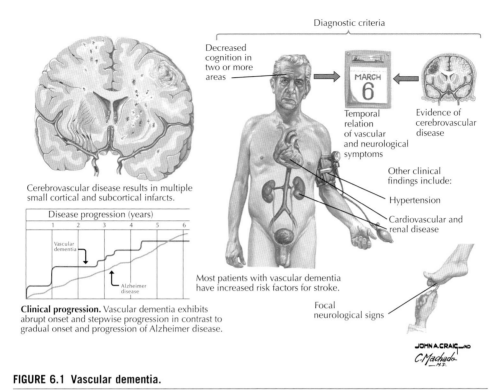

Diagnostic criteria

Decreased cognition in two or more areas

MARCH 6

Temporal relation of vascular and neurological symptoms

Evidence of cerebrovascular disease

Other clinical findings include:

Hypertension

Cardiovascular and renal disease

Cerebrovascular disease results in multiple small cortical and subcortical infarcts.

Disease progression (years)

Vascular dementia

Alzheimer disease

Most patients with vascular dementia have increased risk factors for stroke.

Focal neurological signs

Clinical progression. Vascular dementia exhibits abrupt onset and stepwise progression in contrast to gradual onset and progression of Alzheimer disease.

JOHN A. CRAIG—MD
C. Machado
—M.D.

FIGURE 6.1 Vascular dementia.

A color version of this figure is available online at http://www.expertconsult.com

form of small vessel ischemic disease. If these patients are also included in the definition of vascular dementia, then the majority of patients with dementia would have vascular dementia or vascular cognitive impairment—along with another type of dementia.

We typically classify the cognitively impaired patient with cerebrovascular disease in one of the following ways. If the patient shows no signs of any other etiology of his or her cognitive impairment we would describe him or her as having a "pure vascular dementia" (or "pure vascular cognitive impairment," if not demented). If the patient has a neurodegenerative disease (such as Alzheimer's) and he or she has the average amount of cerebrovascular disease that a non-demented, non-cognitively impaired older adult has, we would describe him or her as simply having that neurodegenerative disease (such as Alzheimer's). If the patient has a neurodegenerative disease (such as Alzheimer's) and he or she has a greater than average amount of cerebrovascular disease—such that it is highly likely that the cerebrovascular disease is making a significant contribution to the patient's dementia—then we would describe him or her as having a "mixed dementia," and would then further specify, for example, "a mixed dementia of Alzheimer's disease plus vascular dementia" (Fig. 6.2). Patients classified in this way with a mixed dementia of cerebrovascular disease plus a neurodegenerative disease probably make up 10–15% of all dementias.

Table 6.1 Comparison between vascular dementia, vascular cognitive impairment, Alzheimer's disease and amnestic mild cognitive impairment

	Vascular dementia	Vascular cognitive impairment	Alzheimer's disease	Amnestic mild cognitive impairment
Cognitive complaints by patient or family	Present	Present	Present	Present
Cognitive deficits	Present	Present, very mild	Present	Present, very mild
Functional impairment	Present	Absent	Present	Absent
Dementia	Present	Absent	Present	Absent
Likely underlying pathology	Cerebrovascular disease	Cerebrovascular disease	Alzheimer's disease	Alzheimer's disease
Deterioration over time	May occur, but may also remain stable	May occur, but may also remain stable	Always occurs	May occur, but may also remain stable or improve
FDA-approved Treatment	None	None	Cholinesterase inhibitors, memantine	None
Recommended treatment	Cholinesterase inhibitors Memantine if apathy SSRI if depression or anxiety	Cholinesterase inhibitors Memantine if apathy SSRI if depression or anxiety	Cholinesterase inhibitors Memantine if apathy SSRI if depression or anxiety	Cholinesterase inhibitors SSRI if depression or anxiety

CRITERIA

There are several published criteria for vascular dementia. However, none of them are particularly helpful. For example, the DSM-IV criteria for vascular dementia are almost identical to the DSM-IV criteria for Alzheimer's disease; it is therefore no surprise that these criteria typically overrepresent patients with a mixed dementia of vascular dementia plus Alzheimer's disease. The NINDS-AIREN criteria (Roman et al., 1993), commonly used in clinical trials, err in the opposite direction, under diagnosing vascular dementia. The sensitivity and specificity using the NINDS-AIREN criteria were 58% and 80% in one study (Gold et al., 1997) and 20% and 93% in another (Gold et al., 2002). Thus, we do not recommend the clinical application of these or other criteria.

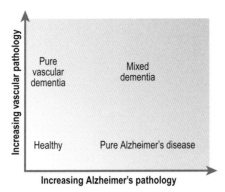

FIGURE 6.2 **The relationship between vascular pathology and clinical diagnosis.**

RISK FACTORS, PATHOLOGY, AND PATHOPHYSIOLOGY

The major risk factors for vascular dementia and vascular cognitive impairment are, of course, the risk factors for cerebrovascular disease in general, with the major ones being hypertension, heart disease, smoking, and diabetes. See Box 6.2 for additional common risk factors.

Cerebrovascular disease can cause cognitive impairment and dementia in a variety of ways, with etiologies including large cortical strokes, small vessel ischemic disease, lacunar infarcts, and other etiologies. These different types of cerebrovascular disease can cause a variety of different types of signs and symptoms depending on where the damage occurs (Fig. 6.3).

BOX 6.2 RISK FACTORS FOR VASCULAR DEMENTIA AND VASCULAR COGNITIVE IMPAIRMENT

Cardiovascular
Clinical strokes or transient ischemic attacks
Hypertension
Atrial fibrillation
Coronary artery disease
Atherosclerosis

Metabolic
Diabetes
Increased cholesterol

Habits
Smoking

Demographics
Old age
Low educational attainment

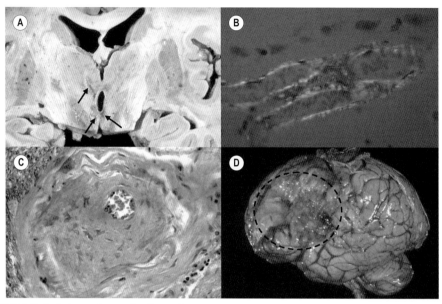

FIGURE 6.3 Pathology of vascular dementia.

Bilateral thalamic lesions are strategic infarcts (A, from a "top of the basilar" stroke, arrows), birefringent cerebral amyloid angiopathy in a small blood vessel (B), large cortical infarct easily visible on the surface of the brain (D, dotted circle), and lipohyalinosis of a small vessel (C). A color version of this figure is avaliable online at http://www.expertconsult.com.

Small vessel ischemic disease (subcortical ischemic vascular disease)

Small vessel ischemic disease (also known as subcortical ischemic vascular disease) is thought to be attributable to two processes, lipohyalinosis and microemboli. Lipohyalinosis is a process in which an eosinophilic material deposits in the connective tissue of the wall of deep penetrating arteries, leading to infarctions. Lipohyalinosis is thought to be secondary to damaged cerebrovascular autoregulation occurring with hypertension and aging. Microemboli can block small penetrating arteries of the brain, leading to infarctions. Microemboli may be due to atheroma, normal or abnormal clotting, and heart disease. Small vessel ischemic disease is very common in older adults. Most individuals aged 70 or older have some small vessel ischemic disease. By itself, a small amount of small vessel ischemic disease does not typically cause noticeable cognitive impairment or dementia. Moderate or large amounts of small vessel ischemic disease, however, can produce cognitive impairment and can cause dementia.

Multi-infarct dementia (also known as cortical vascular dementia and post-stroke dementia)

Multi-infarct dementia (also known as cortical vascular dementia and post-stroke dementia) is typically due to multiple cortical strokes. Cortical strokes are most commonly caused by large emboli, which usually originate from the heart (often related to disrupted flow due to atrial fibrillation or ischemic myocardium), the carotid arteries, or the aorta. Multi-infarct dementia occurs when the patient suffers a number of cortical strokes.

Strategic infarct dementia

Strategic infarct dementia occurs when a focal lesion (or lesions), often quite small, damages a brain region that is critical for cognitive brain function. The lesions are typically lacunar infarcts or embolic strokes, although hypertensive hemorrhages can also damage these regions. There are many critical brain regions where even a small stroke could disrupt cognitive function in this manner, including the medial temporal lobes (hippocampal formation, entorhinal cortex, parahippocampal cortex), angular gyrus, cingulate gyrus, thalamus, fornix, basal forebrain, caudate, and globus pallidus (Table 6.2).

Cerebral amyloid angiopathy

Cerebral amyloid angiopathy is caused by deposits of β-amyloid, predominantly $A\beta_{40}$, in the media of small-to medium-sized arteries in the leptomeninges and superficial cortex, particularly in the parieto-occipital, temporoparietal, and sometimes frontal regions. It is more common in patients with Alzheimer's disease. Thickening and hyalinization of the involved vessel walls may lead to hemorrhage. Hemorrhages typically occur in the superficial cortex and may be multicentric.

Table 6.2 Stroke lesion location and possible signs and symptoms

Lesion location	Possible signs and symptoms
Frontal cortex: left	Word-finding difficulties, Broca's aphasia, poor attention, disinhibition, right hemiparesis
Frontal cortex: right	Poor attention, left neglect, disinhibition, left hemiparesis, can be silent
Basal ganglia: left	Aphasia, right hemiparesis
Basal ganglia: right	Left neglect, left hemiparesis
Temporal cortex: left	Aphasia
Temporal cortex: right	Left neglect
Medial temporal lobe: left or right	Memory loss (left more likely to produce deficits for verbal information, right deficits for non-verbal information)
Parietal cortex: left	Wernicke's aphasia, calculation difficulties
Parietal cortex: right	Confusion, left neglect, can be silent
Thalamus: left	Aphasia, memory loss, disinhibition, right sensory disturbances
Thalamus: right	Left neglect, memory loss, disinhibition, left sensory disturbances
Occipital cortex: left	Visual defects, reading difficulty, confusion, agitation
Occipital cortex: right	Visual defects, confusion, can be silent
Multiple subcortical small vessel strokes	Slowing of cognition, frontal/executive dysfunction, disinhibition, incontinence, weakness, frontal gait

Other

Other types of cerebrovascular disease may also lead to cognitive impairment. Hypoperfusion of the brain may occur regionally if there is a focal stenosis of a major artery or globally if there is cardiovascular insufficiency. Hemorrhages due to hypertension may occur in strategic areas such as the thalamus. There are several relatively rare genetic disorders that can cause vascular cognitive impairment, including CADASIL (cerebral autosomal dominant arteriopathy with subcortical infarcts and leukoencephalopathy), which is due to mutation of the Notch3 gene at the chromosome locus 19p13 (Federico et al., 2005). CADASIL, which may be as common as five in 100,000, typically presents first with migraine and then with multiple subcortical strokes, leading eventually to dementia, motor and sensory deficits, and death (Pantoni et al., 2010).

COMMON SIGNS, SYMPTOMS, AND STAGES

The signs and symptoms that will be present with cognitive impairment due to cerebrovascular disease depend upon both the type of cerebrovascular disease and the particular brain structures affected.

Small vessel ischemic disease

Small vessel ischemic disease most commonly occurs in the subcortical white matter. Because most of the brain's white matter is involved in transferring information to or from the frontal lobes, patients with large amounts of small vessel ischemic disease often show signs and symptoms of frontal subcortical dysfunction. Dysfunction of frontal subcortical regions often leads to difficulty focusing and maintaining attention. Also disrupted is working memory, the ability to keep a number of items in mind and mentally manipulate them. Gait is often affected leading to a "frontal" or "magnetic gait" (called by the French the "*marche à petits pas*," walk of little steps), in which patients describe their feet feeling like they are stuck on the floor. Incontinence is common, even with mild impairment of cognition. Pseudobulbar affect is also often seen (Box 6.3).

Multi-infarct dementia

Multi-infarct dementia, being due to multiple cortical strokes, usually presents with clinical signs and symptoms referable to the particular region of the cortex affected. These cortical strokes are usually detected clinically, but strokes in the right frontal and right parietal

---

BOX 6.3 PSEUDOBULBAR AFFECT

The term "pseudobulbar affect" is often used to indicate the loss of cortical control of emotions, such as when patients show inappropriate laughing and crying. Usually these signs of emotion come out with minimal provocation, although they sometimes occur without any discernible trigger. A common example is that patients may cry when they hear about items on a news broadcast which are sad, but not the sort of thing that would have caused them to come to tears in the past. Pseudobulbar affect is usually caused by disruption of frontal subcortical white matter tracts, which is commonly due to cerebrovascular disease but may also be due to normal pressure hydrocephalus, multiple sclerosis, cerebral palsy, and traumatic brain injury, along with less common disorders.

cortices may first be detected during a work-up for dementia. Common signs and symptoms include poor attention, aphasia, disinhibition, hemiparesis, impairment of vision, and other sensory modalities (Table 6.2).

Strategic infarct dementia

Strategic infarct dementia also typically presents with signs and symptoms referable to the particular region of the brain affected by the infarct. Common signs and symptoms include poor attention, slurred speech (dysarthria), aphasia, incontinence, hemiparesis, and impaired coordination (Table 6.2).

Cerebral amyloid angiopathy

Cerebral amyloid angiopathy is usually present along with concomitant Alzheimer's disease. Thus patients with cerebral amyloid angiopathy often first present with symptoms of Alzheimer's disease, and then the more focal symptoms related to the ensuing hemorrhages become manifest. Several features of cerebral amyloid angiopathy separate it from other cerebrovascular causes of cognitive impairment. First, it has a predilection for affecting the cortex of the temporoparietal–occipital junction. The symptoms resulting from damage to this region can be varied, and may include visual disturbances which may be bizarre (such as multiple fragmented images), Wernicke's aphasia, word-finding difficulties, and visuospatial impairment. Second, despite the fact that the pathology is related to the rupture of blood vessels and hemorrhage, the symptoms can often present over a number of minutes, rather than all at once as often occurs in a hypertensive hemorrhage or embolic stroke.

THINGS TO LOOK FOR IN THE HISTORY

Signs and symptoms of strokes and/or transient ischemic attacks (TIAs) are the most important events to look for in the history. Sudden symptoms are the key: abrupt weakness or numbness of a limb or part of the face, precipitous loss of vision, sudden loss of speech, etc. Most patients with more than average cerebrovascular disease will have a history of one or more of such events. A history of risk factors should also be compiled (Table 6.2).

THINGS TO LOOK FOR ON THE PHYSICAL AND NEUROLOGICAL EXAMINATION

Focal signs suggesting strokes should be sought on the neurological examination, such as a subtle hemiparesis, facial droop, ptosis, neglect, visual field cut, etc. Although non-specific, signs of corticospinal tract dysfunction such as brisk reflexes and extensor plantars (Babinski's sign) are almost invariably present, and usually floridly abnormal. Frontal release signs, including a grasp, snout, and palmomental reflexes, are also commonly present.

PATTERN OF IMPAIRMENT ON COGNITIVE TESTS

Although the specific impairment that will be observed on cognitive tests in a patient with vascular dementia depends upon the specific location and type of the cerebrovascular disease, there are some general principles that are useful. The two aspects of neuropsychological function that are impaired in most patients with cerebrovascular disease are frontal/executive function and the speed of cognition, due to the fact that small vessel ischemic disease typically affects the frontal subcortical white matter tracts.

Attention

Attention is generally impaired in vascular dementia. Difficult tasks for these patients include tasks that require information to be kept "in mind" in working memory, such as counting backwards by 7s or 3s, spelling words backwards or reciting the months of the year backwards.

Language

Word-finding difficulties are extremely common in all types of vascular dementia. True aphasia is uncommon in vascular dementia due solely to small vessel ischemic disease, but is often seen in multi-infarct and strategic infarct dementia.

Memory

Episodic memory shows a "frontal pattern": encoding is often impaired, as is free recall, whereas relative preservation is typically seen when tasks that assist in retrieval, such as cued recall and recognition, are used.

Reasoning and judgment

Reasoning and judgment are typically impaired, both because working memory is reduced, impairing the patient's ability to keep various alternatives and details in mind, and because the frontal lobe's ability to inhibit impulsive responses is impaired.

Visuospatial function

Visuospatial function is typically intact with small vessel ischemic disease, but can be quite impaired with multi-infarct and strategic infarct dementia.

LABORATORY STUDIES

There are no laboratory studies that are useful in either confirming or ruling out vascular dementia. If a vascular dementia is diagnosed, however, a cerebrovascular work-up should be undertaken that will require a number of laboratory studies.

STRUCTURAL IMAGING STUDIES

The key to making a diagnosis of a vascular dementia or vascular cognitive impairment is the structural imaging study. In order to make the diagnosis of *pure* vascular dementia or vascular cognitive impairment there needs to be sufficient cerebrovascular disease present

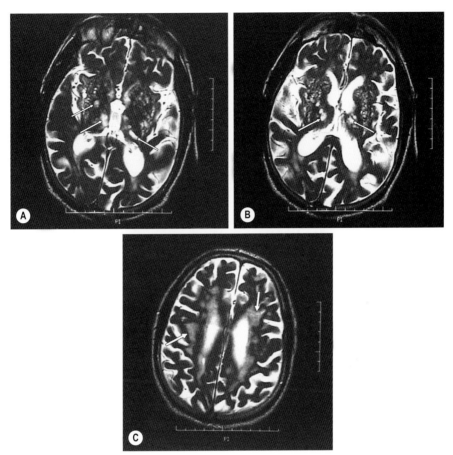

FIGURE 6.4 T2-weighted MRI scan of a patient with pure vascular dementia due to strategic infarcts and small vessel ischemic disease.

Note the multiple bright areas in the deep gray structures of the brain including basal ganglia and thalamus (A and B) and the periventricular subcortical white matter (C) indicating strategic infarcts (thin arrows, not all infarcts indicated) and small vessel ischemic disease (thick arrows, not all disease indicated).

on the CT or MRI scan to explain the degree of cognitive impairment. To make a diagnosis of a *mixed* dementia, with vascular dementia a contributing factor, there needs to be more cerebrovascular disease present on the CT or MRI scan than may be commonly present in an older adult without cognitive impairment. It is, of course, difficult to succinctly articulate exactly how much cerebrovascular disease may be present without significant cognitive impairment. Figures 6.4 and 6.5 show patients with pure vascular dementia.

FUNCTIONAL IMAGING STUDIES

Functional imaging studies are only useful in excluding neurodegenerative diseases such as Alzheimer's disease or frontotemporal dementia.

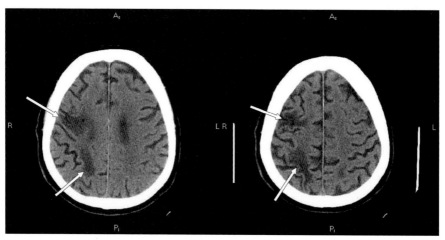

FIGURE 6.5 CT scan of a patient with pure vascular dementia due to multi-infarct dementia.

Note the two large right-hemisphere hypodensities (arrows) due to embolic strokes which extend from subcortical to cortical regions.

DIFFERENTIAL DIAGNOSIS

There are several aspects to consider in the differential diagnosis. First, are the lesions observed in the imaging study due to cerebrovascular disease or some other pathology such as multiple sclerosis or progressive multifocal leukoencephalopathy? Second, is the patient's cerebrovascular disease due to the ordinary causes of stroke such as hypertension, diabetes, and smoking, or to another disorder such as a vasculitis or vasculopathy? Third, as discussed above, does the patient have pure vascular cognitive impairment/vascular dementia, or is it a mixed disorder, vascular plus Alzheimer's disease or plus dementia with Lewy bodies? The answers to these questions are important as they will invariably lead to different treatments.

TREATMENTS (see also Table 6.1)

If the patient has the common scenario of a mixed dementia of vascular dementia plus either Alzheimer's disease or dementia with Lewy bodies, treatment should proceed with medications appropriate to those disorders, such as cholinesterase inhibitors and memantine. If the patient has a pure vascular dementia, although there are no FDA approved treatments, there are a number of studies which have investigated the treatment of vascular dementia. A meta-analysis (Kavirajan & Schneider, 2007) found that all randomized controlled trials for vascular dementia showed improvement on cognitive subscales, although only a few showed improvement on clinical, behavioral, or functional scales. The studies examined included three donepezil (Aricept) (Black et al., 2003; Wilkinson et al., 2003; Roman et al, 2005), two galantamine (Razadyne) (Erkinjuntti et al., 2002; Auchus et al., 2007), one rivastigmine (Exelon) (Moretti et al., 2003), and two memantine (Namenda) (Orgogozo et al., 2002; Wilcock et al., 2002) trials (see also Ballard et al., 2008; Erkinjuntti et al., 2008).

It is our experience that the majority of patients with a pure vascular dementia and resultant memory problems show improvement in their memory with cholinesterase inhibitors. Memantine is also often helpful when problems such as apathy occur. We would therefore recommend a trial of these medications in patients with a pure vascular dementia when those symptoms are present.

Lastly, the underlying cause of the cerebrovascular disease must also be evaluated and treated.

References

Auchus, A.P., Brashear, H.R., Salloway, S., et al., 2007. Galantamine treatment of vascular dementia: a randomized trial. Neurology 69, 448–458.

Ballard, C., Sauter, M., Scheltens, P., et al., 2008. Efficacy, safety and tolerability of rivastigmine capsules in patients with probable vascular dementia: the VantagE study. Curr. Med. Res. Opin. 24, 2561–2574.

Black, S., Roman, G.C., Geldmacher, D.S., et al., 2003. Efficacy and tolerability of donepezil in vascular dementia: positive results of a 24-week, multicenter, international, randomized, placebo-controlled clinical trial. Stroke 34, 2323–2330.

Erkinjuntti, T., Kurz, A., Gauthier, S., et al., 2002. Efficacy of galantamine in probable vascular dementia and Alzheimer's disease combined with cerebrovascular disease: a randomised trial. Lancet 359, 1283–1290.

Erkinjuntti, T., Gauthier, S., Bullock, R., et al., 2008. Galantamine treatment in Alzheimer's disease with cerebrovascular disease: responder analyses from a randomized, controlled trial (GAL-INT-6). J. Psychopharmacol. 22, 761–768.

Federico, A., Bianchi, S., Dotti, M.T., 2005. The spectrum of mutations for CADASIL diagnosis. Neurol. Sci. 26, 117–124.

Gold, G., Giannakopoulos, P., Montes-Paixao, J.C., et al., 1997. Sensitivity and specificity of newly proposed clinical criteria for possible vascular dementia. Neurology 49, 690–694.

Gold, G., Bouras, C., Canuto, A., et al., 2002. Clinicopathological validation study of four sets of clinical criteria for vascular dementia. Am. J. Psychiatry 159, 82–87.

Kavirajan, H., Schneider, L.S., 2007. Efficacy and adverse effects of cholinesterase inhibitors and memantine in vascular dementia: a meta-analysis of randomised controlled trials. Lancet Neurol. 6, 782–792.

Moretti, R., Torre, P., Antonello, R.M., et al., 2003. Rivastigmine in subcortical vascular dementia: a randomized, controlled, open 12-month study in 208 patients. Am. J. Alzheimers Dis. Other Demen. 18, 265–272.

Orgogozo, J.M., Rigaud, A.S., Stoffler, A., et al., 2002. Efficacy and safety of memantine in patients with mild to moderate vascular dementia: a randomized, placebo-controlled trial (MMM 300). Stroke 33, 1834–1839.

Pantoni, L., Pescini, F., Nannucci, S., et al., 2010. Comparison of clinical, familial, and MRI features of CADASIL and NOTCH3-negative patients. Neurology 74, 57–63.

Roman, G.C., Tatemichi, T.K., Erkinjuntti, T., et al., 1993. Vascular dementia: diagnostic criteria for research studies. Report of the NINDS-AIREN International Workshop. Neurology 43, 250–260.

Roman, G.C., Wilkinson, D.G., Doody, R.S., et al., 2005. Donepezil in vascular dementia: combined analysis of two large-scale clinical trials. Dement. Geriatr. Cogn. Disord. 20, 338–344.

Wilcock, G., Mobius, H.J., Stoffler, A., 2002. A double-blind, placebo-controlled multicentre study of memantine in mild to moderate vascular dementia (MMM500). Int. Clin. Psychopharmacol. 17, 297–305.

Wilkinson, D., Doody, R., Helme, R., et al., 2003. Donepezil in vascular dementia: a randomized, placebo-controlled study. Neurology 61, 479–486.

7 Frontotemporal dementia

QUICK START 1: FRONTOTEMPORAL DEMENTIA

Definition	• Frontotemporal dementia is a progressive neurodegenerative disorder with three common clinical presentations and at least four different patterns of pathology (Kipps & Hodges, 2007). The three common clinical presentations are:
	• Behavioral or frontal variant frontotemporal dementia (often abbreviated to bv-FTD or fv-FTD)
	• Semantic dementia or temporal variant frontotemporal dementia (often abbreviated to SD or tv-FTD)
	• Progressive non-fluent aphasia (often abbreviated to PNFA).
	• The term primary progressive aphasia (often abbreviated to PPA) can be used for both patients who present with semantic dementia and those who present with progressive non-fluent aphasia.
Prevalence	• Frontotemporal dementia is found in 5–10% of cases of dementia.
	• Frontotemporal dementia tends to affect younger individuals, with approximately three-quarters of the cases presenting from ages 45 to 65, and the remaining quarter presenting after age 65.
	• Up to 10% of patients with motor neuron disease (amyotrophic lateral sclerosis or ALS) also show signs and symptoms of frontotemporal dementia.
Genetic risk	• Up to 40% of cases of frontotemporal dementia are familial with an autosomal dominant pattern.
	• A small percentage have a mutated tau gene on chromosome 17.
Cognitive and behavioral symptoms	• In behavioral variant frontotemporal dementia there are changes in personality and social conduct, including apathy, loss of insight, disinhibition, lack of empathy, inappropriate social remarks, abnormal eating behaviors, and neglect of self-care.
	• In semantic dementia there is a loss of memory for words, starting with anomia, continuing with impaired comprehension of words, and ultimately leading to impaired comprehension of objects as well.
	• In progressive non-fluent aphasia there is a reduction in the ability to produce speech characterized by word-finding difficulty, speaking in short sentences, reduced phrase length, and difficulty pronouncing words, similar to that of a patient with Broca's aphasia.
	• Although brief cognitive measures such as the Mini-Mental State Examination (MMSE) are sometimes normal in all presentations of frontotemporal dementia, neuropsychological testing will often show dysfunction of tests of attention, response inhibition, frontal/executive function, and language.

Continued

   Memory Loss: A Practical Guide for Clinicians.

QUICK START 1: FRONTOTEMPORAL DEMENTIA—Cont'd

Diagnostic criteria
- Core components: (a) insidious onset and gradual progression, (b) early decline in social interpersonal conduct, (c) early emotional blunting, (d) early loss of insight.
- Supportive diagnostic features:
  - Behavioral disorder: (a) decline in personal hygiene and grooming, (b) mental rigidity and inflexibility, (c) distractibility and impersistence, (d) hyperorality and/or dietary change, (e) utilization behavior (sees an object and feels compelled to use it).
  - Speech and language disorder: altered speech output including (a) aspontaneity of speech, (b) economy of speech, (c) stereotypy of speech, (d) echolalia, (e) perseveration, (f) mutism.

Treatment
- There are no FDA approved medications to treat frontotemporal dementia.
- The treatment of frontotemporal dementia consists of supportive management.
- Many medications, including SSRIs and atypical antipsychotics, are used to treat the symptoms.

Top differential diagnoses
- Alzheimer's disease, vascular dementia, corticobasal degeneration, progressive supranuclear palsy, Huntington's disease, as well as other causes of frontal lobe dysfunction (such as a frontal tumor). If Parkinsonism is present consider frontotemporal dementia with Parkinsonism, dementia with Lewy bodies, and vascular dementia.

PREVALENCE, PROGNOSIS, AND DEFINITION (Fig. 7.1)

Frontotemporal dementia is a progressive neurodegenerative disorder with three common clinical presentations and at least four different patterns of pathology. Unfortunately, no correlation has been observed between clinical phenotype and underlying pathology. The three common clinical presentations are:

1. behavioral or frontal variant frontotemporal dementia (often abbreviated to bv-FTD or fv-FTD)
2. semantic dementia or temporal variant frontotemporal dementia (often abbreviated to SD or tv-FTD)
3. progressive non-fluent aphasia (often abbreviated to PNFA).

The term primary progressive aphasia (often abbreviated to PPA) can be used for both patients who present with semantic dementia and those who present with progressive non-fluent aphasia. Note that, after a few years, many patients with a frontotemporal dementia with one initial presentation show signs and symptoms of the other types of frontotemporal dementias as well.

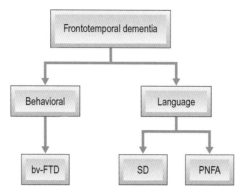

FIGURE 7.1 One classification scheme for frontotemporal dementias.

bv-FTD, behavioral variant frontotemporal dementia; PNFA, progressive non-fluent aphasia; SD, semantic dementia.

From Kipps, C.M., Hodges, J.R., 2007. Frontotemporal dementia syndromes. In: Growdon, J.H., Rossor, M. (Eds.), The Dementias 2, Butterworth-Heinemann, Philadelphia, PA, pp. 112–140.

In studies of memory clinics, frontotemporal dementia has been found in 5–10% of cases, with our experience closer to 5%. Frontotemporal dementia tends to affect younger individuals, with approximately three-quarters of the cases presenting from ages 45 to 65, the remaining one-quarter presenting after age 65.

CRITERIA

The Lund–Manchester criteria (Anonymous, 1994) are the first and most often cited for frontotemporal dementia (Box 7.1). However, we and most in this field diagnose patients with one of the three common clinical variants, and use more informal criteria to do so.

RISK FACTORS, PATHOLOGY, AND PATHOPHYSIOLOGY

Other than family history there are no known risk factors for frontotemporal dementia. If a family history of dementia, psychiatric illness, Parkinson's disease, or amyotrophic lateral sclerosis are all considered positive indicators, one may conclude from various studies that up to 40% of cases of frontotemporal dementia are familial with an autosomal dominant pattern. The best studied familial frontotemporal dementia syndrome is that of familial frontotemporal dementia with Parkinsonism linked to chromosome 17. Individuals with this disorder have a mutation in the tau gene located in the chromosome 17q21–22 region. Other genetic abnormalities that have been associated with frontotemporal dementia include that of progranulin (chromosome 17q21), valosin-containing protein (chromosome 9p12–13), charged multivesicular body protein (chromosome 3), pre-senilin (chromosome 14), and an unidentified protein from the region of chromosome 9p13.3–21.3.

BOX 7.1 MODIFIED LUND–MANCHESTER CRITERIA FOR FRONTOTEMPORAL DEMENTIA

I. Core components:
  a. Insidious onset and gradual progression.
  b. Early decline in social interpersonal conduct.
  c. Early emotional blunting.
  d. Early loss of insight.

II. Supportive diagnostic features:
  a. Behavioral disorder
    i. Decline in personal hygiene and grooming
    ii. Mental rigidity and inflexibility
    iii. Distractibility and impersistence
    iv. Hyperorality and/or dietary change
    v. Utilization behavior (sees an object and feels compelled to use it).
  b. Speech and language disorder
    i. Altered speech output
      1. aspontaneity of speech
      2. economy of speech
      3. stereotypy of speech
      4. echolalia
      5. perseveration
      6. mutism.
  c. Physical signs
    i. Primitive reflexes
      1. grasp
      2. snout
      3. palmomental
    ii. Incontinence
    iii. Akinesia
    iv. Rigidity
    v. Tremor.
  d. Investigations
    i. Neuropsychology
      1. Impairment on tests sensitive to frontal lobe functions
      2. No amnesia (when frontal lobe and semantic functions are excluded)
      3. No perceptual deficits
    ii. Brain imaging
      1. frontal and/or anterior temporal lobe abnormality
    iii. EEG
      1. generally normal.

There are at least four common pathologies observed in patients diagnosed with frontotemporal dementia. Many frontotemporal dementias show tau-positive inclusions. These include classic Pick's disease which has tau- and ubiquitin-positive spherical cortical inclusions, familial FTD with characteristic tau-positive inclusions in neurons and glial cells, and argyrophilic grain disease. Many patients with frontotemporal dementias, particularly those with motor neuron disease but also those without it, also show ubiquitin-positive inclusions. Neuronal filament inclusions are sometimes observed. Microvacuolar degeneration and gliosis lacking distinctive inclusions can also be seen. See Figures 7.2 and 7.3 for two of the more common pathologies.

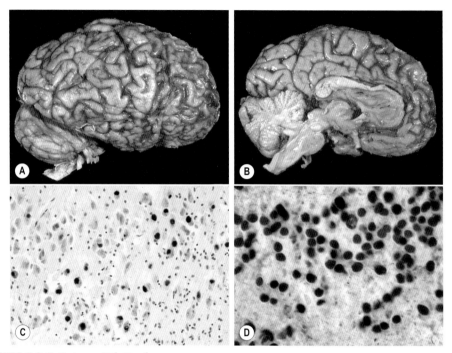

FIGURE 7.2 Pathology of Pick's disease.

Severe atrophy can be clearly seen in the frontal lobes and also the anterior portion of the temporal lobe (A and B). Microscopically, Pick bodies—tau-immunoreactive rounded inclusions in neurons—can be seen (C and D). A color version of this figure is avaliable online at http://www.expertconsult.com.

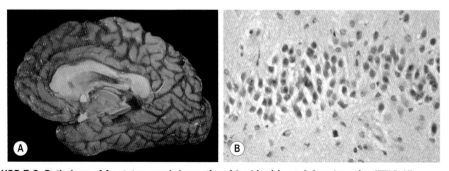

FIGURE 7.3 Pathology of frontotemporal dementia with ubiquitin-staining deposits (FTLD-U).

Note the atrophy of the front part of the brain (A, left side of figure), shrinking the gyri and making the vessels appear more prominent. (B) Ubiquitin-staining inclusions in neurons in the dentate gyrus of the hippocampus. A color version of this figure is avaliable online at http://www.expertconsult.com.

COMMON SIGNS, SYMPTOMS, AND STAGES
Behavioral variant frontotemporal dementia

In behavioral variant frontotemporal dementia there is insidious onset of gradual changes in personality and social conduct. Although changes in personality and social conduct can occur in many other dementias as well, in behavioral variant frontotemporal dementia these changes occur early in the disease process and are prominent. Apathy is probably one of the most common signs, although other dementias also commonly present with apathy. Insight is also generally lost very early. Early disinhibition is one of the more pathognomonic signs, and may manifest itself by inappropriate social remarks, improper remarks of a sexual nature, and poorly concealed use of pornography. Empathy for others is typically lacking. Abnormal eating behaviors can manifest in many different ways, ranging from dramatic changes in food preferences (particularly sweets), poor manners, gluttonous behavior, and eating inappropriate things. For example, one of our patients ate a raw steak and an entire jar of mayonnaise. Stereotypic and ritualistic behaviors such as pacing the same route, using the same verbal phrases, are common (e.g., another patient would repetitively walk right up to people and loudly state, "You're handsome!"). Neglect of self-care is common, and may be related to apathy. To reiterate, although all of these signs and symptoms could be present with Alzheimer's disease as well (as the frontal lobes become involved), they are early manifestations in behavioral variant frontotemporal dementia, but late manifestations of Alzheimer's disease.

It is also interesting to note that the particular behavioral abnormalities that a patient presents with may relate to the different brain regions which are involved. For example, on a particular clinic day we happened to evaluate two very different patients with behavioral variant frontotemporal dementia. One patient showed signs and symptoms of ventromedial frontal lobe dysfunction: he was rude, disinhibited, and socially inappropriate, although he was perfectly able to achieve normal eye contact and relate to whomever he was speaking to. This patient came to the attention of his physicians because he began soliciting sexual acts from his daughter-in-law, quite an uncharacteristic thing for him to do! The second patient showed signs and symptoms of dorsolateral frontal lobe dysfunction: he was unable to make normal eye contact, he showed signs of apathy, slowness of movement, and performed no activity unless he was specifically asked (and he then was happy to comply). This second patient presented with extreme difficulty and slowness in doing simple things like shaving, and would walk out of the house holding items like shaving cream.

Semantic dementia

Semantic dementia could be described as a loss of memory for words. The disorder often starts as problems with word-finding and naming difficulties (anomia), but progresses to include impaired word comprehension and ultimately impaired comprehension of objects as well. The naming deficit in semantic dementia is often referred to as a two-way naming deficit, because patients have difficulty naming an object when shown its picture, and also describing an object when given its name. They have difficulty in word-to-picture matching, identifying the right color for objects (e.g., yellow for banana), and knowing which objects belong together (e.g., dental floss with toothbrush rather than hairbrush). This difficulty occurs because these patients lose the meaning of what things are. It is as if they lived in a culture without bananas or dental floss, and so therefore they would not know the right color for the banana, or what the floss is used for. (For additional explanation, see Appendix C: *Our current understanding of memory*.) All manifestations of the behavioral variant of frontotemporal dementia may also be seen, although these typically occur later in patients with semantic dementia.

Progressive non-fluent aphasia

In progressive non-fluent aphasia there is a reduction in the ability to produce speech from a number of causes, including word-finding difficulty, speaking in short sentences, and difficulty in pronouncing words, similar to that of a patient with Broca's aphasia. These patients are often said to have speech apraxia, meaning that they are impaired in the motor planning and sequencing of the lips, tongue, and breath necessary for articulate speech. The ability to converse becomes reduced over time, with the patient eventually becoming monosyllabic or mute. Although patients with both semantic dementia and progressive non-fluent aphasia have early word-finding difficulties, the characteristic manifestation in semantic dementia is that of circumlocution, whereas long pauses in speech are more common with progressive non-fluent aphasia. It is also notable that most patients with progressive non-fluent aphasia are aware of their language difficulties, which are understandably quite frustrating for them (Table 7.1)

Table 7.1 Language deficits in semantic dementia and progressive non-fluent aphasia

Feature	Semantic dementia	Progressive non-fluent aphasia
Reduced speech	Not seen (except pauses for word-finding)	Severe
Repetition impairment	None	Severe
Semantic errors	Moderate	Not seen
Anomia	Severe	Moderate
Impaired word comprehension	Severe	Not seen
Impaired sentence comprehension	Mild	Moderate

After Kipps, C.M., Hodges, J.R., 2007. Frontotemporal dementia syndromes. In: Growdon, J.H., Rossor, M. (Eds.), The Dementias 2, Butterworth-Heinemann, Philadelphia, PA, pp. 112–140.

THINGS TO LOOK FOR IN THE HISTORY

As described above there are different presentations of frontotemporal dementia (Fig. 7.4). Nevertheless these different presentations of frontotemporal dementia share many common signs, and as a group they differ from other dementias, such as Alzheimer's disease.

Incontinence is common early in frontotemporal dementia, and often presents in a very different manner than that of early Alzheimer's disease. Although in both disorders there is urgency, patients with Alzheimer's disease will rush to the bathroom and be embarrassed if they have an accident, whereas patients with frontotemporal dementia will often be indifferent to having an accident, allowing themselves to be soiled wherever they are. Many patients will subsequently refuse to be cleaned up. One patient we cared for with early

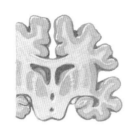

Atrophy of frontal and/or
temporal areas

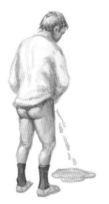

Bizarre, uninhibited
socially inappropriate
behavior

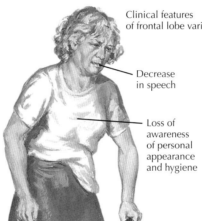

Clinical features
of frontal lobe variant

Decrease
in speech

Loss of
awareness
of personal
appearance
and hygiene

Oral fixation:
increased eating
causes weight
gain

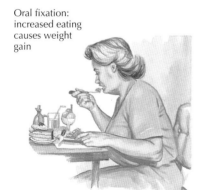

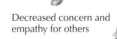

Decreased concern and
empathy for others

FIGURE 7.4 Frontotemporal dementia.

A color version of this figure is available online at http://www.expertconsult.com

behavioral variant frontotemporal dementia and a perfect score on the MMSE refused to change his pants after a urinary accident, claiming "it will dry"! Another patient was found happily watching TV—despite there being feces all over the living room.

Problems in driving are also common in frontotemporal dementia and also often present differently than in Alzheimer's disease. In Alzheimer's disease the first problem is invariably that the patient becomes lost, even when traveling familiar routes. In frontotemporal dementia the problem is more likely to be driving on the wrong side of the road, or other abnormal and risky behavior leading to accidents.

Sequencing problems are very common in frontotemporal dementia, making it difficult for patients to perform tasks like brushing their teeth, showering, making coffee, or preparing a sandwich. Often steps are missing or mixed up. One of our patients would make a sandwich with the bread on the inside and the meat on the outside. Another decided to paint the house upon returning from church, but did not change out of his suit into appropriate painting clothes until he had finished painting.

It is remarkable the number of patients with frontotemporal dementia who, when watching TV, believe that the persons or characters on it are either personally relevant for their life or actually talking directly to them. One patient we cared for thought that the events happening on a soap opera were events happening to her own children. Another patient believed that the political messages on the TV during a campaign season were all directed to him and he talked back to the TV.

Another characteristic behavior of frontotemporal dementia (particularly the behavioral variant) is sexual disinhibition. Many patients spend more time with pornography than previously. One patient we evaluated now showed more interest in sexual activity with his wife—making advances and requesting sexual activity—than in their 35+ years of marriage. Another patient began to try to pick up men from a restaurant—despite the fact that she was having dinner with her husband at the time! And we commented above about the patient who requested sexual favors from his daughter-in-law. Although patients with Alzheimer's disease will sometimes exhibit sexual disinhibition, in frontotemporal dementia it occurs earlier in the disease process and is typically more prominent than in Alzheimer's disease.

Memory problems are commonly mentioned by family, although they have a different flavor than memory problems in Alzheimer's disease. In frontotemporal dementia the memory problems tend to be related to poor frontal lobe function. Patients show difficulties in learning new information because they have difficulties paying attention, and thus information needs to be repeated a number of times to be learned. Once learned, information is generally retained in memory, although there is often difficulty accessing it because of poor frontally mediated memory search processes. Patients with frontotemporal dementia thus do much better on tests of multiple choice than free recall. Also related to their frontal lobe dysfunction, these patients show prominent distortions of memory, frequently mixing up details or confusing two or more memories.

THINGS TO LOOK FOR ON THE PHYSICAL AND NEUROLOGICAL EXAMINATION

There are no particular signs on the physical or neurological examination to suggest a frontotemporal dementia. Although one might suspect that frontal release signs such as the snout, grasp, and palmomental reflexes are more common in frontotemporal dementia, in our experience we have not found this to be the case.

The patient with frontotemporal dementia should, however, be carefully examined for any signs of motor neuron disease. It is now recognized that up to 10% of patients with motor neuron disease also show signs and symptoms of frontotemporal dementia. Thus, so-called "mixed signs" of upper and lower motor neuron dysfunction should be sought for, including brisk reflexes, extensor plantars, fasciculations, and muscle wasting.

PATTERN OF IMPAIRMENT ON COGNITIVE TESTS

The first point that should be noted is that, in many cases of frontotemporal dementia, the standard cognitive testing may be normal until quite late in the disease. This point is particularly true for brief measures such as the Mini-Mental State Examination (MMSE). Thus, additional tests specifically evaluating frontal lobe function must be performed whenever a frontotemporal dementia is suspected. And, perhaps because the frontal lobes are so large and mediate such a diverse group of cognitive and behavioral functions, different patients may show impairment on different tests even within the same variant, so (unfortunately) there is not a single frontal lobe test that can be used to make the diagnosis.

In behavioral variant frontotemporal dementia helpful tests include the Wisconsin Card Sorting Test, verbal fluency to letters, the Trailmaking Test Part B, the Delis–Kaplan Executive Function System (D-KEFS), and the Cambridge Neuropsychological Test Automated Battery (CANTAB). Although memory is often relatively spared, memory may be impaired secondary to problems with attention, encoding, retrieval, source memory, memory distortions, and other frontal aspects of memory.

In semantic dementia impairments are prominent on tests of semantic memory. These include verbal fluency to categories, picture naming, and the generation of definitions to words or pictures. The Pyramids and Palm Trees test was developed specifically to evaluate patients for semantic dementia; in this test patients are asked which of two pictures best go with a third picture (Fig. 7.5). In this way semantic information can be assessed in a non-verbal way, to help distinguish disorders which affect solely language from those affecting semantic information. (Very early patients with semantic dementia may perform normally on the Pyramids and Palm Trees test, but in later stages almost all patients show abnormalities.)

In progressive non-fluent aphasia it is important to do similar tests to those used in semantic dementia, to ensure that underlying semantic abilities are intact. Thus these patients invariably perform normally on the Pyramids and Palm Trees test. Aphasia batteries that include tests of speech production, comprehension, repetition, reading, and writing are helpful, such as the Boston Diagnostic Aphasia Examination. Early on, the difficulty is usually problems in producing speech, although later difficulty understanding spoken and written language occurs. Particularly challenging for these patients is comprehending syntactically complex questions such as, "The lion was killed by the tiger, which one is dead?" and "Pick up the cup after writing with the pen." Often referral for neuropsychological testing will be helpful in evaluating these patients.

LABORATORY STUDIES

There are no routine laboratory studies to support or refute the diagnosis of frontotemporal dementia. Genetic testing for frontotemporal dementia with Parkinsonism linked to chromosome 17 is becoming more readily available, which may be helpful in evaluating a

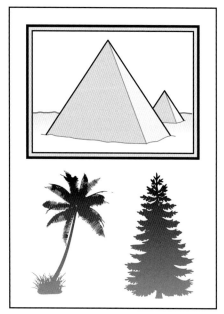

FIGURE 7.5 The Pyramids and Palm Trees test.

The goal of the test is for the patient to correctly point out which of the two lower pictures is most associated with the upper picture.

patient for possible frontotemporal dementia who has a family history of either frontotemporal dementia or Parkinsonism. Electromyogram and nerve conduction studies are essential when motor neuron disease is suspected.

STRUCTURAL IMAGING STUDIES

Although the structural imaging scan may be normal at the time of presentation, most cases of frontotemporal dementia show frontal and anterior temporal lobe atrophy at some point in the course of their disease. In behavioral variant frontotemporal dementia the atrophy tends to be most prominent in the frontal lobes. In semantic dementia the atrophy is most often found in anterior temporal lobes, left somewhat greater than right. And in progressive non-fluent aphasia, the atrophy is invariably more left- than right-sided, and may include more posterior left peri-Sylvian regions than the other disorders.

FUNCTIONAL IMAGING STUDIES

Functional imaging studies such as SPECT and PET typically show decreased function in the same regions as those that show atrophy on structural scans, although abnormalities are often present on these functional scans for several years prior to the atrophy being noted (Fig. 7.6). Thus, such imaging will often show frontal hypofunction for behavioral variant

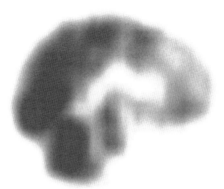

FIGURE 7.6 Mid-sagittal slice of a SPECT scan in a patient with behavioral frontotemporal dementia.
Note the reduced activity in the front of the brain (right side of image) relative to more posterior regions.

frontotemporal dementia, left greater than right anterior temporal lobe hypofunction for semantic dementia, and left peri-Sylvian hypofunction in progressive non-fluent aphasia. The difficulty with these functional imaging studies is that they will sometimes be normal or ambiguous early in the course of the illness.

DIFFERENTIAL DIAGNOSIS

Because Alzheimer's disease is so common, when suspecting a frontotemporal dementia one must always consider the possibility that it is an atypical case of Alzheimer's disease (Table 7.2). Alzheimer's disease should be especially considered when the patient is over the age of 65, as only one-quarter of cases of frontotemporal dementia—but most cases of Alzheimer's disease—present over age 65.

Other etiologies that can cause frontal/executive or behavioral dysfunction must also be considered. Cortical basal degeneration is typically associated with frontal/executive dysfunction on neuropsychological tests, although these patients rarely have the behavioral manifestations seen in frontotemporal dementia.

There are many causes of frontal/executive dysfunction due to subcortical dysfunction. These include vascular dementia, Huntington's disease, normal pressure hydrocephalus, and multiple sclerosis.

When Parkinsonism is present along with cognitive and/or behavioral symptoms, in addition to frontotemporal dementia with Parkinsonism linked to chromosome 17, the differential diagnosis must include dementia with Lewy bodies, progressive supranuclear palsy, cortical basal degeneration, and vascular dementia.

Lastly, when it is clear that the patient is suffering from a frontotemporal dementia, it is always important to look for evidence of motor neuron disease. The history may include weakness in the hands or dropping items, and the neurological examination will typically show scattered evidence of atrophy, fasciculations, weakness, and brisk reflexes.

Table 7.2 Similarities and differences between Alzheimer's disease and frontotemporal dementia

	Alzheimer's disease	Behavioral variant frontotemporal dementia	Semantic dementia	Progressive non-fluent aphasia
Age of onset	Typically > 65	Typically < 65	Typically < 65	Typically < 65
Cognitive deficits	Memory deficits prominent, along with multiple other cognitive areas	Cognition relatively undisturbed early in the disease; progressive cognitive decline in the middle and late stages	Speech fluent but loss of word meaning; other areas of cognition relatively intact early in the disease, cognitive deficits in multiple areas developing later	Reduced speech output but word meaning preserved; other areas of cognition relatively intact early in the disease, cognitive deficits in multiple areas developing later
Behavioral symptoms	Absent early in the disease; apathy, agitation, and other symptoms as the disease progresses	Socially inappropriate behavior early in the disease	Absent early in the disease, but may become inappropriate as the disease progresses	Absent early in the disease, but may become inappropriate as the disease progresses

TREATMENTS

Frontotemporal dementias are difficult to manage. The treatment consists of supportive management. Non-pharmacological treatments include the use of redirection, music, and calm voices. Speech therapy can sometimes be helpful for patients with language disturbances. Patients with frontotemporal dementia show a significant deficit of serotonin, and it is therefore not surprising that selective serotonin reuptake inhibitors are often of help. Studies have suggested that irritability, agitation, and abnormal eating behavior are improved by this class of medications.

Unfortunately, as the disease progresses patients with frontotemporal dementia almost always require additional medications to control agitation and aggression. Atypical antipsychotics are most often used as first-line medications to control these unwanted behaviors. It should be noted that these medications carry "black-box warnings" from the FDA because these medications (along with traditional neuroleptic medications) alter glucose metabolism and have been associated with an increased risk of cardiovascular disease and stroke in the older adult. We would therefore recommend that these medications be used with caution in patients with frontotemporal and other dementias, and that the clinician discuss the risks of these medications openly with the family and documents that discussion in the medical record. Some of the other common side-effects caused by this class of medication include sedation and Parkinsonism. The three atypical antipsychotics that we most frequently use are risperidone (Risperdal), quetiapine (Seroquel), and olanzapine (Zyprexa) (see Chapter 22 for important additional information). Risperidone causes the least sedation of the three, and is often our first-line medication for daytime agitation. Quetiapine causes the most sedation, and is therefore particularly useful for night-time agitation. Olanzapine is a useful second-line medication although its side-effect profile, including its effect on glucose metabolism, is not as favorable as those of risperidone and quetiapine.

Other medications that may be useful include the sedating antidepressant trazodone. No clinical trials of medications have demonstrated cognitive improvement in patients with frontotemporal dementia. It is not unreasonable, however, to try a small dose of memantine or a cholinesterase inhibitor, particularly early in the course of the disease. Similarly, stimulants might be helpful. One study found that 20 mg of dextroamphetamine improved behavioral symptoms when compared with quetiapine (Huey et al., 2008). We are quite cautious with cholinesterase inhibitors and stimulants as these classes of medications can sometimes "activate" a patient with frontotemporal dementia and make behavior worse; nonetheless some patients do appear to show cognitive and behavioral improvement. We have also found that a number of patients do appear to receive benefit from memantine.

QUICK START 2: TREATMENT OF FRONTOTEMPORAL DEMENTIA

Medication class	Medication and FDA approval status	Summary of benefits	Common side-effects
Selective serotonin reuptake inhibitors	Sertraline (Zoloft) and escitalopram (Lexapro); off-label use	Improvement of irritability, agitation, and abnormal eating behavior	Gastrointestinal upset and sexual dysfunction
Atypical antipsychotics	Risperidone (Risperidal) and quetiapine (Seroquel); off-label use	Control of agitation and aggression	Altered glucose metabolism, risk of cardiovascular disease, Parkinsonism, sedation

---

References

Anonymous, 1994. Clinical and neuropathological criteria for frontotemporal dementia. The Lund and Manchester Groups. J. Neurol. Neurosurg. Psychiatry 57, 416–418.

Huey, E.D., Garcia, C., Wassermann, E.M., et al., 2008. Stimulant treatment of frontotemporal dementia in 8 patients. J. Clin. Psychiatry 69, 1981–1982.

Kipps, C.M., Hodges, J.R., 2007. Frontotemporal dementia syndromes. In: Growdon, J.H., Rossor, M. (Eds.), The Dementias 2, Butterworth-Heinemann, Philadelphia PA, pp. 112–140.

Progressive supranuclear palsy

QUICK START: PROGRESSIVE SUPRANUCLEAR PALSY

Definition	• Progressive supranuclear palsy (often abbreviated to PSP) is a neurodegenerative disease due to the accumulation of hyperphosphorylated tau protein isoforms in the brain. • Its main features include abnormalities of vertical eye movements (supranuclear palsy), along with postural instability with backwards falling, gait like "a drunken sailor," axial rigidity, frontal lobe signs and symptoms, and difficulty swallowing and eventually talking (pseudobulbar palsy).
Prevalence	• Progressive supranuclear palsy has a prevalence of five per 100,000. • The mean age of onset of the disease is 66 years. • The prognosis ranges from 6 to 9 years from diagnosis to death.
Genetic risk	• There are no known genetic or other risk factors.
Cognitive and behavioral symptoms	• Early cognitive and affective symptoms may include slowing of all aspects of mental processing, executive dysfunction, irritability, irascibility, apathy, introversion, and depression.

Diagnostic criteria	• A degenerative disorder with onset in middle age or later with supranuclear palsy including down-gaze abnormalities and at least two of the following cardinal features:
	  • Postural instability and falls backwards
	  • Axial rigidity and dystonia
	  • Pseudobulbar palsy
	  • Bradykinesia and rigidity
	  • Frontal lobe signs
	    – Slow thinking (bradyphrenia)
	    – Perseveration
	    – Grasp
	    – Utilization behavior.
	• Atrophy of the midbrain in patients with progressive supranuclear palsy has been frequently observed on MRI; the midbrain reduction in size can be measured on either film or electronic images.

Treatment	• There are no FDA approved medications to treat progressive supranuclear palsy. • Treatment consists of supportive management. • Symptomatic treatments to consider include levodopa/carbidopa (Sinemet), memantine, and amantadine.

Continued

 Memory Loss: A Practical Guide for Clinicians.

QUICK START: PROGRESSIVE SUPRANUCLEAR PALSY—Cont'd

Top differential diagnoses	• Corticobasal degeneration, dementia with Lewy bodies, vascular dementia, frontotemporal dementia (particularly with Parkinsonism linked to chromosome 17 or with amyotrophic lateral sclerosis), Creutzfeldt–Jakob disease, normal pressure hydrocephalus, Huntington's disease, multiple sclerosis, medication side-effects.

PREVALENCE, PROGNOSIS, AND DEFINITION

Progressive supranuclear palsy (often abbreviated to PSP and sometimes referred to as the Steele–Richardson–Olszewski syndrome) is a neurodegenerative disease of the brain due to the accumulation of hyperphosphorylated tau protein isoforms in the brain. Its main feature is an abnormality of vertical eye movements (supranuclear palsy), along with postural instability with falls, axial rigidity, frontal lobe signs and symptoms, and difficulty swallowing and eventually talking (pseudobulbar palsy; Box 8.1). It has a prevalence of five per 100,000. The mean age of onset of the disease is 66 years, with a usual prognosis ranging from 6 to 9 years from diagnosis to death. The disease received increased attention in the popular press when the comedian Dudley Moore was diagnosed with it in 1999.

CRITERIA AND DIAGNOSIS

The cardinal feature of progressive supranuclear palsy is an abnormality of vertical eye movements (Box 8.2). Because up-gaze is sometimes impaired in normal aging, abnormalities of down-gaze are particularly sought for as confirmatory clinical signs when this diagnosis is being entertained. Published clinical criteria by Lees (1987) can be found in Box 8.3. These research criteria (the Revised National Institutes of Neurological Disorders and Stroke–Society of Progressive Supranuclear Palsy Consensus Criteria for Clinical Diagnosis) focus only on the eye movement abnormalities and the postural instability and falls; these criteria are less sensitive but more specific, assuring that subjects who enter clinical trials truly have progressive supranuclear palsy.

BOX 8.1 WHAT DOES "PSEUDOBULBAR PALSY" MEAN?

If a patient has a "pseudobulbar palsy," it indicates that there is dysfunction of part of the brain that mimics dysfunction of the lower part of the brainstem, the medulla. A "pseudobulbar palsy" refers to dysfunction of the part of the brain above the medulla that controls movements of the tongue, pharynx, and larynx. Thus, the patient with a pseudobulbar palsy typically exhibits slurred and otherwise abnormal speech (dysarthria), and difficulty eating and swallowing (dysphagia).

BOX 8.2 WHAT DOES "SUPRANUCLEAR PALSY" MEAN?

A "supranuclear palsy" causing eye movement abnormalities means that there is dysfunction of the part of the brain that controls voluntary eye movements above (*supra* in Latin) the level of the oculomotor nucleus (in the midbrain, the upper part of the brainstem). This type of palsy affects mainly voluntary eye movements, while involuntary movements are relatively spared. (Involuntary movements may be controlled by a group of neurons called the superior colliculus.) Testing for a supranuclear palsy involves comparing eye movements for voluntary and involuntary gaze. Testing for voluntary gaze may be easily accomplished by having the patient look rapidly between two points (often called "saccades"), usually between the thumb on one hand and the index finger on the other ("Look at my thumb, look at my finger," and so on). Testing for involuntary gaze is best performed by having the patient stare at a stationary point while you gently move their head up and down and back and forth, thus moving their eyes in their head. In a supranuclear palsy the rapid, voluntary eye movements will be abnormal while the involuntary movements will be normal (or relatively normal) demonstrating that the eye movement problem is in the voluntary gaze centers, above the oculomotor nucleus.

BOX 8.3 DIAGNOSTIC CRITERIA FOR THE CLINICAL DIAGNOSIS OF PROGRESSIVE SUPRANUCLEAR PALSY

A degenerative disorder with onset in middle age or later with supranuclear palsy including down-gaze abnormalities and at least two of the following cardinal features:
- Postural instability and falls backwards
- Axial rigidity and dystonia
- Pseudobulbar palsy
- Bradykinesia and rigidity
- Frontal lobe signs
  - Slow thinking (bradyphrenia)
  - Perseveration
  - Grasp
  - Utilization behavior

Selected supportive signs
- Other ocular abnormalities
- Rest tremor
- Dystonia of limbs and face
- Cerebellar ataxia
- Dysphagia
- Dyspraxia
- Respiratory dyskinesias (inspiratory gasps, tachypnea)
- Echolalia and palilalia
- Myoclonus
- Emotional lability (pseudobulbar affect)

Adapted from Lees, A.J., 1987. The Steele-Richardson-Olszewski syndrome (progressive supranuclear palsy). In: Marsden, C.D., Fahn, S. (Eds.), Movement Disorders 2, Butterworth-Heinemann, London, pp. 272–287.

RISK FACTORS, PATHOLOGY, AND PATHOPHYSIOLOGY

There are no known risk factors for developing progressive supranuclear palsy. The disorder is associated with the accumulation of hyperphosphorylated tau protein isoforms in the brain. Neuropathological diagnostic criteria for progressive supranuclear palsy

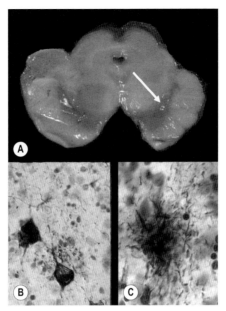

FIGURE 8.1 Pathology in progressive supranuclear palsy.

(A) Pallor of the substantia nigra (should be black) and atrophy of the midbrain, particularly in the anterior–posterior dimension (up and down in this figure). Tangles (B) and a tufted astrocyte (C). A color version of this figure is avaliable online at http://www.expertconsult.com.

include the presence of numerous neurofibrillary tangles and neuropil threads in a number of subcortical regions, such as globus pallidus, subthalamic nucleus, substantia nigra, pons, corpus striatum, oculomotor nucleus, medulla oblongata, and dentate cerebellar nuclei. The tangles are composed of 12- to 20-nm straight filaments, tend to be rounded, and have been termed "globose." Tau immunostaining has shown that tau in progressive supranuclear palsy is primarily made up of a four-repeat tau, whereas in frontotemporal dementia the tau is predominantly composed of a three-repeat tau. Atrophy of midbrain, pontine tegmentum, and globus pallidus is common in progressive supranuclear palsy (Fig. 8.1).

COMMON SIGNS, SYMPTOMS, AND STAGES

One useful way to think about progressive supranuclear palsy is that it is a disorder of several aspects of the nervous system, any or all of which may be affected depending upon the relative distribution of pathology. All clinical diagnoses of progressive supranuclear palsy must include some abnormality of eye movements. Other signs and symptoms of the disorder will be present in varying degrees; these include disorders of movement (postural instability with backwards falls, axial rigidity and dystonia, bradykinesia and rigidity), pseudobulbar palsy (difficulty swallowing and talking), and frontal/executive cognitive deficits. Over time, the features that the patient presented with typically worsen, and other symptoms may occur (but not invariably).

Some more common signs and symptoms that are seen as the disorder progresses are as follows:

- The gait, sometimes described as that of a drunken sailor, becomes more abnormal.
- Impulsiveness may lead to suddenly rising from sitting, increasing risk of falls.
- Balance becomes more impaired.
- Fractures and bruises are common due to falls.
- Sloppy eating is attributable to the combination of loss of dexterity, swallowing difficulties, and difficulty looking down at the plate of food.
- In the severe stages the patient is typically confined to a wheelchair, and more severe chewing and swallowing difficulties, drooling, coughing, spluttering, and choking are common.
- Death is typically due to aspiration pneumonia.

THINGS TO LOOK FOR IN THE HISTORY

Testimony to the fact that progressive supranuclear palsy is a difficult disorder to diagnose is the common occurrence of a delay in diagnosis of 3 years or more. The most important feature to look for in the history is that of backward falls. Early cognitive and affective symptoms may include irritability, irascibility, apathy, introversion, and depression. Inappropriate sexual behavior may also be present. The patient may complain of visual symptoms including blurred vision, difficulty focusing, dry eyes, photophobia, and double vision. Navigating stairs is usually difficult. These visual symptoms frequently lead to appointments with optometrists or ophthalmologists, often resulting in new eyeglasses prescriptions (which of course do not alleviate symptoms). The patient may also note difficulties walking, speaking, or swallowing, as well as fatigue, dizziness, and clumsiness.

THINGS TO LOOK FOR ON THE PHYSICAL AND NEUROLOGICAL EXAMINATION

The most important feature to look for on the neurological examination is a supranuclear vertical gaze disturbance, as described in Box 8.2. It should be emphasized that, although there must be at least a slowing or disruption of vertical or horizontal eye movements, an actual reduction in the degree of downward gaze is not necessary. Other common ocular abnormalities include spontaneous involuntary eyelid closure, reduced spontaneous blink rate (0–4 per minute), and a mild drooping of the eyelid (ptosis). It is likely from these latter symptoms that patients with progressive supranuclear palsy are often described as having a slightly astonished and worried look, felt to be attributable to the patient compensating for the mild drooping of the eyelids by raising their eyebrows, in combination with the decreased blink rate (Fig. 8.2).

Other features to look for on the neurological examination are abnormalities of gait, postural reflexes, axial rigidity, snout, grasp, dystonia, and myoclonus. Impairment of gait and postural reflexes leads to loss of balance and staggering when walking, with frequent falls. On rising from a chair the patient may extend the neck and trunk and spontaneously topple backwards. Axial rigidity can be assessed by passively and gently moving the head and bending the neck forward and backward.

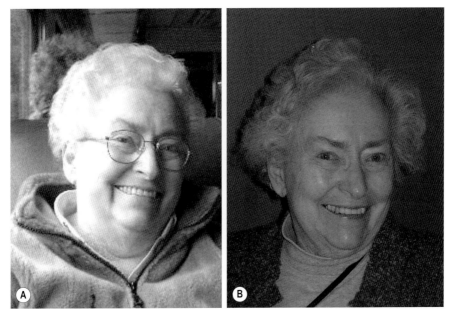

FIGURE 8.2 Changes in facial expression due to progressive supranuclear palsy.

Note the somewhat astonished look of the patient after she was diagnosed with progressive supranuclear palsy (B), compared with how she looked several years earlier (A). A color version of this figure is avaliable online at http://www.expertconsult.com.

PATTERN OF IMPAIRMENT ON COGNITIVE TESTS

The first thing that should be noted is that not all patients with progressive supranuclear palsy demonstrate cognitive deficits. One study found that approximately one-third of patients examined showed moderate cognitive impairment, one-third showed mild impairment, and one-third showed no clinically significant cognitive impairment (Maher et al., 1985).

Two main aspects of cognition are commonly impaired in patients with progressive supranuclear palsy. First there is a slowing of mental processing, often termed "bradyphrenia." This slowing will obviously produce impairment on any timed test, including verbal fluency to letters and categories, the Trailmaking Tests parts A and B, and others.

The second aspect of cognition which is impaired is executive function. As described in detail in Chapter 2: *Evaluating the patient with memory loss* there are a number of tests available to measure executive function. Patients with progressive supranuclear palsy have been observed to show impairment on many of these, including the Tower of London Task, the Addenbrookes Cognitive Examination, the Frontal Assessment Battery, and tests of "set-shifting" such as the Trailmaking Test part B. Tests of set-shifting require the patient to shift back and forth between two or more cognitive sets. For example, in the Trailmaking Test part B the patient must shift between going up the alphabet and counting forwards. Tests of memory, by contrast, will be either normal (in the early stages) or abnormal owing to poor executive function, showing poor encoding and free recall with relatively normal recognition. When executive function becomes severely impaired, other aspects of cognition will also show impairment.

LABORATORY STUDIES

There are no laboratory, genetic, or cerebrospinal fluid studies that are helpful in either confirming or ruling out progressive supranuclear palsy.

STRUCTURAL IMAGING STUDIES

Atrophy of the midbrain in patients with progressive supranuclear palsy has been frequently observed on MRI. One study found that whereas the average midbrain diameter of healthy individuals was $117 \, mm^2$, the average midbrain diameter was significantly smaller in progressive supranuclear palsy ($56 \, mm^2$). Patients with Parkinson's disease and the Parkinsonian syndrome multiple system atrophy also showed smaller midbrains than healthy individuals on average (103 and $97 \, mm^2$, respectively), although their size was still much larger than those with progressive supranuclear palsy (Oba et al., 2005). When viewed from a midline sagittal perspective, the shrunken midbrain with a relatively normal pons leads to what has been called the "hummingbird" sign. Warmuth-Metz et al. (2001) found that patients with PSP had midbrain anterior–posterior diameters ranging from 11 to 15 mm (average 13.4 mm), much smaller than both controls (range 17–20 mm, average 18.2 mm) and patients with Parkinson's disease (range 17–19 mm, average 18.5 mm). Although midbrain measurement does not have 100% sensitivity or specificity, it should always be obtained as supportive data if the diagnosis of progressive supranuclear palsy is suspected. In our experience, anterior–posterior midbrain measurement can be performed by the radiologist if requested, and it is also fairly easily measured either on the film itself or using the viewing software when viewing the images from a CD. The midbrain is usually present on two MRI slices, and we measure both (Fig. 8.3).

FUNCTIONAL IMAGING STUDIES

The usefulness of functional imaging studies such as SPECT or FDG-PET is mainly to evaluate the patient in whom you suspect progressive supranuclear palsy for other neurodegenerative diseases such as Alzheimer's and frontotemporal dementia. Although they are not routinely used to make the diagnosis of progressive supranuclear palsy, one study using standard SPECT (^{99m}Tc-HMPAO) found that abnormalities of anterior cingulate distinguished this disorder from both healthy individuals and those with Parkinson's disease (Varrone et al., 2007).

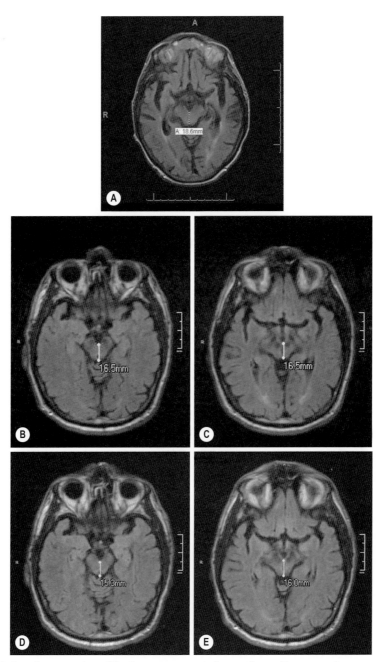

FIGURE 8.3 Anterior–posterior midbrain measurements in a patient with progressive supranuclear palsy compared with a patient with Alzheimer's disease.

(A) An 81-year-old patient with Alzheimer's disease, with notable temporal lobe atrophy but normal midbrain measurement. (B–C) A patient with progressive supranuclear palsy when he first presented to an outside neurologist at age 69. (D–E) The same patient imaged on the same MRI scanner 1 year later at age 70, showing remarkable midbrain shrinkage within 1 year.

DIFFERENTIAL DIAGNOSIS

The differential diagnosis of progressive supranuclear palsy, from the standpoint of a patient presenting with a cognitive impairment, involves considering other etiologies that can cause some combination of cognitive impairment (especially executive dysfunction), behavioral changes, eye movement abnormalities, slurred speech (dysarthria), difficulty swallowing (dysphagia), rigidity, dystonia, or Parkinsonism (Table 8.1). Such disorders include the following:

- dementia with Lewy bodies
- vascular dementia
- frontotemporal dementia including
  - frontotemporal dementia with Parkinsonism linked to chromosome 17
  - frontotemporal dementia with amyotrophic lateral sclerosis
- prion disease including Creutzfeldt–Jakob disease
- hydrocephalus including normal pressure hydrocephalus
- Huntington's disease
- multiple sclerosis
- medication side-effects including those of neuroleptics and anti-emetics.

Table 8.1 Comparison between progressive supranuclear palsy and other conditions with cognitive and sensory/motoric symptoms

	Progressive supranuclear palsy	Corticobasal degeneration	Dementia with Lewy bodies
Cognitive deficits	Early cognitive and affective symptoms may include slowing of all aspects of mental processing and executive dysfunction. Cognitive symptoms are rarely the first symptoms	Cognitive testing demonstrates frontal and parietal cognitive dysfunction with relative preservation of memory. Speech may be disrupted owing to apraxia or non-fluent aphasia	More prominent deficits in visuospatial, attentional, and executive function with memory deficits as a less prominent complaint
Functional deficits	Present	Present	Present
Dementia	Eventually	Eventually	Present
Behavioral symptoms	Irritability, irascibility, apathy, introversion, and depression	Insight and accompanying depression	Visual hallucinations often present early in the disease
Motor and sensory symptoms	Backward falls, postural instability, and disrupted voluntary vertical (downward) gaze are present early in the disease	Focal and asymmetric signs and symptoms are the cardinal features of corticobasal degeneration, including asymmetric apraxia, cortical sensory loss, and unilateral visual or sensory neglect	Parkinsonian symptoms often present early in the disease

TREATMENTS

There are no FDA approved treatments for progressive supranuclear palsy. Symptomatic treatments that are worth trying include levodopa/carbidopa (Sinemet), memantine, and amantadine. Botulinum toxin may be used to treat spasms and dystonia. Atropine 1% eye drops can be administered sublingually to help reduce drooling.

References

Maher, E.R., Smith, E.M., Lees, A.J., 1985. Cognitive deficits in the Steele-Richardson-Olszewski syndrome (progressive supranuclear palsy). J. Neurol. Neurosurg. Psychiatry 48, 1234–1239.

Oba, H., Yagishita, A., Terada, H., et al., 2005. New and reliable MRI diagnosis for progressive supranuclear palsy. Neurology 64, 2050–2055.

Varrone, A., Pagani, M., Salvatore, E., et al., 2007. Identification by [99mTc]ECD SPECT of anterior cingulate hypoperfusion in progressive supranuclear palsy, in comparison with Parkinson's disease. Eur. J. Nucl. Med. Mol. Imaging 34, 1071–1081.

Warmuth-Metz, M., Naumann, M., Csoti, I., et al., 2001. Measurement of the midbrain diameter on routine magnetic resonance imaging: a simple and accurate method of differentiating between Parkinson disease and progressive supranuclear palsy. Arch. Neurol. 58, 1076–1079.

Corticobasal degeneration

QUICK START: CORTICOBASAL DEGENERATION

Definition
- Corticobasal degeneration is a neurodegenerative disease of the brain caused by the accumulation of hyperphosphorylated tau isoforms and characterized by asymmetric cortical dysfunction.
- Clinically there are difficulties with motor control of a limb (apraxia), cognitive dysfunction, rigidity, a jerky postural tremor, myoclonus, dystonia, and a gait disorder.

Prevalence
- It is a relatively rare disorder, with the prevalence being about two per 100,000.
- The age of onset ranges from 53 to 73 (mean 61) years, with a prognosis of about 2–8 years.

Genetic risk
- There are no known genetic or other risk factors.

Cognitive and behavioral symptoms
- Focal and asymmetric signs and symptoms are the cardinal features of corticobasal degeneration, including asymmetric apraxia, cortical sensory loss, and unilateral visual or sensory neglect.
- An "alien limb"—a limb with "a mind of its own"—is a pathognomonic but uncommon sign.
- Speech may be disrupted owing to apraxia or non-fluent aphasia.
- Cognitive testing demonstrates frontal and parietal cognitive dysfunction with relative preservation of memory.

Diagnostic criteria
- Core features:
  - Insidious onset
  - Progressively degenerative course
  - Cortical dysfunction including one or more of the following:
    - Asymmetric apraxia
    - Asymmetric myoclonus
    - Alien limb phenomenon
    - Cortical sensory loss
    - Visual or sensory neglect
    - Speech disorder owing to apraxia or non-fluent aphasia
  - Extrapyramidal dysfunction including one or more of the following:
    - Asymmetric limb (appendicular) rigidity relatively unresponsive to levodopa (Sinemet)
    - Asymmetric limb (appendicular) dystonia.
- Supportive investigations:
  - Testing demonstrating focal cognitive dysfunction with relative preservation of memory

Continued

QUICK START: CORTICOBASAL DEGENERATION—Cont'd

	• Structural brain imaging studies (CT or MRI) showing focal or asymmetric atrophy, maximal in parietal and frontal cortex
	• Functional imaging studies (SPECT or PET) showing focal or asymmetric hypofunction, maximal in parietal and frontal cortex, although basal ganglia and/or thalamus may also be involved.
Treatment	• There are no US Food and Drug Administration-approved medications to treat corticobasal degeneration; treatment is supportive.
	• Antidepressants should be used to treat depression, which is often present.
	• Dystonia may be relieved with botulinum toxin.
	• Clonazepam may be helpful for myoclonus.
Top differential diagnoses	• Frontotemporal dementia, primary progressive aphasia, progressive supranuclear palsy, dementia with Lewy bodies, Alzheimer's disease, vascular dementia.

PREVALENCE, PROGNOSIS, AND DEFINITION

Corticobasal degeneration is a neurodegenerative disease of the brain characterized by asymmetric cortical dysfunction, often affecting motor control of a limb, along with cognitive dysfunction, rigidity, a jerky postural tremor, myoclonus, dystonia, and a gait disorder. Speech may be disrupted owing to apraxia or non-fluent aphasia. Like progressive supranuclear palsy, it is caused by the accumulation of hyperphosphorylated tau isoforms. It is a relatively rare disorder with a prevalence of about two per 100,000. From one autopsy series, the mean age of onset was 61 years, ranging from 53 to 73 years, with an average prognosis from diagnosis to death of about 5.5 years, ranging from 2 to 8 years (Murray et al., 2007).

CRITERIA

Focal and asymmetric signs and symptoms are the cardinal features of corticobasal degeneration. Published clinical criteria can by found in Box 9.1. See Boxes 9.2–9.5 for additional explanations.

BOX 9.1 DIAGNOSTIC CRITERIA FOR CORTICOBASAL DEGENERATION

Core features

- Insidious onset
- Progressively degenerative course
- Cortical dysfunction including one or more of the following:
  - Asymmetric apraxia
  - Alien limb phenomenon
  - Cortical sensory loss
  - Visual or sensory neglect
  - Asymmetric myoclonus
  - Speech disorder owing to apraxia or non-fluent aphasia

Continued

BOX 9.1 DIAGNOSTIC CRITERIA FOR CORTICOBASAL DEGENERATION—Cont'd

- Extrapyramidal dysfunction including one or more of the following:
  - Asymmetric limb (appendicular) rigidity relatively unresponsive to levodopa (Sinemet)
  - Asymmetric limb (appendicular) dystonia

Supportive investigations

- Cognitive testing demonstrating focal cognitive dysfunction with relative preservation of memory
- Structural brain imaging studies (CT or MRI) showing focal or asymmetric atrophy, maximal in parietal and frontal cortex
- Functional imaging studies (SPECT or PET) showing focal or asymmetric hypofunction, maximal in parietal and frontal cortex, although basal ganglia and/or thalamus may also be involved

Adapted from Lees, A.J., 2007. Progressive supranuclear palsy and corticobasal degeneration. In: Growdon, J.H., Rossor, M.N. (Eds.), The Dementias 2. Butterworth Heinemann, Philadelphia, PA, pp. 141–164.

BOX 9.2 "ALIEN LIMB"?

The alien limb phenomenon is not common, but it is a striking, pathognomonic symptom when it occurs. The affected limb is often described as "having a mind of its own," and patients report having little or no control over it. It may rise up in the air, or take hold of objects, clothes, and people. Occasionally it may interfere with the function of the unaffected limb.

BOX 9.3 APRAXIA

A patient is said to have an apraxia when he or she is unable to perform a purposeful, coordinated movement despite normal strength and sensation. The patient's actions often appear clumsy and uncoordinated. Apraxias come in a variety of types. Some of the more common are as follows.

- *Limb-kinetic apraxia* refers to the loss of the ability to make precise independent finger movements, such as the pincer grasp that is needed to pick up a small coin off a flat surface.
- Patients with *ideomotor apraxia* make errors in spatial movement, orientation, and/or timing of previously learned skilled movements. For example, when pantomiming cutting paper with scissors, he or she may not keep the scissors correctly oriented to the paper.
- In *conduction apraxia*, patients show more difficulty imitating a skilled movement (such as a salute) than performing the movement to command.
- *Dissociation apraxia* refers to the inability to pantomime to command, despite the ability to imitate and use objects perfectly.
- Although the term *ideational apraxia* has been used to describe a variety of apraxias, its current meaning is an inability to correctly sequence a series of acts that lead to a goal (such as making a sandwich).
- Patients with *conceptual apraxia* show errors in trying to use or pantomime using tools correctly, such that they may show hammering when asked to demonstrate the use of a screwdriver. Many of these patients also show deficits in semantic memory, having lost the meaning of these items.

BOX 9.4 CORTICAL SENSORY LOSS

Patients with cortical sensory loss show normal primary sensory abilities, but demonstrate deficits in their ability to use this information to make appropriate judgments. These patients therefore are able to feel a light touch: they can distinguish sharp from dull, warm from cold, etc., but they are unable to identify a coin by feeling it (stereognosis) or a number when it is drawn in their hand (graphesthesia).

BOX 9.5 NEGLECT

Patients with neglect tend to ignore the region of space on the opposite side (contralateral) of a brain lesion. Neglect is often tested by presenting stimuli on both sides of the body simultaneously and ascertaining whether patients ignore stimuli on one side of the body. It is important, however, to exclude a problem with the sensory modality itself, by testing each side of the body separately. Note that it is sometimes difficult to tell whether the problem is attributable to profound neglect mimicking a primary sensory deficit or to mild sensory loss mimicking neglect. Neglect is usually associated with a right-hemisphere lesion; left neglect is therefore much more common than right neglect. Neglect is most often associated with anatomical lesions such as strokes and tumors. It is one of the characteristics of corticobasal degeneration that the neglect experienced by the patient may be so complete as to mimic that of a large stroke or tumor.

RISK FACTORS, PATHOLOGY, AND PATHOPHYSIOLOGY

There are no known risk factors for developing corticobasal degeneration. A characteristic of this disorder is that the distribution of pathology and atrophy is asymmetric. Cortical regions affected are around the main sulci of the brain: parasagittal, peri-Rolandic, and peri-Sylvian. Subcortical structures affected include substantia nigra, and variably the globus pallidus, subthalamic nucleus, and thalamus. Under the microscope, the pathology consists of swollen achromatic neurons in amygdala and limbic structures, as well as ballooned neocortical achromatic neurons in specific layers (III, V, and VI) in frontal and parietal lobes (Fig. 9.1). Hippocampal and temporal lobe regions are least affected. As in progressive supranuclear palsy, corticobasal degeneration is associated with the accumulation of hyperphosphorylated tau protein isoforms in the brain.

COMMON SIGNS, SYMPTOMS, AND STAGES

Corticobasal degeneration classically starts with an impaired limb, which may present as an "alien limb" (Box 9.2), but more often it presents as a stiff, clumsy, and useless hand. Retrospective autopsy studies show, however, that more patients actually present with cognitive, speech, behavioral, or gait abnormalities than those who present with limb abnormalities. Limb abnormalities are likely relatively specific for corticobasal degeneration but are not sensitive enough to allow one to rely upon this sign to detect the disorder. Common presenting and early symptoms may include the following:

- useless limb
- focal apraxias
- sensory symptoms including numbness and tingling
- rigidity
- a jerky postural tremor
- myoclonus
- dystonia
- speech disturbance
- executive dysfunction
- behavioral disorder.

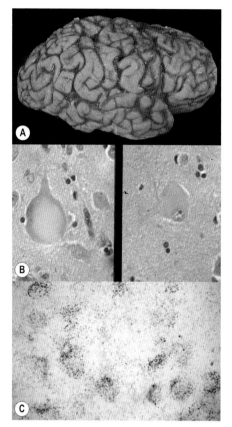

FIGURE 9.1 Pathology of corticobasal degeneration.

(A) Atrophy of the frontal lobe. (B) Swollen and ballooned achromatic neurons. (C) Astrocytic plaques. A color version of this figure is avaliable online at http://www.expertconsult.com.

Over time the affected limbs become more rigid, with rapid movements such as pronation/supination and alternating finger tapping becoming impaired. Eventually even passive stretch may not be possible. Dystonia may become prominent, with the hand often becoming a clenched fist or having hyperextension of one or more fingers. Myoclonus is often seen in the fingers, which may increase with sensory stimulation and finger movements. Although all four limbs are commonly involved in the later stages, asymmetry is usually maintained.

THINGS TO LOOK FOR IN THE HISTORY

The characteristic feature that should be sought in the history is that of asymmetric limb dysfunction. The limb dysfunction may consist of rigidity, apraxia, dystonia, myoclonus, alien limb phenomena, or some combination thereof. By history the apraxia will often present as a loss of a previously acquired function, such as being unable to fold laundry or use a screwdriver (Box 9.3). Other features to look for in the history include postural instability and a speech disturbance. The speech disturbance is usually of the non-fluent variety, and often includes word-finding difficulties and decreased fluency of speech, resembling (or causing) primary progressive aphasia. Some families have reported that patients often confuse yes/no responses, nodding their head when they mean "no," and shaking their head when they mean "yes." The most common neuropsychiatric symptoms in corticobasal degeneration are depression, fatigue, and irritability—symptoms all too common in many kinds of dementia. Memory complaints are common, but when recognition memory is tested in the clinic it is found to be relatively preserved. Thus, *complaints* of memory are very consistent with corticobasal degeneration, whereas *impairment* of recognition memory on testing is unusual in this disorder.

THINGS TO LOOK FOR ON THE PHYSICAL AND NEUROLOGICAL EXAMINATION

The examination of the limbs, and in particular the hands, is critical when suspecting corticobasal degeneration. Asymmetry of findings in the limbs should be expected. In addition to looking for signs of alien limb, the arms and hands should be examined for signs of rigidity, dystonia, myoclonus, and jerky action tremor. (Note that a pill-rolling rest tremor has never been described in corticobasal degeneration; such a tremor would strongly suggest Parkinson's disease or dementia with Lewy bodies.) Eye movement abnormalities, including supranuclear gaze palsies, may be found in up to one-third of patients (Murray et al., 2007), making it somewhat difficult to differentiate corticobasal degeneration from progressive supranuclear palsy. Cortical sensory loss is often present, making it difficult for patients to identify a coin by feeling it (stereognosis) or a number when it is drawn in their hand (graphesthesia), despite normal primary sensory function (Box 9.4). Naming and other aspects of language should be tested, looking for a pattern of non-fluent aphasia. Comprehension difficulties, when present, are most likely to be due to difficulty understanding grammatically complex sentences. When suspecting corticobasal degeneration, praxis should be carefully tested (Box 9.3). Ideomotor apraxia is most common, such that patients are often unable to correctly pantomime using tools such as scissors, hammer, or screwdriver.

PATTERN OF IMPAIRMENT ON COGNITIVE TESTS

The dementia of corticobasal degeneration differs from that of Alzheimer's disease. In Alzheimer's disease medial temporal lobe dysfunction is most prominent, leading to memory difficulties, whereas in corticobasal degeneration frontal and parietal dysfunction are common, thus leading to difficulties with executive function, visuospatial function, language, and praxis. Difficulties with calculations are common; caregivers report that patients are impaired at handling money. Neglect may also occur (Box 9.5). Episodic memory is relatively preserved. Neuropsychological tests that show prominent impairment include reverse digit span, word fluency to letters and animals, Stroop test, Pyramid and Palm Trees test, and visuospatial constructions. One aspect of corticobasal degeneration that may help to distinguish it from frontotemporal dementia is that insight is often preserved in corticobasal degeneration, perhaps leading to the frequently observed depression in this disorder.

LABORATORY STUDIES

There are no laboratory, genetic, or cerebrospinal fluid studies that are helpful in either confirming or ruling out corticobasal degeneration.

STRUCTURAL IMAGING STUDIES

There is no pathognomonic pattern of atrophy which can by itself distinguish corticobasal degeneration from other types of dementia. Structural imaging of corticobasal degeneration does, however, typically show much asymmetric posterior frontal and parietal atrophy. One study found, in fact, that atrophy in corticobasal degeneration was greater than that observed in Alzheimer's disease, dementia with Lewy bodies, frontotemporal dementia, and progressive supranuclear palsy (Whitwell et al., 2007). In one likely case we have seen, the atrophy was so asymmetric and severe that a casual glance at the CT scan suggested multiple strokes; upon closer inspection, however, these "holes" in the brain were caused by severe focal areas of atrophy.

FUNCTIONAL IMAGING STUDIES

The usefulness of functional imaging studies such as SPECT or FDG-PET is mainly to differentiate corticobasal degeneration from other neurodegenerative diseases such as Alzheimer's and frontotemporal dementia. Typically, the patient with corticobasal degeneration will show marked asymmetry of frontal and parietal blood flow and metabolism on SPECT and FDG-PET imaging. The usefulness of nuclear medicine imaging in corticobasal degeneration using dopamine transporter ligands is currently being researched.

DIFFERENTIAL DIAGNOSIS

It is worth stating that it is difficult to correctly diagnosis this disorder. Autopsy studies have shown that on average only half of those patients premorbidly diagnosed with corticobasal degeneration meet pathological criteria for the disorder, and, conversely, only half of those patients with pathologically confirmed corticobasal degeneration were correctly diagnosed premorbidly. In a study published in 2007 only six of 15 pathologically proven cases were suspected of having corticobasal degeneration (Murray et al., 2007). The most common misdiagnoses were frontotemporal dementia, primary progressive aphasia, and progressive supranuclear palsy. Alzheimer's disease is much less likely to be mistaken for corticobasal degeneration. A more complete differential diagnosis is shown in Box 9.6. (see also Table 8.1).

TREATMENTS

There are no FDA approved treatments for corticobasal degeneration. Antidepressants should be used to treat depression, which is often present. Dystonia may be relieved with botulinum toxin. Clonazepam may be helpful for myoclonus.

BOX 9.6 DIFFERENTIAL DIAGNOSIS OF CORTICOBASAL DEGENERATION

Primary differential diagnosis

- Frontotemporal dementia
- Primary progressive aphasia
- Progressive supranuclear palsy
- Dementia with Lewy bodies

Other conditions to consider

- Alzheimer's disease
- Vascular dementia
- Prion disease
- Spinocerebellar atrophy 8
- Progressive multifocal leukodystrophy
- Sudanophilic leukodystrophy (Pelizaeus–Merzbacher disease)
- Neurosyphilis
- Familial idiopathic basal ganglia calcification
- Marchiafava–Bignami disease

References

Murray, R., Neumann, M., Forman, M.S., et al., 2007. Cognitive and motor assessment in autopsy-proven corticobasal degeneration. Neurology 68, 1274–1283.

Whitwell, J.L., Jack, C.R., Jr., Parisi, J.E., et al., 2007. Rates of cerebral atrophy differ in different degenerative pathologies. Brain 130, 1148–1158.

10 Normal pressure hydrocephalus

QUICK START: NORMAL PRESSURE HYDROCEPHALUS

Definition	• Normal pressure hydrocephalus (often referred to as NPH) is a relatively rare disorder characterized by enlargement of the ventricles, a gait disorder, incontinence, and cognitive impairment.
	• It is thought to result from low-grade scarring or obstruction of the ventricular system or subarachnoid pathways.
Prevalence	• It is a relatively rare disorder, making up between 1% and 5% of patients referred to a memory clinic.
Genetic risk	• There are no known genetic or other risk factors.
Cognitive and behavioral symptoms	• The most common cognitive and behavioral presentation is that of a frontal subcortical disturbance including apathy, abulia, poor attention, and slowing of processing.
Diagnostic criteria	• Normal pressure hydrocephalus should be suspected when the triad of symptoms of cognitive impairment, gait disorder, and urinary incontinence are present in the setting of enlarged ventricles.
	• The frontal gait disturbance in normal pressure hydrocephalus, sometimes called a "magnetic gait" or a "*marche à petits pas*" (walk of little steps), is typically the most prominent symptom and is usually the earliest in onset.
	• Urinary incontinence generally occurs late in normal pressure hydrocephalus, and is associated with urinary urgency.
	• A CT or MRI scan showing enlargement of the ventricles and rounding of the ventricular contours, with or without periventricular abnormalities due to trans-ependymal flow of cerebrospinal fluid, is essential to making the diagnosis.
	• A lumbar puncture to withdraw 30–50 ml of CSF with pre- and post-lumbar puncture gait evaluations can help to determine both diagnosis and possible response to treatment.
	• Referral to a neurosurgeon for an evaluation including a lumbar drain or continuous ventricular pressure monitoring may be helpful.
Treatment	• A ventricular–peritoneal shunt provides the definitive treatment.
Top differential diagnoses	• Because many disorders can cause cognitive impairment, a gait disorder, and urinary incontinence, and virtually all dementias lead to dilatation of the ventricles, the differential diagnosis must be carefully considered.

PREVALENCE, PROGNOSIS, AND DEFINITION

Normal pressure hydrocephalus is a relatively rare disorder characterized by enlargement of the ventricles, a gait disorder, incontinence, and cognitive impairment. Although some studies have suggested that up to 5% of patients with dementia have normal pressure hydrocephalus, other studies have found the prevalence to be closer to 1%, which is consistent with our experience of patients referred to a memory disorders clinic (for a review see Tanaka et al., 2009).

CRITERIA

Normal pressure hydrocephalus should be suspected when the so-called "triad" of symptoms (cognitive impairment, gait disorder, and urinary incontinence) is present in the setting of enlarged ventricles. However, it cannot be stated strongly enough that many disorders can cause cognitive impairment, a gait disorder, and urinary incontinence, and virtually all neurodegenerative diseases lead to ex-vacuo dilatation of ventricles (enlarged ventricles due to loss of brain tissue), so the differential diagnosis of these symptoms and signs must be carefully considered. Some frequently used criteria for diagnosing normal pressure hydrocephalus are shown in Box 10.1.

RISK FACTORS, PATHOLOGY, AND PATHOPHYSIOLOGY

Normal pressure hydrocephalus is thought to result from low-grade scarring or obstruction of the ventricular system or subarachnoid pathways. Thus, although most cases are idiopathic, other causes include subarachnoid hemorrhage, head trauma, tumor, prior surgery, aqueductal stenosis, meningitis, and even lumbar puncture. The basic idea is that one of these etiologies causes enough scarring and/or obstruction to increase pressure and to damage the myelinated fibers surrounding the ventricles, but an equilibrium is reached such that the pressure is not raised enough to present as high-pressure hydrocephalus (Fig. 10.1).

COMMON SIGNS, SYMPTOMS, AND STAGES

The gait disturbance in normal pressure hydrocephalus is typically the most prominent symptom and is usually the earliest in onset. The gait disorder is of a frontal type, and has been described as a "magnetic gait" or a *"marche à petits pas"* (walk of little steps), and is somewhat different from shuffling. It is very unsteady. There are a number of different problems that can occur with a frontal gait, including a gait apraxia, spasticity, and unsteadiness. Patients may describe a loss of strength in their legs that may not be due to weakness of any individual muscles. Some patients may complain of difficulty lifting their feet off the ground, feeling like their feet are stuck to the floor.

Cognitive impairment generally presents next. A number of cognitive disturbances can occur, but the most common presentation is that of a frontal subcortical disturbance. Normal pressure hydrocephalus puts pressure on and ultimately damages periventricular white matter tracts. Because most of the brain's white matter is involved in transferring information to or from the frontal lobes, patients with normal pressure hydrocephalus often

BOX 10.1 CRITERIA FOR PROBABLE NORMAL PRESSURE HYDROCEPHALUS

I. History must include:
   a. Insidious onset
   b. Age 40 years or older
   c. Duration of symptoms greater than 3 months
   d. No evidence of an antecedent event known to cause hydrocephalus
   e. Progression of symptoms over time
   f. No other neurological, psychiatric, or medical condition that can explain the presenting signs and symptoms.

II. Brain imaging:
   a. (CT or MRI) must show
      i. Ventricular enlargement not solely due to atrophy or congenital enlargement
      ii. No visible obstruction of cerebrospinal fluid flow
      iii. Callosal angle of 40 degrees or greater (rounding of the ventricular contours)
      iv. Evidence of periventricular trans-ependymal flow of cerebrospinal fluid
      v. Aqueductal or fourth ventricular flow void on MRI.
   b. Supportive brain imaging (CT or MRI) findings include
      i. Prior brain imaging study showing smaller ventricular size
      ii. Radionuclide cisternogram showing delayed clearance of radiotracer
      iii. Cine MRI showing increased ventricular flow
      iv. SPECT-acetazolamide challenge showing decreased perfusion not altered by acetazolamide.

III. Clinical findings of gait/balance disturbance plus either cognitive impairment or urinary symptoms or both:
   a. Gait disturbance that includes at least two of the following (not entirely attributable to other conditions)
      i. Decreased step height
      ii. Decreased step length
      iii. Decreased cadence (speed of walking)
      iv. Increased trunk sway during walking
      v. Widened standing base
      vi. Toes turned outward on walking
      vii. Spontaneous or provoked retropulsion
      viii. En bloc turning (needing 3+ steps for turning 180 degrees)
      ix. Impaired walking balance, tested by 2+ corrections needed for tandem gait of eight steps.
   b. Cognitive impairment that includes at least two of the following (not entirely attributable to other conditions)
      i. Psychomotor slowing (increased latency of response)
      ii. Decreased fine motor speed
      iii. Decreased fine motor accuracy
      iv. Difficulty dividing or maintaining attention
      v. Impaired memory recall, especially for recent events
      vi. Executive dysfunction, including impairment in multistep procedures, working memory, abstractions, similarities, and insight
      vii. Behavioral or personality changes.
   c. Urinary incontinence not entirely attributable to other conditions consisting of either
      i. Episodic urinary incontinence
      ii. Persistent urinary incontinence
      iii. Urinary and fecal incontinence
      Or any two of the following
      iv. Frequent perception of the need to void
      v. Urinary frequency
      vi. Nocturia greater than two times per night.

IV. Physiological
   a. CSF opening pressure of 70–245 mmH$_2$0 (5–18 mm Hg)

Adapted from Relkin, N., Marmarou, A., Klinge, P., et al., 2005. Diagnosing idiopathic normal-pressure hydrocephalus. Neurosurgery 57, S4–S16.

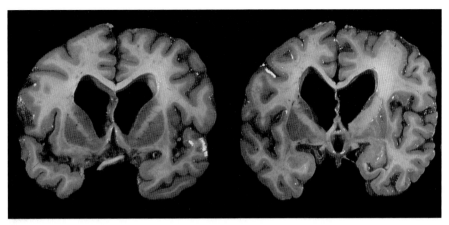

FIGURE 10.1 Gross pathology of a patient with normal pressure hydrocephalus.

Note the large ventricles but little hippocampal or cortical atrophy (Compare with Figure 3.9; see how it looks like the normal brain except for the enlarged ventricles). A color version of this figure is avaliable online at http://www.expertconsult.com.

show signs and symptoms of frontal subcortical dysfunction. Attention is often severely affected. Most cognitive processes are slow, and some, such as memory, require additional trials in order to reach normal performance. Changes in behavior, including a slowing of thought and action that may progress to apathy and abulia, are often observed.

Incontinence generally occurs late in normal pressure hydrocephalus. Urge incontinence is usually seen, such that the patient only has a very short time between when he or she feels the need to empty their bladder and when it empties. Fecal incontinence is rarely seen.

THINGS TO LOOK FOR IN THE HISTORY

The history will typically be that of a progressive gait disorder of the type described above, followed by changes in behavior and cognition including apathy, abulia, slowness, and poor attention. Patients are generally very easily distracted and may have difficulty focusing on tasks. Memory problems will typically be secondary to poor attention. Urinary incontinence typically occurs later as the third major symptom.

THINGS TO LOOK FOR ON THE PHYSICAL AND NEUROLOGICAL EXAMINATION

Observation of the gait is the most important aspect of the neurological examination. As discussed above it will usually present as a frontal, unsteady, apraxic, and/or spastic gait. The deep tendon reflexes are generally increased, and an extensor plantar (Babinski's sign) may be present in one or both feet. Frontal release signs may also be present such as the snout, grasp, and palmomental reflexes (see Chapter 2: *Evaluating the patient with memory loss* for details). Hand tremors, poor fine finger movements, and poor handwriting may also be seen. In order to distinguish normal pressure hydrocephalus from other disorders, efforts should also be made to look for signs of other disorders, such as Parkinson's disease and progressive supranuclear palsy.

PATTERN OF IMPAIRMENT ON COGNITIVE TESTS

The frontal subcortical white matter damage in normal pressure hydrocephalus causes impairment on a variety of cognitive tests. In general the pattern is similar to that described above for vascular dementia. Attention is invariably impaired. Working memory tasks, such as keeping information in mind and/or manipulating it, are also commonly impaired. Cognition tends to be generally slow. Word-finding difficulties are prominent, but true aphasia is not. Episodic memory performance shows a frontal pattern: encoding is often impaired, as is free recall, whereas recognition is relatively preserved. Visuospatial tasks may or may not be impaired.

LABORATORY STUDIES

There are no laboratory studies to either support or rule out the diagnosis of normal pressure hydrocephalus.

STRUCTURAL IMAGING STUDIES

A structural imaging study supportive of a diagnosis of normal pressure hydrocephalus is essential in making the diagnosis (Fig. 10.2). The imaging study, either a CT or MRI, will invariably show enlargement of the ventricles, rounding of the ventricular contours, the presence of periventricular abnormalities—particularly around the frontal horns, and relatively normal-sized subarachnoid spaces. The periventricular abnormalities are due to trans-ependymal flow of cerebrospinal fluid, that is, cerebrospinal fluid that has pushed its way into the white matter. The importance of relatively normal-sized subarachnoid spaces is to differentiate ex-vacuo dilatation of the ventricular system due to atrophy from true ventricular enlargement. In comparison with Alzheimer's disease, the ventricular enlargement in normal pressure hydrocephalus will be out of proportion to the amount of cortical atrophy. One way to think about this issue is that the brain will do what is

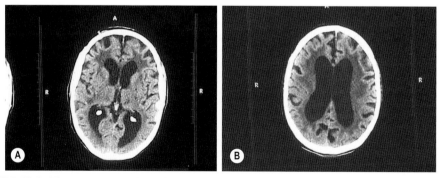

FIGURE 10.2 CT scan from a patient with normal pressure hydrocephalus.

In this example there is some cortical atrophy, but note the overly large, "ballooned-out" expansion of the ventricular system in both slices. Note also the trans-ependymal cerebrospinal fluid that appears hypo-dense anterior to the frontal horns of the lateral ventricles (A) and surrounding the ventricles (B). This patient improved dramatically after a diagnostic lumbar puncture, and subsequently received a ventricular–peritoneal shunt.

necessary to keep a constant volume. In Alzheimer's disease, because of the loss of cells in the cortex there is atrophy in the cortex. The ventricular enlargement fills the space, thus the term *ex-vacuo* dilatation. In normal pressure hydrocephalus there is no initial loss of neural tissue (except for minimal shrinkage due to aging), thus the increased ventricular size is out of proportion to the cortical loss.

LUMBAR PUNCTURE

After a structural imaging study, the most important test is a lumbar puncture. Measuring the opening pressure is important, as some patients with suspected normal pressure hydrocephalus will actually have high-pressure hydrocephalus.

The next step is to withdraw a large volume of cerebrospinal fluid, between 30 and 50 ml, to see if the gait improves after the fluid is withdrawn. Gait should be measured between two points on the floor (around 30 feet apart), and a number of trials (around 3–10) should be undertaken, until a reliable measurement is obtained. If possible, a videotape of the gait pre- and post-lumbar puncture provides both a record of the timing and also a valuable way to evaluate other aspects of gait, such as stride length, apraxia, and the like. If the gait improves after a single large-volume lumbar puncture, the diagnosis is confirmed, and, more importantly, the patient will likely respond to treatment by shunting (see Treatments below). If there is no definite response from a single large-volume lumbar puncture, serial large-volume lumbar punctures can be performed daily for several days. Improvement of gait after 3 days of lumbar puncture also predicts a good response to shunting.

OTHER STUDIES

If the lumbar puncture tests are non-diagnostic, a number of other tests can be used to work towards confirming the diagnosis and predicting response to treatment. MRI has been used to measure the flow of cerebrospinal fluid through the Sylvian aqueduct; increased flow has been reported in those who ultimately had a good response to shunting. Continuous pressure monitoring for 24–48 hours can be performed using a frontal ventricular catheter, lumbar catheter, or epidural transducer; elevated baseline cerebrospinal fluid pressure or pressure waves also suggest a good response to shunting. Improvement in gait with a lumbar drain also predicts a good response to shunting. Cisternography (in which an intrathecal injection of either a radioactive isotope or contrast material is performed and the flow pattern of cerebrospinal fluid is observed) is less frequently performed.

DIFFERENTIAL DIAGNOSIS

The differential diagnosis of normal pressure hydrocephalus is quite broad. Any disorder that damages the periventricular frontal subcortical white matter tracts can lead to the clinical triad of gait disorder, cognitive impairment, and urinary incontinence. Vascular dementia and multiple sclerosis should always be considered, as these disorders frequently damage these periventricular frontal subcortical white matter tracts. Lyme disease can also damage this region of the brain. Other disorders that should be considered include disorders that affect gait and cognition, such as Parkinson's disease, dementia with Lewy bodies, progressive supranuclear palsy, and corticobasal degeneration. Disorders of cognition such as frontotemporal dementia (with or without motor neuron disease/amyotrophic lateral sclerosis) and Huntington's disease should also be considered. Alzheimer's disease must be considered; because it is so common unusual presentations may occur. Any cause of pre-existing enlarged ventricles (e.g., from congenital hydrocephalus, cerebral palsy, traumatic brain injury) plus a degenerative disease, such as Alzheimer's, can mimic normal pressure hydrocephalus. To complicate matters, sometimes patients can have both normal pressure hydrocephalus and Alzheimer's disease; in such cases both disorders must be treated. Lastly, other causes of hydrocephalus, such as carcinomatous meningitis, should be considered.

TREATMENTS

The treatment for normal pressure hydrocephalus is a shunt to help remove excess cerebrospinal fluid from the ventricular system. The most common type shunts fluid from the lateral ventricle (usually on the right to avoid language centers on the left) to the peritoneum. The typical approach is either right frontal or right parieto-occipital. Whereas high-pressure hydrocephalus almost always improves with treatment, studies suggest that between 46% and 63% of patients with normal pressure hydrocephalus improve (Relkin et al., 2005). Complications of treatment also occur; in one study with an improvement rate of 61% there was a complication rate of 35% (Black, 1980). In another study there was improvement in 79% of patients and complications in 32% (Eide & Sorteberg, 2010). The most common complications were subdural collections, shunt malfunction, headaches, and postoperative seizures.

References

Black, P.M., 1980. Idiopathic normal-pressure hydrocephalus. Results of shunting in 62 patients. J. Neurosurg. 52, 371–377.

Eide, P.K., Sorteberg, W., 2010. Diagnostic intracranial pressure monitoring and surgical management in idiopathic normal pressure hydrocephalus: a 6-year review of 214 patients. Neurosurgery 66, 80–91.

Relkin, N., Marmarou, A., Klinge, P., et al., 2005. Diagnosing idiopathic normal-pressure hydrocephalus. Neurosurgery 57, S4–S16.

Tanaka, N., Yamaguchi, S., Ishikawa, H., et al., 2009. Prevalence of possible idiopathic normal-pressure hydrocephalus in Japan: the Osaki-Tajiri project. Neuroepidemiology 32, 171–175.

Creutzfeldt–Jakob disease

QUICK START: CREUTZFELDT–JAKOB DISEASE

Definition
- Creutzfeldt–Jakob disease (CJD) is one of several prion transmissible neurodegenerative diseases characterized by a rapid cognitive decline which can progress to akinetic mutism over weeks.
- Creutzfeldt–Jakob disease is the most common type of prion disease; prion diseases are also called transmissible spongiform encephalopathies.
- Prion diseases have a specific neuropathology characterized by spongiform changes, neuronal death, astrocytosis, and accumulation of a pathological protein (PrP^{Sc}) in the brain and sometimes other organs.
- Other forms of Creutzfeldt–Jakob disease include familial (fCJD), iatrogenic (iCJD), and variant (vCJD) forms.
- Variant Creutzfeldt–Jakob disease is similar biochemically and histopathologically to bovine spongiform encephalopathy (aka "mad cow disease").

Prevalence
- Sporadic Creutzfeldt–Jakob disease has an incidence of approximately one per million.
- The usual age of onset of sporadic Creutzfeldt–Jakob disease is from 45 to 75 years; variant Creutzfeldt–Jakob disease often presents in younger individuals.

Genetic risk
- Prion diseases are transmissible because an inoculation with the pathological protein can cause the disease in another individual.
- There are a number of mutations of the gene PRNP (located on the short arm of chromosome 20), which codes for the pathological protein (PrP^{Sc}), leading to familial, autosomal dominant Creutzfeldt–Jakob disease.

Cognitive, behavioral, and other symptoms
- Cognitive and behavioral changes include impairment of memory and executive function, as well as depression and sometimes personality changes.
- Cerebellar signs and myoclonus are frequent, and can worsen over a period of days.

Diagnostic criteria
- Electroencephalographic recordings often show a characteristic periodic sharp-wave complex.
- MRI is currently the test of choice to evaluate a patient for possible Creutzfeldt–Jakob disease.
- Creutzfeldt-Jakob disease can be confirmed neuropathologically by biopsy or at autopsy.

Treatment
- Treatment for Creutzfeldt–Jakob disease is supportive.

Continued

QUICK START: CREUTZFELDT–JAKOB DISEASE—Cont'd

Top differential diagnoses
- Slow progression: common degenerative diseases
  - Dementia with Lewy bodies
  - Frontotemporal dementia
  - Corticobasal degeneration
  - Progressive supranuclear palsy
  - Alzheimer's disease (particularly when associated with cerebral amyloid angiopathy)
- Rapidly progressing dementias
  - Cerebrovascular disease
  - Vasculitis
  - Autoimmune disease
  - Collagen vascular and granulomatous disease
  - Infectious disease
  - Malignancies
  - Paraneoplastic disorders
  - Toxic and metabolic disorders
  - Psychiatric disorders

PREVALENCE, PROGNOSIS, AND DEFINITION

Creutzfeldt–Jakob disease (CJD) is the most common type of prion disease. Prion diseases, also called transmissible spongiform encephalopathies, are progressive neurodegenerative diseases characterized by a specific neuropathology and a rapid cognitive decline which can progress to akinetic mutism over weeks (Box 11.1). Cerebellar signs and myoclonus are frequent. Electroencephalographic (EEG) recordings often show a characteristic periodic sharp-wave complex. Sporadic Creutzfeldt–Jakob disease has an incidence of approximately one per million, with a usual age of onset from 45 to 75 years. Other forms of Creutzfeldt–Jakob disease include familial (fCJD), iatrogenic (iCJD), and variant (vCJD). Age of onset of variant Creutzfeldt–Jakob disease is in general younger, sometimes presenting in the second decade of life. Creutzfeldt–Jakob disease can be confirmed neuropathologically by biopsy or at autopsy.

BOX 11.1 PRIONS

Prions are unconventional agents that consist of proteinaceous infectious particles that produce transmissible spongiform diseases in the brain. The first known prion disease, scrapie, was identified in sheep more than 200 years ago. Scrapie was demonstrated to be transmissible when it was transferred from affected sheep to healthy sheep and goats. Since that time other prion diseases have been described including Creutzfeldt–Jakob disease, kuru, Gerstmann–Straussler–Schenker disease, and fatal familial insomnia.

Kuru was rampant among the South Fore people of New Guinea. It was the practice in these communities to consume dead relatives as a mark of respect and mourning. Carelton Gadjusek (who was awarded the Nobel Prize for his work) connected the spread of kuru to the practice of cannibalism and with the elimination of this practice kuru disappeared within a generation. Prions were later characterized as the common culprit in these diseases by Stanley Prusiner, who was also awarded a Nobel Prize for his work.

RISK FACTORS, PATHOLOGY, AND PATHOPHYSIOLOGY

Prion diseases are transmissible neurodegenerative diseases characterized by spongiform changes, neuronal death, astrocytosis, and accumulation of a pathological protein (PrP^{Sc}) in the brain as well as other organs to a lesser extent (Fig. 11.1). Prion diseases are transmissible because an inoculation with the pathological protein can cause the disease in another individual. Iatrogenic cases have been attributed to transplantation of human brain tissues or human pituitary hormones from individuals with unrecognized prion diseases. Patients with familial Creutzfeldt–Jakob disease have been found to have mutations in the gene that codes for the PrP^{Sc} protein.

Variant Creutzfeldt–Jakob disease is similar biochemically and histopathologically to bovine spongiform encephalopathy, often referred to in the lay press as "mad cow disease." A number of these cases in the United Kingdom have been attributed to ingesting beef contaminated with bovine spongiform encephalopathy.

CLINICAL PRESENTATION

Patients with Creutzfeldt–Jakob disease present with a rapid cognitive and motor decline that can progress to akinetic mutism within weeks. Myoclonus, cerebellar signs (such as ataxia), as well as pyramidal abnormalities (such as weakness) may all occur. Myoclonus occurring as a heightened startle response to sound or light is often present in the middle to late stages. The vast majority of patients show a significant cognitive decline, including

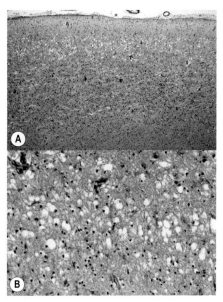

FIGURE 11.1 Pathology of Creutzfeldt–Jakob disease.

Note spongiform changes, i.e., the clear spaces, which can be visualized at both low power (A) and high power (B). A color version of this figure is avaliable online at http://www.expertconsult.com.

abnormalities of memory and executive function in addition to depression and/or other changes in personality. More variability is seen with visual disturbances and naming, with only some patients showing impairment (Cordery et al., 2005).

LABORATORY STUDIES AND ELECTROENCEPHALOGRAPHY

Laboratory studies can play only a supportive role in the diagnosis of Creutzfeldt–Jakob disease. Although the EEG classically shows diffuse slowing with periodic triphasic complexes, this is a nonspecific sign of generalized brain dysfunction and is not always present until the disease is evident clinically. Similarly, the elevation of the 14–3–3 protein in the cerebral spinal fluid is a sign of rapid neuronal injury, and is neither sensitive nor specific for Creutzfeldt–Jakob disease.

Brain biopsy can often provide a definitive diagnosis. However, the diagnostic specificity of MRI now rivals that of brain biopsy. Moreover, brain biopsy poses the risk of transmission to operating room personnel because standard surgical sterilization methods do not remove prion proteins.

Definitive diagnosis of variant Creutzfeldt–Jakob disease can often be made by a biopsy and examination of the tonsils, which has been shown to contain the PrP^{Sc} protein in germinal centers.

STRUCTURAL IMAGING STUDIES

Characteristic abnormalities on the MRI scan are probably the most helpful non-invasive diagnostic findings. Because neurons are rapidly dying, most cases show FLAIR and diffusion MRI abnormalities in cortical and deep gray matter structures including basal ganglia (caudate and putamen) and thalamic involvement (Kong et al., 2008). One study found that those patients with more diffusion abnormalities in basal ganglia had a more rapid progression to akinetic mutism (Yi et al., 2008).

DIFFERENTIAL DIAGNOSIS

When suspecting a case of Creutzfeldt–Jakob disease that is progressing relatively slowly over months, the differential diagnosis includes common degenerative diseases such as dementia with Lewy bodies, frontotemporal dementia, corticobasal degeneration, progressive supranuclear palsy, and Alzheimer's disease (particularly when associated with cerebral amyloid angiopathy). Vascular dementia can also be confused with Creutzfeldt–Jakob disease. See Box 11.2 for the differential diagnosis of rapidly progressing dementias (for review, see Geschwind et al., 2008).

TREATMENTS

Treatment for Creutzfeldt–Jakob disease is supportive. Although a number of therapies aimed at ameliorating the underlying disorder have been tried, none have proved to be effective. In the majority of cases Creutzfeldt–Jakob disease is rapidly fatal, with most patients dying from the disease within a year of diagnosis, often within weeks to months.

```
┌─────────────────────────────────────────────────────────────────────────┐
│ BOX 11.2 DIFFERENTIAL DIAGNOSIS OF RAPIDLY PROGRESSING DEMENTIAS          │
├─────────────────────────────────────────────────────────────────────────┤
```

- Cerebrovascular disease
- Autoimmune disease (e.g., Hashimoto's encephalopathy)
- Vasculitis
- Collagen vascular and granulomatous diseases (e.g., sarcoid)
- Infectious disease
  - HIV
  - Opportunistic infections in HIV and other immunocompromised states
    - Cryptococcus
    - JC virus
    - Mycobacteria
  - Syphilis
  - Lyme disease
  - Subacute sclerosing panencephalitis
  - Whipple's disease
- Malignancies
  - Primary central nervous system lymphoma
  - Intravascular lymphoma
  - Lymphomatoid granulomatosis
- Paraneoplastic disorders (e.g., limbic encephalitis)
- Toxic metabolic disorders
  - Heavy metals (e.g., bismuth from Pepto-bismol®)
  - Vitamin deficiencies (e.g., Wernicke's encephalopathy)
- Metabolic disorders (e.g., metachromatic leukodystrophy)
- Psychiatric disorders

References

Cordery, R.J., Alner, K., Cipolotti, L., et al., 2005. The neuropsychology of variant CJD: a comparative study with inherited and sporadic forms of prion disease. J. Neurol. Neurosurg. Psychiatry 76, 330–336.

Geschwind, M.D., Shu, H., Haman, A., et al., 2008. Rapidly progressive dementia. Ann. Neurol. 64, 97–108.

Kong, A., Kleinig, T., Van der Vliet, A., et al., 2008. MRI of sporadic Creutzfeldt-Jakob disease. J. Med. Imaging Radiat. Oncol. 52, 318–324.

Yi, S.H., Park, K.C., Yoon, S.S., et al., 2008. Relationship between clinical course and diffusion-weighted MRI findings in sporadic Creutzfeldt-Jakob disease. Neurol. Sci. 29, 251–255.

CHAPTER

12 Other disorders

QUICK START: OTHER DISORDERS

Depression and anxiety
- Although depression and/or anxiety may cause memory loss, many patients with memory loss and depression and/or anxiety have mild cognitive impairment or Alzheimer's disease.

Medication side-effects
- Medication side-effects are one of the most common causes of memory complaints and cognitive dysfunction

Disrupted sleep
- Disrupted sleep is one of the most common causes of memory problems we see in patients younger than age 60.
- Sleep is needed in order to sustain attention when learning new information.
- Recent evidence suggests that sleep is necessary to consolidate memories from temporary to long-term storage.

Hormones?
- The literature is mixed regarding whether peri- or post-menopausal status is related to alterations in memory.
- There are no randomized controlled trials of hormone replacement therapy showing a cognitive benefit.

Metabolic disorders
- Almost any medical disorder that makes a patient ill can cause memory loss and/or impair other aspects of cognition.
- Metabolic disorders affect attention, wax and wane, and may unmask an incipient dementia.

Diabetes
- Diabetes can cause memory loss and other cognitive problems from cerebrovascular disease and hypoglycemia.

Alcohol abuse and alcoholic Korsakoff's syndrome
- About half of the 18 million problem drinkers in the USA develop some cognitive deficits.
- Most patients with alcoholism complain of memory deficits.
- Patients with alcoholic Korsakoff's syndrome show severe anterograde and some retrograde amnesia.

Lyme disease
- Lyme neuroborreliosis is uncommon but highly treatable, and should be considered in those who live in an area endemic for Lyme who are at risk for deer tick exposure by, for example, taking walks in the woods.
- The memory problems are typically secondary to difficulties with focusing and sustaining attention, leading to difficulties in encoding (learning).

Hippocampal sclerosis
- Hippocampal sclerosis is defined as severe gliosis and loss of neurons in the CA1 region of the hippocampus and neighboring regions.

Continued

QUICK START: OTHER DISORDERS—Cont'd

	• Hippocampal sclerosis may occur by itself or with a wide variety of other diseases, including temporal lobe epilepsy, multiple sclerosis, Alzheimer's disease, cardiovascular disease, frontotemporal dementia, and amyotrophic lateral sclerosis.
	• Clinically, we suspect that a patient may have hippocampal sclerosis if he or she shows evidence of memory dysfunction without other cognitive deficits, and the patient does not progress over time.
Chronic traumatic encephalopathy: Dementia pugilistica	• Repetitive head injury has been associated with chronic traumatic encephalopathy, a progressive dementia, years later in life.
	• Common signs and symptoms are memory problems, behavioral and personality changes, Parkinsonism, and speech and gait abnormalities.
	• Head trauma has also been associated with Alzheimer's disease later in life, particularly associated with an APOE ε4 allele.
Subdural and epidural hematomas	• Subdural and epidural hematomas may cause a number of symptoms, including drowsiness, inattention, hemiparesis, or seizures, depending upon the size, age, and composition of the fluid collection.
Vitamin B12 deficiency	• Symptoms of B12 deficiency include memory loss, psychosis including hallucinations and delusions, fatigue, irritability, depression, and personality changes.
	• B12 deficiency should be suspected when the patient is elderly, a vegetarian, taking certain medications (e.g., metformin), or has had intestinal infections.
Seizures	• Seizures are an uncommon cause of memory problems but must be considered both because they are treatable and because they can lead to disability and death if they were to occur, for example, while driving a car.
	• Partial complex seizures should be suspected in patients of any age in whom there is a history of "episodes" of memory loss that may be quite profound in the setting of otherwise good memory and normal cognitive testing.
Hashimoto's encephalopathy	• Hashimoto's encephalitis is a rare, rapidly progressing, treatable autoimmune disorder associated with chronic lymphocytic Hashimoto's thyroiditis.
	• It often begins with psychiatric symptoms such as depression, personality changes, or psychosis, and then progresses with cognitive decline and one or more of a variety of signs and symptoms including myoclonus, ataxia, pyramidal and extrapyramidal signs, stroke-like episodes, altered levels of consciousness, confusion, and seizures.
	• Patients with Hashimoto's encephalitis can be euthyroid, hypothyroid, or hyperthyroid.

In this chapter we present additional disorders that can cause memory loss and other cognitive impairment. Although some of these disorders are common, because none are causes of dementia per se, we touch on them here just briefly to round out the differential diagnosis of memory loss. These disorders are presented in the order which roughly corresponds to how often we see them in our clinic.

DEPRESSION AND ANXIETY

It is quite common that we will see a patient with memory loss who was treated with an antidepressant rather than a cholinesterase inhibitor by their primary care physician. The typical scenario is that the patient noticed that they were beginning to lose their memory, was concerned that they might be developing Alzheimer's disease, and understandably felt quite concerned, anxious, and depressed about their memory loss. The physician, correctly picking up on their anxiety and depression, prescribed an antidepressant. In our experience it is much more likely that a patient who is over the age of 65 and presents with both memory loss and depression has depression due to the memory loss, rather than the other way around (Boxes 12.1 and 12.2). In fact, studies suggest that 20–40% of patients with dementia also have major depression, and up to 70% of patients have some depressive symptoms (Cummings et al., 1995; Tractenberg et al., 2003).

The relationship between Alzheimer's disease and depression is both complex and controversial (for a review see Panza et al. 2010). Studies have suggested that (1) a history of depression earlier in life is a risk factor for Alzheimer's disease and (2) symptoms of depression are common in the few years preceding the diagnosis of Alzheimer's disease, prompting some researchers to hypothesize that it is an early symptom of Alzheimer's disease, especially in individuals with no lifetime history of depression.

BOX 12.1 RULE OF THUMB?

It used to be a rule of thumb that patients who do not think that they have memory problems have Alzheimer's disease, whereas patients who are worried about their memory problems are aging normally or are depressed. Now we believe that it is much more likely that patients who are worried about their memory problems actually have mild cognitive impairment or early Alzheimer's disease (see Chapters 3 and 4).

BOX 12.2 PSEUDODEMENTIA?

The term "pseudodementia" has been used to signify any "functional" psychiatric illness that mimics dementia, and more specifically the symptoms of dementia caused by depression (Brown, 2005). This term has been helpful historically in enabling clinicians to be aware that cognitive impairment can be secondary to depression, and in reminding them to consider depression in the differential diagnosis of memory loss. Today, however, the problem is much more likely to be the other way around: clinicians need to be reminded that memory loss due to a neurological disorder (such as Alzheimer's disease) can cause depression and thus these neurological disorders should be considered in the differential diagnosis of depression. We therefore believe that the term "pseudodementia" has had its day. Perhaps for patients with mild cognitive impairment who present with depression we should consider using the term "pseudodepression"...

The history is one important clue to help determine whether the memory loss or the depression is primary. It would be extremely unlikely that a 75-year-old patient without a prior history of major depression would now develop a first episode of major depression severe enough to cause memory problems. On the other hand, a patient with a life-long history of major depression severe enough to lead to multiple hospitalizations and medication trials may certainly be experiencing another episode of depression at age 75, causing his or her memory loss.

Some of the most common cognitive disturbances due to depression include poor energy, motivation, and attention. Frontal/executive and speed of processing deficits are often found on neuropsychological testing. Memory problems are typically secondary to these disturbances. Depression and anxiety disrupt the "file clerk" of the memory system, whereas Alzheimer's disease disrupts the "file cabinet." In other words, the patient with depression has difficulty placing (storing, encoding) information in the memory (the file clerk isn't doing its job), but, once it is stored, the brain mechanisms that maintain the memory are intact (the file cabinet is fine). (See Appendix C: *Our current understanding of memory*, for more on the filing analogy of memory.) Thus, patients with depression may appear to have a "frontal pattern" of memory loss, often performing poorly in learning (encoding) and free recalling information off the top of their head, while performing relatively normally when choosing previously studied items from a list. Another pattern that is sometimes present in patients with depression is that they experience more difficulty remembering things in the past than the present. This pattern is thought to occur because it is more effortful for a person whose memory is normal to recall items from the distant past than to recall events that occurred yesterday. This pattern is just the opposite of that of most patients with Alzheimer's disease, in which the patient recalls the past easily but cannot remember what happened yesterday.

In treating a patient who has both memory loss and depression, we always recommend treating the underlying disorder first. This may seem obvious, but many clinicians suggest treating the depression first regardless of whether it is primary or secondary. In our experience the depression secondary to awareness of memory loss typically improves when the memory improves. Similarly, the cognitive impairments secondary to depression generally improve when the depression is treated. Each patient may still benefit from a medication to treat the secondary symptom. For example, the patient with memory loss and secondary depression may still benefit from an SSRI medication (sertraline (Zoloft), citalopram (Celexa), and escitalopram (Lexapro) being our favorites. Each of these medications has been approved for the treatment of both depression and anxiety. See Chapter 22 for more on the pharmacological treatment of depression.

MEDICATION SIDE-EFFECTS

Medication side-effects are one of the most common causes of cognitive dysfunction. In our experience, attention is the most common cognitive function to become affected, followed by memory, and then language. There are too many medications which interfere with cognition to individually list them all. Note that even a relatively safe class of medication from a cognitive perspective may still contain a few individual drugs that can cause confusion. Box 12.3 lists some classes and properties of medications that can lead to cognitive dysfunction.

BOX 12.3 COMMON CLASSES OR PROPERTIES OF MEDICATIONS CAUSING COGNITIVE DYSFUNCTION

- **Allergy/antihistamines/common cold medications**
- **Analgesics including migraine medications**
- Antiarrhythmics
- **Anticholinergic**
- Anticonvulsants
- Antidiarrheals
- Antiemetics
- Anesthetics
- **Antipsychotics/dopamine antagonists**
- **Antispasmodics/incontinence medications**
- Asthma/pulmonary medications
- **Barbiturates**
- **Benzodiazepines**
- Beta-blockers
- **Cancer chemotherapy**
- **Corticosteroids**
- Digoxin
- Dopamine (Sinemet)/dopamine agonists
- **Muscle relaxants**
- **Opioids (narcotics)**
- **Sedating medications of any class**
- **Sleeping medications of any class**
- Stimulants/stimulating medications of any class
- Tricyclic antidepressants

Note: Worst offenders are in **bold**. This is not an exhaustive list. Please consult the Physicians Desk Reference or other source when determining whether a particular medication may be causing cognitive impairment in your patient.

DISRUPTED SLEEP

Disrupted sleep is one of the most common causes of memory problems we see in patients younger than age 60. Sleep can disrupt memory in two main ways. First, sleep is necessary for good attention. In order to encode or learn new information, being able to focus and sustain attention is critical. Second, there is increasing evidence that our consolidation of memory—memories going from temporary to more long-term storage—requires sleep (Stickgold, 2005, 2006.) Thus, poor sleep makes it difficult to learn new information and to retain that information in long-term storage.

Disrupted sleep may be due to a sleep disorder such as insomnia, sleep apnea, periodic limb movements of sleep, and restless leg syndrome. Sleep may be disrupted by depression. And sleep may be commonly disrupted by poor sleep hygiene—that is, poor scheduling or management of sleep.

Shift workers, including nurses, factory workers, and others, are one group that is prone to memory disorders because of poor sleep hygiene. However, in our experience even more common than shift workers are individuals of any age who simply have too many things to do in their day to allow enough time for adequate sleep. When we are referred individuals with memory problems who are in their 30s or 40s, we always ask about sleep problems in several different ways. When asked, "Do you have any problems with sleep?" the response is usually no. But when asked to briefly take us through their day, a common response often goes something like the following. "I'm up at 5 a.m. to exercise, shower and get myself ready for work at 6, get the kids up and get them ready for school at 7, and then leave for work at 8. I come home from work around 6 p.m., make dinner, help the kids with their homework, and get them ready for bed by 9. Then I usually spend an hour or two finishing up work for the office, and then at 10 or 11 I have an hour or two to spend some time with my spouse talking or watching TV, till we go to bed after the evening news around 11:30 (or later if *The Tonight Show* has someone good on)." While this may sound like a perfectly normal schedule, this individual is only allowing themselves between 5 and 5 ½ hours of sleep a night. For the average individual who is best with 8–9 hours of sleep, one can often get away with 7 hours without noticeable cognitive consequences. But trying to reduce sleep further often causes difficulty with attention and memory.

HORMONES?

Another possible cause of memory problems in individuals younger than age 60 is a decrease in gonadotropin hormones. For women this is most commonly due to perimenopausal status; for either women or men this can be secondary to treatment for cancer or other disorders. The literature on this topic is quite mixed, with some studies demonstrating memory impairment and other studies not, and at least one literature review suggests that the natural transition to menopause is not associated with objective change in episodic memory (Henderson, 2009). Nonetheless, many individuals who come to us in the clinic are quite clear about their subjective experience that their memory is not as good as it was previously, which they relate to a change in their hormone status.

Regarding treatment, the literature again shows mixed results, with some studies finding improvement with hormone replacement therapy and others not, and again at least one literature review suggests no improvement (Henderson, 2009). Most importantly, however, large randomized controlled trials have now shown no evidence for improvement and instead worsening of cognition and increased risk for dementia with hormone replacement therapy (Craig et al., 2005; Henderson, 2009; Coker et al., 2010).

In summary, despite historical claims that hormone replacement therapy has cognitive benefit, we now know from randomized controlled trials that there is no evidence for this claim, and indeed there are increased risks for dementia and other disorders. As such, we do not recommend hormone replacement therapy for postmenopausal women solely as a treatment for memory problems.

METABOLIC DISORDERS

Almost any medical disorder that makes a patient ill can cause memory loss and/or impair other aspects of cognition. Common disorders that impair cognition include renal failure, liver failure, congestive heart failure, hypercapnea from chronic obstructive pulmonary disease, hypercalcemia, and many others. There are several clues that can help the clinician to know that the cognitive impairment is secondary to a metabolic disorder and not secondary to a primary cause of dementia.

The first clue is that dementias are progressive, whereas metabolic disorders tend to wax and wane. For example, if the patient with congestive heart failure becomes confused when his heart failure acutely worsens but then is completely back to normal when the heart failure is better, the confusion is unlikely due to a dementia. A similar scenario can happen with other metabolic disorders such as with liver failure. We have treated a 65-year-old man who has liver disease secondary to chronic alcohol use. When his liver failure was severe (and it was severe enough to require extended hospitalization) he was terribly confused, and even after he left the hospital and his liver function tests returned to just about normal, his cognition was still not what it used to be. This continued cognitive impairment in the setting of near normal liver function tests led his family to worry that he was now developing a dementia on top of everything else. Over a period of months, however, his cognitive function improved rather than worsened, and this was one reason that we knew that the patient was still recovering from his liver failure, and was not developing a dementia.

The second clue that cognitive impairment is due to a metabolic disorder is that the impairment in cognition is virtually always poor attention. Patients with a metabolic disorder show extreme difficulties in paying attention, both on formal cognitive testing and in observing them at the bedside or in the clinic. Simple tasks, such as counting backwards from 20 to 1, reciting the months of the year backwards, or spelling the word "WORLD" backwards, are quite difficult for these patients. Memory problems are prominent, but these memory problems are secondary to poor attention. The ability to learn new information is severely impaired during the time when the patient is confused with poor attention, often leading to the patient having no memory of the time that they were confused.

The last thing to note here is that a patient may have an incipient dementia that is made apparent by a metabolic disorder—the so-called "unmasking effect." For example, a 74-year-old patient with no clinical complaints of memory loss by either herself or her family may have a small amount of Alzheimer's pathology in the brain. Under normal circumstances this pathology is "silent," that is, it produces no clinical signs or symptoms. If this patient develops hypercalcemia, however, she may show signs of inattention and memory loss that are attributable both to the hypercalcemia and to the small amount of Alzheimer's pathology in the brain. Thus, her cognitive dysfunction may be worse than that of another 74-year-old with hypercalcemia but without the Alzheimer's pathology. When the hypercalcemia is successfully treated, her cognition returns to normal. How do we know that she has underlying Alzheimer's pathology? We know that she has underlying Alzheimer's pathology if several months or years later she now develops the signs and symptoms of Alzheimer's disease when she does not have hypercalcemia or another metabolic disorder.

DIABETES

Diabetes can cause memory loss and other cognitive problems in several different ways. The two most common and concerning are from cerebrovascular disease and hypoglycemia. Along with hypertension, increased cholesterol, and smoking, diabetes predisposes the patient to cerebrovascular disease. These effects are discussed in Chapter 6: *Vascular dementia and vascular cognitive impairment*. Hypoglycemia can also damage the brain. A variety of cognitive, behavioral, and personality changes can be seen (Gold et al., 1994). Although the specific pathophysiology has not been worked out, hypoglycemia damages both gray and white matter, meaning that both neurons and myelinated axons and dendrites suffer injury (Ma et al., 2009). In our experience there is the not surprising correlation between how tightly the glucose is trying to be maintained and how frequently episodes of hypoglycemia and subsequent cognitive impairment occur. We would therefore recommend that control of glucose not be so tight such that hypoglycemic episodes are frequent. Tight control is of course particularly dangerous when the patient is not aware of his or her hypoglycemia.

ALCOHOL ABUSE AND ALCOHOLIC KORSAKOFF'S SYNDROME

About half of the 18 million problem drinkers in the USA develop cognitive deficits (Oscar-Berman & Marinkovic, 2007). Most of these develop mild neuropsychological difficulties which improve within a year of abstinence. Approximately 2 million alcoholics, however, develop life-long disabling conditions that require custodial care. Factors that contribute to alcohol's effect on the brain include older age, comorbid health conditions, and positive family history.

The brain structures most vulnerable to dysfunction and damage in alcoholism include the frontal lobes, limbic system, and cerebellum. Other structures showing either atrophy or reduced blood flow on MRI include the other regions of the cerebral cortex, corpus callosum, hippocampus, and the amygdala. Additional structures damaged in alcoholic Korsakoff's syndrome will be discussed below.

Alcohol's acute effects on the brain include both stimulating effects in low doses and depressant effects in higher doses. Neuropsychologically there is a reduction in working memory, planning, other executive functions, visuospatial ability, and interhemispheric processing speed. Attention and vigilance can be reduced at blood alcohol levels as low as 0.02–0.03%, much lower than legal intoxication levels. Regarding behavior, alcohol intoxication increases the likelihood of aggressive behaviors secondary to impulsivity, disinhibition, social or sexual inappropriateness, and impairments in decision-making and executive function. Alcoholics frequently make poor decisions, including decisions regarding their alcohol consumption. Changes in emotion and personality are also seen, including a diminished ability to recognize emotional facial expressions and emotional spoken prosody (tone of voice). Personality traits are often described in terms of "disinhibition," impulsivity, aggression, and a lack of concern for the consequences of inappropriate behaviors. On the neurological examination the most common problems are with gait and balance, typically associated with cerebellar dysfunction. (Cerebellar function is what is typically evaluated in field sobriety tests.)

Common comorbid medical conditions that, in combination with alcoholism, are most likely to result in greater cognitive dysfunction include head injury, liver disease, cardiovascular disease, fetal alcohol syndrome, and malnutrition leading to thiamine (vitamin B1) deficiency. Frequent comorbid psychiatric conditions that can worsen cognition include depression, schizophrenia, and other drug use.

Neurobehavioral functioning can improve within 3–4 weeks of abstinence, accompanied by recovery of metabolic functions and partial reversal of brain shrinkage in some patients. Frontal lobe blood flow returns to normal after approximately 4 years. Most neurocognitive deficits resolve within 7 years, with the exception of visuospatial processing deficits, which may not recover.

Patients with alcohol-induced persisting amnestic disorder, more commonly known as the alcoholic Korsakoff's syndrome, show severe anterograde amnesia (inability to remember new information) as well as some retrograde amnesia (loss of previously acquired information). These patients are permanently unable to remember new information for more than the time the information is being kept in mind—typically just a few seconds. Patients with Korsakoff's syndrome live in the past, and generally retain many older memories formed prior to the onset of their alcohol-related brain damage. The damaged areas of the brain include the mamillary bodies, basal forebrain, hippocampus, fornix, and medial and anterior nuclei of the thalamus. Although damage to the mamillary bodies is commonly thought to be the cause of the memory deficit in this syndrome, at least one study suggests that it is actually damage to the anterior nucleus of the thalamus that is most closely correlated with the memory deficit (Harding et al., 2000). In addition to memory deficits, patients with Korsakoff's syndrome are abnormally sensitive to proactive interference, have restricted attention, retarded perceptual processing abilities, are impaired on tests of fluency and cognitive flexibility, and show perseverative responding. They are also ataxic.

The cerebellum in particular deserves mention. Alcoholism is associated with marked cerebellar atrophy, particularly of the cerebellar vermis. The cerebellum is now understood to be important for normal cognitive and behavioral function (Schmahmann & Sherman, 1998; Schmahmann & Caplan, 2006), particularly executive function including cognitive flexibility, allocation of attentional resources, set shifting ability, inhibition of perseverative errors, abstraction, planning, and inhibition of irrelevant information. Thus, damage to the cerebellum may also be responsible for some of the cognitive and behavioral impairment seen in patients with alcoholism.

Most patients with alcoholism complain of memory deficits. If their alcoholism is mainly affecting frontal/executive function, then the memory deficit will be of a "frontal" variety; that is, difficulty learning new information and freely recalling it, but if enough effort is used new information can be learned and retrieved. If their alcoholism has led to Korsakoff's syndrome, then their memory deficit will be similar to that of a patient with Alzheimer's disease or other hippocampal injury; that is, new information may not be able to be learned, regardless of the effort employed. It is sometimes difficult to distinguish patients with alcoholism and Alzheimer's disease from patients with alcoholism and Korsakoff's syndrome, particularly at a single visit. Both will have frontal executive and episodic memory dysfunction. Over time, however, things become clearer. As long as the patient abstains from drinking, over time the patient with Korsakoff's syndrome will be stable, whereas the patient with Alzheimer's disease will deteriorate.

LYME DISEASE

Lyme neuroborreliosis, caused by Lyme disease affecting the central nervous system, is an uncommon but highly treatable cause of memory problems. The memory problems are typically secondary to difficulties with focusing and sustaining attention, leading to difficulties in encoding (learning).

Lyme disease should be considered in those who live in an area endemic for Lyme who are at risk for deer tick exposure by, for example, taking walks in the woods. Exposure to Lyme disease can be determined from a positive serum IgG. A positive serum IgM indicates active infection. Traditionally, a positive IgA in the cerebral spinal fluid confirms the diagnosis of Lyme neuroborreliosis, although newer techniques have focused on poly-merase chain reaction of specific Lyme DNA sequences in the cerebrospinal fluid (Stanek & Strle, 2009).

HIPPOCAMPAL SCLEROSIS

Hippocampal sclerosis is defined as severe gliosis and loss of neurons in the CA1 region of the hippocampus and neighboring regions such as the subiculum (Duyckaerts et al., 2009) (Fig. 12.1). Hippocampal sclerosis may occur by itself or with a wide variety of other diseases including temporal lobe epilepsy, multiple sclerosis, Alzheimer's disease, cardio-vascular disease, frontotemporal dementia, and amyotrophic lateral sclerosis. Autopsy stud-ies have tended to look at the prevalence of hippocampal sclerosis with other disorders, such as with temporal lobe epilepsy or dementia, making an overall prevalence difficult to determine. One large study of 1000 elderly patients with dementia found that 28 (2.8%) had hippocampal sclerosis in addition to other dementia pathologies (Attems & Jellinger, 2006). Twenty patients also had Alzheimer's disease pathology (out of 650 cases; 3.1%), six had vascular pathology consistent with vascular dementia, one had frontotemporal dementia pathology, and one had Lewy body pathology. In this series there was no difference cognitively at the end of life between those patients who had Alzheimer's disease alone and those who had Alzheimer's disease and hippocampal sclerosis.

Clinically, we suspect that a patient may have hippocampal sclerosis without another cause of memory loss if he or she shows evidence of memory dysfunction without other cog-nitive deficits, and the patient does not progress over time. For example, a patient may come in with complaints of memory loss, and is found by history and neuropsychological examination to have an isolated problem with memory and not meet criteria for dementia. This patient will

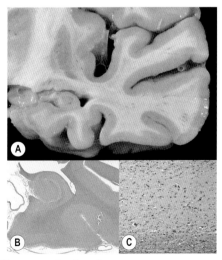

FIGURE 12.1 Pathology of hippocampal sclerosis.

Gross (A) and low- (B) and high- (C) power views of hippocampal sclerosis showing atrophy and loss of neurons. A color version of this figure is avaliable online at http://www.expertconsult.com.

typically be diagnosed with mild cognitive impairment, amnestic type. If this patient remains stable over several years without progression, hippocampal sclerosis may be the correct diagnosis. The differential diagnosis would include other causes of stable, non-progressive memory loss, such as alcoholic Korsakoff's syndrome (although, of course, Korsakoff's syndrome would also require protracted alcohol abuse; see above).

CHRONIC TRAUMATIC ENCEPHALOPATHY: DEMENTIA PUGILISTICA

There is increasing evidence that head trauma may be associated with encephalopathy and dementia later in life. The exact pathogenesis of how head trauma at one point in life can cause dementia decades later is complex and is still being determined. We do know that, in addition to causing an encephalopathy that is maximal at the time of the head injury and generally improves (though not necessarily back to baseline), repetitive head injury has recently been associated with progressive neurofibrillary degeneration of the brain (McKee et al., 2009). Thus, repetitive head injury can cause a progressive dementia years later in life. Chronic traumatic encephalopathy is associated with memory problems, behavioral and personality changes, Parkinsonism, as well as speech and gait abnormalities. The pathology includes extensive tau-immunoreactive neurofibrillary tangles, astrocytic tangles, as well as spindle- and thread-shaped neurites throughout the brain, and gross atrophy of cerebral hemispheres, medial temporal lobe, thalamus, mammillary bodies, and brainstem, with ventricular dilation and a fenestrated cavum septum pellucidum. Deposition of β-amyloid (Alzheimer's pathology) most commonly occurs as diffuse plaques and is present in less than half of the cases (Fig. 12.2).

Although the research is ongoing, it appears that multiple concussions, such as those that may occur in the course of playing contact sports, provide sufficient head trauma to cause chronic traumatic encephalopathy (Box 12.4).

Head trauma has also been associated with Alzheimer's disease later in life, particularly associated with an APOE ε4 allele. As discussed in Chapter 3: *Alzheimer's disease*, one study found a 10-fold increase in Alzheimer's disease in individuals with traumatic head injury and an APOE ε4 allele, but no increase in the disease was seen in individuals with traumatic head injury without an APOE ε4 allele (Mayeux et al., 1995).

SUBDURAL AND EPIDURAL HEMATOMAS

Subdural and epidural hematomas may cause a number of symptoms, including drowsiness, inattention, hemiparesis, or seizures, depending upon the size, age, and composition of the fluid collections. Subdural hematomas are when blood accumulates between the brain and the dura, lining the sulci and gyri of the brain with blood. Epidural hematomas are between the dura and the skull, and often appear in the shape of a lens. As the brain atrophies or shrinks with normal aging or with a neurodegenerative disease (such as Alzheimer's disease), the bridging veins between the dura and the brain become relatively longer. The dura may also start to pull away from the skull. Thus, the effect of the brain shrinking makes it much more likely that even a minor fall involving the head can lead to a subdural or epidural hematoma. These hematomas are even more likely in some dementias—such as progressive supranuclear palsy—which predispose the patient to falls. In Alzheimer's disease

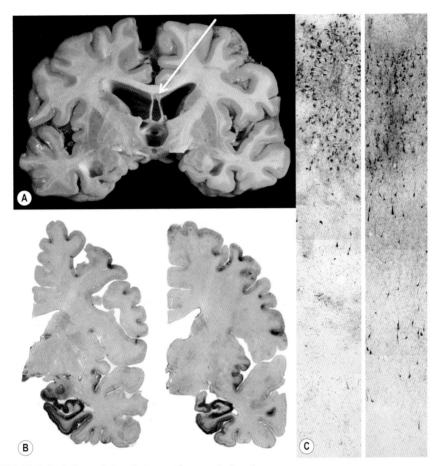

FIGURE 12.2 Pathology of chronic traumatic encephalopathy.

Gross pathology (A) shows atrophy of cerebral hemispheres, medial temporal lobes, ventricular dilatation, and a fenestrated cavum septum pellucidum (arrow). Whole-mount 50-μm-thick coronal sections show dense deposition of tau protein in medial temporal lobe structures, with less dense deposition elsewhere in the cortex in two cases (B). Microscopic views of the same two cases showing prominent perivascular collections of neurofibrillary and astrocytic tangles evident in the superficial cortical layers with lesser involvement of the deep laminae (C). Note that this pathology is different from that of Alzheimer's disease (see Chapter 3). A color version of this figure is avaliable online at http://www.expertconsult.com.

and other dementias with prominent memory loss, there is also the problem that the patient may fall but not remember to tell anyone. We have often seen patients who present with bruises to the face and cannot tell their caregivers or doctors how they came about.

VITAMIN B12 DEFICIENCY

Vitamin B12 deficiency should always be looked for when a patient presents with memory loss, since it is generally reversible with treatment. Many neuropsychiatry symptoms have been observed, and many in patients who do not have a megaloblastic anemia. These

---

BOX 12.4 CONTACT SPORTS THAT HAVE BEEN ASSOCIATED WITH MULTIPLE CONCUSSIONS

- **Boxing**
- **Football**
- **Wrestling**
- **Rugby**
- **Soccer**
- Hockey
- Lacrosse
- Skiing
- Karate
- Horseback riding
- Parachuting

Note: sports in **bold** have been associated with chronic traumatic encephalopathy at autopsy. From McKee, A.C., Cantu, R.C., Nowinski, C.J., et al., 2009. Chronic traumatic encephalopathy in athletes: progressive tauopathy after repetitive head injury. J. Neuropathol. Exp. Neurol. 68, 709–735.

---

include memory loss, psychosis including hallucinations and delusions, fatigue, irritability, depression, and personality changes.

Vitamin B12 deficiency should be suspected when the patient is a vegetarian (particularly vegan), and in older adults since inability to absorb B12 due to atrophic gastritis is common in the elderly. Some medications (e.g., metformin) can also interfere with B12 dietary absorption, as can a number of intestinal infections.

Diagnosis of B12 deficiency can be performed in a number of ways. We typically screen patients for B12 deficiency with a serum B12 level. However, if the suspicion is strong and the B12 level is low normal we will follow up with serum levels of methylmalonic acid, which is more sensitive.

Treatment is of course supplementation with vitamin B12, either orally (if due to a dietary deficiency such as a vegan diet) or parenterally (if due to poor absorption such as in atrophy gastritis). It is important to monitor serum B12 and/or methylmalonic acid to assure that levels are returning to normal. Cognition should return to normal with treatment.

SEIZURES

Seizures are an uncommon cause of memory problems but must be considered both because they are a very treatable disorder and because they can lead to disability and death if they were to occur, for example, while driving a car. Because generalized tonic–clonic seizures are rarely a secret, undiagnosed seizures that cause memory problems are generally partial complex seizures—partial seizures that interfere with consciousness without generalizing.

Sometimes the amnesia caused by the seizure can be profound, such as in the case of transient epileptic amnesia, in which patients have an inability to form any new memories for several hours. More commonly partial complex seizures intermittently impair consciousness causing patients to have difficulty focusing their attention such that their encoding (learning) is intermittently reduced. This intermittent deficit in encoding can lead to intermittent problems with memory that may sound quite similar to those of a patient with amnestic mild cognitive impairment or even mild Alzheimer's disease.

Partial complex seizures should be suspected in patients of any age in whom there is a history of "episodes" of memory loss that may be quite profound in the setting of otherwise good memory and normal cognitive testing. These seizures should also be considered in patients younger than 65 years of age. Diagnosis can sometimes be made by history alone if a partial complex seizure is observed. If the seizures are frequent enough, the diagnosis can be confirmed by ambulatory EEG monitoring. Epileptiform activity on the routine EEG can also suggest the diagnosis.

HASHIMOTO'S ENCEPHALOPATHY

Hashimoto's encephalopathy is a rare but treatable autoimmune disorder associated with chronic lymphocytic Hashimoto's thyroiditis (Geschwind et al., 2008). It often begins with psychiatric symptoms such as depression, personality changes, or psychosis, and then progresses with cognitive decline and one or more of a variety of signs and symptoms including myoclonus, ataxia, pyramidal and extrapyramidal signs, stroke-like episodes, altered levels of consciousness, confusion, and seizures. Because it produces a rapidly progressing dementia it is most commonly mistaken for Creutzfeldt–Jakob disease. Seizures, hallucinations, and delusions are common. Women represent 85% of patients with Hashimoto's encephalitis. The course tends to be fluctuating. Patients with Hashimoto's encephalitis can be euthyroid, hypothyroid, or hyperthyroid, although the diagnosis cannot be made until the patient is euthyroid. Elevated levels of either anti-thyroglobulin or anti-thyroperoxidase in the appropriate clinical context suggest the diagnosis. EEG is non-specific and can be confused with Creutzfeldt–Jakob disease, as can the cerebrospinal fluid examination because both show increased protein. MRI often shows increased T2-weighted signal in the subcortical mesial temporal white matter, which may resolve after treatment.

The etiology of Hashimoto's encephalitis is not clear, but it is thought to be due to the presence of a shared antigen in the brain and the thyroid. More than 90% of patients respond well to immunosuppression. The typical treatment is with high-dose steroids followed by a long, slow taper. Some patients may have persistent symptoms or a fluctuating course. Plasmapheresis has also been used.

References

Attems, J., Jellinger, K.A., 2006. Hippocampal sclerosis in Alzheimer disease and other dementias. Neurology 66, 775.

Brown, W.A., 2005. Pseudodementia: Issues in diagnosis. Applied Neurology 40–43.

Coker, L.H., Espeland, M.A., Rapp, S.R., et al., 2010. Postmenopausal hormone therapy and cognitive outcomes: the Women's Health Initiative Memory Study (WHIMS). J. Steroid Biochem. Mol. Biol. 118, 304–310.

Craig, M.C., Maki, P.M., Murphy, D.G., 2005. The Women's Health Initiative Memory Study: findings and implications for treatment. Lancet Neurol. 4, 190–194.

Cummings, J.L., Ross, W., Absher, J., et al., 1995. Depressive symptoms in Alzheimer disease: assessment and determinants. Alzheimer Dis. Assoc. Disord. 9, 87–93.

Duyckaerts, C., Delatour, B., Potier, M.C., 2009. Classification and basic pathology of Alzheimer disease. Acta Neuropathol. 118, 5–36.

Geschwind, M.D., Shu, H., Haman, A., et al., 2008. Rapidly progressive dementia. Ann. Neurol. 64, 97–108.

Gold, A.E., Deary, I.J., Jones, R.W., et al., 1994. Severe deterioration in cognitive function and personality in five patients with long-standing diabetes: a complication of diabetes or a consequence of treatment? Diabet. Med. 11, 499–505.

Harding, A., Halliday, G., Caine, D., et al., 2000. Degeneration of anterior thalamic nuclei differentiates alcoholics with amnesia. Brain 123, 141–154.

Henderson, V.W., 2009. Aging, estrogens, and episodic memory in women. Cogn. Behav. Neurol. 22, 205–214.

Ma, J.H., Kim, Y.J., Yoo, W.J., et al., 2009. MR imaging of hypoglycemic encephalopathy: lesion distribution and prognosis prediction by diffusion-weighted imaging. Neuroradiology 51, 641–649.

Mayeux, R., Ottman, R., Maestre, G., et al., 1995. Synergistic effects of traumatic head injury and apolipoprotein-epsilon 4 in patients with Alzheimer's disease. Neurology 45, 555–557.

McKee, A.C., Cantu, R.C., Nowinski, C.J., et al., 2009. Chronic traumatic encephalopathy in athletes: progressive tauopathy after repetitive head injury. J. Neuropathol. Exp. Neurol. 68, 709–735.

Oscar-Berman, M., Marinkovic, K., 2007. Alcohol: effects on neurobehavioral functions and the brain. Neuropsychol. Rev. 17, 239–257.

Panza, F., Frisardi, V., Capurso, C., et al., 2010. Late-life depression, mild cognitive impairment, and dementia: possible continuum? Am. J. Geriatr. Psychiatry 18, 98–116.

Schmahmann, J.D., Sherman, J.C., 1998. The cerebellar cognitive affective syndrome. Brain 121 (Pt 4), 561–579.

Schmahmann, J.D., Caplan, D., 2006. Cognition, emotion and the cerebellum. Brain 129, 290–292.

Stanek, G., Strle, F., 2009. Lyme borreliosis: a European perspective on diagnosis and clinical management. Curr. Opin. Infect. Dis. 22, 450–454.

Stickgold, R., 2005. Sleep-dependent memory consolidation. Nature 437, 1272–1278.

Stickgold, R., 2006. Neuroscience: a memory boost while you sleep. Nature 444, 559–560.

Tractenberg, R.E., Weiner, M.F., Patterson, M.B., et al., 2003. Comorbidity of psychopathological domains in community-dwelling persons with Alzheimer's disease. J. Geriatr. Psychiatry Neurol. 16, 94–99.

Goals of treatment

13

In our experience, treatment of Alzheimer's disease and other forms of dementia is best carried out in a partnership between the patient, his or her caregiver(s), and the clinician. As with most diseases, when the diagnosis of Alzheimer's disease is made, the first question that is asked is: "What can be done?" As we explain to our patients and families, there are many aspects to treatment ranging from counseling and education to medication that, when skillfully combined, lead to the best outcomes.

TALKING ABOUT TREATMENTS FOR ALZHEIMER'S DISEASE

Patients for whom we prescribe a cholinesterase inhibitor, memantine (Namenda), or a combination of the two often ask how these medications work and what else can be done. We typically have a discussion with these patients and their families that attempts to incorporate the following points.

- Alzheimer's disease is a brain disease. In the most basic sense, brain cells are dying. As you lose brain cells, the abilities to which these cells contribute are also lost. For example, early in the course of the disease individuals with Alzheimer's disease lose cells in a brain structure called the hippocampus. The hippocampus is critical to the formation of new memories and this is why one of the first signs of Alzheimer's disease is difficulty remembering new information. (We sometimes show a photograph or a model of the brain with the hippocampus (such as in Figs 3.9 and 3.12) and we generally show the patient their CT or MRI scan and indicate the hippocampus and other regions of atrophy to show where brain cells have been lost.)
- Unlike many other organs in the body, brain cells do not regenerate, so, once a brain cell is lost, it is gone forever.
- As more brain cells die, the disease progresses and more abilities are lost.
- The goal of treatment is to treat with medications that will help the remaining brain cells—even those that may be diseased—function more efficiently. This improved efficiency can help to compensate for the ongoing loss of brain cells.
- The two most commonly used types of medication to accomplish this goal are cholinesterase inhibitors and memantine (Namenda).
- Cholinesterase inhibitors help brain cells that use the neurotransmitter acetylcholine to function more efficiently.
- Memantine (Namenda) helps brain cells that use the neurotransmitters glutamate and dopamine to function more efficiently.
- Acetylcholine, glutamate, and dopamine are all important in human memory.

Following this discussion, patients and families typically grasp the notion that the disease is progressive and that by using these approved medications we are attempting to treat the symptoms of the disease such as memory deficits, but we are not treating the underlying cause, that is, the death of neurons. If at this point they ask if there is anything else that might be done, we discuss the opportunity to participate in clinical trials. Because Alzheimer's is a fatal disease, as in the field of oncology, we believe that the best care allows patients to participate in clinical trials of novel medications if they so choose.

STRATEGIES TO TREAT THE SYMPTOMS OF ALZHEIMER'S DISEASE

In the following chapters we discuss several different strategies to treat Alzheimer's disease. In Chapters 14 and 15 we discuss the cholinesterase inhibitors and memantine (Namenda), respectively. In Chapter 16 whether vitamins, herbs, supplements, and anti-inflammatory medications are helpful is discussed. In Chapter 17 some of the possible future treatments of Alzheimer's disease are explored. And finally Chapter 18 presents some non-pharmacological strategies to help compensate for memory loss.

TREATING COGNITION AND TREATING BEHAVIOR

Patient JH is a 73-year-old retired high school music teacher who has been having memory and related problems for about a year. He recognizes his memory problems and is anxious to be treated. He lives with his wife and has two children who live nearby. He seems to be in generally good spirits with no symptoms of anxiety or depression. There is no sign of agitation. He sleeps well and his appetite and energy level are unchanged. There are no psychiatric symptoms such as hallucinations, delusions or thought disorder. His primary deficit is in recent memory; he forgets conversations by the next day and cannot remember to take his medications. He also has some recent word-finding problems. We diagnosed him with Alzheimer's disease and then had a discussion with the patient, his wife, and his daughter regarding treatments.

Patient EB is an 84-year-old woman who is living with her two nieces. She moved to the United States at age 22, never married, and worked in the fashion industry in New York, retiring at age 65. She has memory problems (denies having conversations which she had and constantly repeats questions), problems with executive functioning (she has great difficulty managing her finances and has inappropriately given away money), and visuospatial functioning (she can become lost walking in her neighborhood). She also entirely denies any cognitive deficits and does not understand why she needs to live with her nieces. She is agitated and this agitation is expressed by constantly berating her nieces, denying her problems, and attempting to wander in the neighborhood. Her nieces are extremely frustrated in attempting to care for her. We diagnosed her with Alzheimer's disease and then had a discussion with the patient and her nieces regarding treatments.

Although both of these patients have the same diagnosis, it is clear that they each present with different treatment needs. Both patients are experiencing cognitive problems, the hallmark of Alzheimer's disease, that require treatment. But patient EB also has what has come to be known as the behavioral and psychological symptoms of dementia (BPSD; Finkel, 2001, 2002). These behavioral and psychiatric symptoms can manifest in a variety of ways, including hallucinations, delusions, depression, anxiety, and agitation (which can also be expressed in a variety of ways; see Chapter 19: *Evaluating the behavioral and psychological symptoms of dementia*). Although it does not occur in all cases of dementia, by some estimates 50–90% of Alzheimer's disease patients will experience one or more behavioral and psychiatric symptoms during the course of the disease. Some symptoms, such as depression, occur relatively early in the disease, whereas other symptoms, such as agitation and delusions, tend to occur later in the disease. Whenever they occur, in many cases these behavioral and psychiatric symptoms are more distressing to the family and patient than the cognitive problems and as such demand treatment. In some cases behavioral and psychiatric symptoms can be treated with behavioral techniques, but often medication is necessary. We will consider diagnosing and treating these symptoms in more detail in Section IV: *Behavioral and Psychological Symptoms of Dementia*. For now we simply want to acknowledge the presence of this important aspect of Alzheimer's disease treatment. In this section we will focus on treating the cognitive aspect of the disease.

References

Finkel, S.I., 2001. Behavioral and psychological symptoms of dementia: a current focus for clinicians, researchers, and caregivers. J. Clin. Psychiatry 62 (Suppl. 21), 3–6.

Finkel, S.I., 2002. Behavioral and psychological symptoms of dementia. Assisting the caregiver and managing the patient. Geriatrics 57, 44–46.

14 Cholinesterase inhibitors

QUICK START: CHOLINESTERASE INHIBITORS

Mechanism of action and cognitive benefit	• Cholinesterase inhibitors increase the concentration of acetylcholine at the synapse and improve memory, attention, mood, and behavior. • Cholinesterase inhibitors are efficacious and well tolerated.

Indications and recommendations	• For Alzheimer's disease in mild, moderate, and severe stages, we recommend using one of the following once-a-day cholinesterase inhibitor formulations:
	  • Donepezil (generic & Aricept) pill or oral dissolving tablet
	  • Galantamine (generic, formerly Razadyne and Reminyl) extended-release (ER) pill
	  • Rivastigmine (Exelon) patch.
	• In general, titrate to highest recommended dose that is tolerated.

Common side effects	• Some common and important side-effects are (listed in approximate order of prevalence):
	  • Gastrointestinal: loss of appetite, nausea, vomiting, diarrhea
	  • Vivid dreams at night
	  • Dehydration
	  • Rash
	  • Bradycardia
	  • Peptic ulcer disease
	  • Seizures
	  • Other: anorexia and weight loss, rhinorrhea, salivation, muscle cramps, fasciculations.
	• Cholinesterase inhibitors should not be used with some conditions and medications (see text).

Judging efficacy	• It is important to set appropriate expectations as to the magnitude of the average improvement observed with cholinesterase inhibitors: • Most patients improve equivalent to "turning the clock back" 6–12 months. • To determine whether the cholinesterase inhibitor is working, ask the patient, ask the family, and evaluate the patient's cognition and function 2–3 months after starting the medication.

Off-label uses	• We also recommend a trial of cholinesterase inhibitors in the following disorders:
	  • Mild cognitive impairment
	  • Dementia with Lewy bodies (Parkinson's disease dementia)
	  • Vascular dementia.

CHOLINESTERASE INHIBITORS IN ALZHEIMER'S DISEASE

There are currently four cholinesterase inhibitors approved by the US Food and Drug Administration (FDA) for the treatment of Alzheimer's disease (Table 14.1): tacrine (Cognex, no longer marketed), donepezil (generic and Aricept), rivastigmine (Exelon), and galantamine (generic, formerly marketed as Razadyne and Reminyl). These drugs all work in essentially the same way: they bind to and reversibly inhibit acetylcholinesterase, the enzyme responsible for metabolizing acetylcholine in the synapse (Fig. 14.1). By doing this they increase the level of acetylcholine in the synapse. By increasing the level of acetylcholine in the synapse, the cholinesterase inhibitors are hypothesized to improve cognition. Although no one understands exactly how that happens, one hypothesis is as follows. In most regions of the brain, any individual neuron will receive input from tens or hundreds of other neurons. Because in Alzheimer's disease neurons—particularly cholinergic neurons—are dying, there are fewer cholinergic neurons from which to receive input. The idea is that if the acetylcholine from the remaining cholinergic neurons can bind to the synaptic receptor more times before the acetylcholine is broken down, these remaining neurons will be able to compensate for those neurons which are damaged or dead. There are two basic decisions that a clinician must make regarding the cholinesterase inhibitors:

1. Should I prescribe a cholinesterase inhibitor for my patient with Alzheimer's disease or other dementia?
2. If so, which one should I prescribe?

SHOULD I PRESCRIBE A CHOLINESTERASE INHIBITOR?

As with any medication, the decision to prescribe or not to prescribe is made on an individual basis for each patient and is based on a risk/benefit analysis. Let us consider the pros and cons of this class of medication.

Cholinesterase inhibitors are well tolerated

In our experience, supported by published clinical trials, cholinesterase inhibitors are tolerated by more than 90% of patients. The most common side-effects, occurring in about 10% of patients, are gastrointestinal in nature including loss of appetite, upset stomach, mild nausea, and loose stools. These side-effects are due to muscarinic cholinergic receptors in the gut. In the majority of cases, these gastrointestinal side-effects subside in a few days and are not of any notable distress to the patients. In a small percentage of cases, the gastrointestinal side-effects are more serious and include nausea and vomiting or diarrhea. In these cases the patient should either stop taking the medication or reduce the dose. The gastrointestinal side-effects will then fully resolve within a few days. It is next worth trying at least one other cholinesterase inhibitor, as some patients experience more side-effects with one medication than with another. Unfortunately, patients who experience significant nausea, vomiting, or diarrhea with two or more of these medications are probably not good candidates for cholinesterase inhibitors. Some clinicians may try to manage these side-effects with antiemetic agents, but we have not found this to be a particularly helpful strategy (Table 14.2). In general, we suggest that patients take the medication in the evening so that, if they experience mild gastrointestinal side-effects during the peak concentrations (these generally occur within 2–6 hours after taking cholinesterase inhibitors), they can sleep through them.

Table 14.1 FDA-approved medications for the treatment of Alzheimer's disease (AD)

Drug	Mechanism of action	Half-life metabolism/ elimination	Dosing (therapeutic doses in italics)	Common side-effects	Comment	FDA approved	Demonstrated efficacy
Donepezil (generic & Aricept)	Inhibits acetylcholinesterase	70–80 h liver; CYP450: 2D6; 3A4 /urine and feces	Once daily • *5 mg QD 4 weeks* • *10 mg QD 3 months* • *23 mg QD (for moderate to severe patients)*	Nausea, vomiting, anorexia, diarrhea	Generally well tolerated. Also comes in same strength oral dissolving tablet	Alzheimer's disease. 5 mg QD: mild to moderate; 10 mg QD: mild, moderate, and severe; 23 mg QD: moderate to severe	Cognition (memory, attention), mood, behavior
Rivastigmine (Exelon) capsule	Inhibits acetylcholinesterase (also inhibits butylcholinesterase)	2 h plasma; CYP450 /urine 97%, feces 0.4%	Twice daily • *1.5 mg BID 4 weeks* • *3 mg BID 4 weeks* • *4.5–6 mg BID*	Nausea, vomiting, anorexia, diarrhea; side-effects more frequent than with others	Side-effects less if taken with food and titrated slowly	Mild, moderate Alzheimer's disease	Cognition (memory, attention) mood, behavior
Rivastigmine (Exelon) patch	Inhibits acetylcholinesterase (also inhibits butylcholinesterase)	2 h but in continuous release patch plasma; CYP450 /urine 97%, feces 0.4%	Once daily • *4.6 mg/24 h QD patch 4 weeks* • *9.5 mg/24 h QD patch*	Nausea, vomiting, anorexia, diarrhea; side-effects equal to or less than others	Well tolerated. Patch should be removed slowly and carefully to reduce skin irritation	Mild, moderate Alzheimer's disease and Parkinson's disease dementia	Cognition (memory, attention) mood, behavior

Drug	Mechanism	Pharmacokinetics	Dosing	Side effects	Notes	Indication	Effect measures
Galantamine (generic, formerly Razadyne and Reminyl)	Inhibits acetylcholinesterase (also has allosteric nicotinic modulation)	5–7 h liver partially; CYP450: 2D6; 3A4 /urine 95%, feces 5%	Twice daily • 4 mg BID 4 wks • 8 mg BID 4 wks • 12 mg BID	Nausea, vomiting, anorexia, diarrhea 12 mg dose side-effects more frequent	12 mg dose highly efficacious; side-effects less if taken with food	Mild, moderate Alzheimer's disease	Cognition (memory, attention) mood, behavior
Galantamine (extended release) (generic, formerly Razadyne and Reminyl)	Inhibits acetylcholinesterase (also has allosteric nicotinic modulation)	5–7 h, released immediately and 12 hours later (metabolism/ elimination as galantamine)	Once daily • 8 mg QD 4 wks • 16 mg QD 4 wks • 24 mg QD	Nausea, vomiting, anorexia, diarrhea 24 mg dose side-effects more frequent	24 mg dose highly efficacious; side-effects less if taken with food	Mild, moderate Alzheimer's disease	Cognition (memory, attention) mood, behavior
Memantine (Namenda)	Glutamate antagonist (also dopamine agonist)	60–80 h liver minimally; CYP450 /urine	Twice daily • 5 mg QAM 1wk • 5 mg BID 1 wk • 10 mg QAM, 5 mg QPM 1wk • 10 mg BID	Confusion, drowsiness	Can be taken with acetylcholinesterase inhibitors	Moderate, severe Alzheimer's disease	Cognition (attention, alertness) mood, behavior

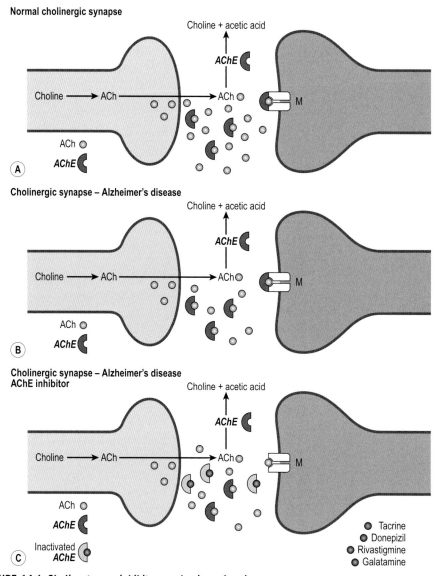

Normal cholinergic synapse

Cholinergic synapse – Alzheimer's disease

**Cholinergic synapse – Alzheimer's disease
AChE inhibitor**

- Tacrine
- Donepizil
- Rivastigmine
- Galatamine

FIGURE 14.1 Cholinesterase inhibitor mechanism of action.

(A) Normal cholinergic synapse with muscarinic receptor (M). Note the large number of acetylcholine (ACh) molecules. Acetylcholinesterase (AChE) breaks down acetylcholine into choline and acetic acid. (B) Cholinergic synapse in Alzheimer's disease (AD). Because the neurons that produce acetylcholine in the nucleus basalis of Mynert are being damaged and destroyed by Alzheimer's disease pathology, there are many fewer molecules of acetylcholine available. (C) The cholinesterase inhibitors tacrine, donepezil, rivastigmine, and galantamine reversibly inhibit acetylcholinesterase such that more molecules of acetylcholine are available in the synapse.

Table 14.2 Selected side-effects of cholinesterase inhibitors and possible management techniques

Side-effect	Possible management technique
Loss of appetite	Take at night or reduce dose
Nausea	Take at night or reduce dose
Vomiting	Reduce dose
Diarrhea	Can try over-the-counter *Imodium A-D* or the like once or twice a week to reduce bowel movements to 1 or 2 per day. Or reduce dose
Vivid dreams	Take in the morning or reduce dose
Dizziness	Depends upon the cause; investigate swiftly whether this could be a sign of bradycardia (slowing of the heart rate)
Dehydration	Determine cause, increase hydration, and/or reduce dose
Insomnia	Take in the morning or reduce dose
Headache	Reduce dose
Rhinorrhea (runny nose)	Reduce dose
Salivation	Reduce dose
Muscle cramps	Increase water intake, increase electrolyte intake including eating bananas (for potassium) and taking over-the-counter magnesium oxide, or reduce dose
Fasciculations	Reduce dose
Rash	Discontinue immediately. Can later try another cholinesterase inhibitor
Bradycardia (slowing of the heart rate)	Discontinue immediately, and immediately initiate an inpatient cardiac evaluation including continuous cardiac monitor
Seizure	If single brief seizure: reduce dose and initiate seizure evaluation. If multiple or prolonged: discontinue immediately and initiate seizure evaluation

Note: This table contains some of the common and/or serious side-effects that our patients have experienced and some strategies that we have found to be successful in dealing with these side-effects. It is not meant to be an exhaustive list nor a substitute for clinical judgment. When in doubt regarding a serious side-effect, discontinue the cholinesterase inhibitor and fully evaluate the patient.

A second common side-effect is vivid dreams. These dreams are not nightmares; in general they are the dreams the patient normally has, just more vivid. These are brought about by the role of brainstem cholinergic systems in producing rapid eye movement (REM) sleep (dream sleep). Vivid dreams are generally characterized by our patients as being extremely realistic and lifelike. In some instances patients find these disturbing; in other cases they are neutral about them; and occasionally they even find them enjoyable. In cases where patients find these unpleasant, vivid dreams can usually be minimized or eliminated by moving the dosing of the medication to earlier in the day. This will cause the peak concentration of the medication to be during waking hours and the troughs at night.

Other less common side-effects reported in the clinical trials of cholinesterase inhibitors are dizziness, insomnia, and headache. Other side-effects of note in our clinical experience (and also reported in controlled studies) are rhinorrhea (runny nose), increased salivation, muscle cramping, fasciculations, rash, and rarely seizures or a slowing of the heart rate (one of our patients developed syncope and ultimately required a pacemaker). We recommend caution in prescribing cholinesterase inhibitors when patients have any of the

---

BOX 14.1 SERIOUS REACTIONS AND CONDITIONS THAT EITHER CONTRAINDICATE OR REQUIRE CAUTION WHEN PRESCRIBING CHOLINESTERASE INHIBITORS

- Hypersensitivity to the specific drug or class of medications
- Hypersensitivity to cholinergic medications such as succinylcholine
- Syncope/cardiac conduction disorders/sick sinus syndrome – can cause bradycardia or heart block
- Seizures and seizure disorders – can lower seizure threshold
- Asthma and chronic obstructive pulmonary disease – can increase secretions and/or cause bronchospasm
- Peptic ulcer disease – can worsen peptic ulcer disease
- Concomitant use of non-steroidal anti-inflammatory drugs – can increase risk of peptic ulcer disease
- Urinary obstruction
- Hepatic impairment – can raise cholinesterase inhibitor levels
- Renal impairment – can raise cholinesterase inhibitor levels (particularly for galantamine)

Note: This box contains some of the more serious side-effects, cautions, and contraindications of the cholinesterase inhibitors that have been reported. It is not meant to be an exhaustive list nor a substitute for clinical judgment. When in doubt regarding a serious side-effect, discontinue the cholinesterase inhibitor and fully evaluate the patient. When in doubt regarding whether to start a medication, consult expert colleagues or do not start the cholinesterase inhibitor.

Adapted from www.online.epocrates.com, Aricept, Razadyne ER, and Exelon, accessed 8/15/2009.

---

conditions in Box 14.1. Cholinesterase inhibitors may interact with many other medications. Although in our experience few of these interactions are clinically important, it is important to be aware of them (Box 14.2).

Cholinesterase inhibitors are efficacious

Comprehensive reviews of the efficacy of cholinesterase inhibitors generally conclude that the drugs have modest benefits in some, but not all, patients. For example, one comprehensive review carried out by the Cochrane Collaboration (Birks, 2006) concluded that, in patients with mild, moderate, or severe dementia due to Alzheimer's disease, those treated with donepezil (Aricept), rivastigmine (Exelon), or galantamine (Razadyne) showed benefit on objective measures compared with patients treated with placebo. Additionally, clinicians who were blinded to the results of these objective cognitive tests judged patients on cholinesterase inhibitors to be doing better than patients on placebo.

This conclusion is certainly consistent with our clinical experience using these drugs in thousands of patients. We have found that in most, but not all, of our patients there is benefit in terms of both cognitive function and daily activities. When we talk to the caregivers, their most common description of the patient taking these medications is that not only do these medications improve memory but also that the patient is "more with it." By this they mean that they are more engaged in family activities, they are more likely to participate in day-to-day activities in the home such as setting the table or walking the dog, and they are more likely to engage in conversation in social situations. How much improvement should we and caregivers expect to see? Both studies (for review see Cummings, 2004) and our experience suggest that for the majority of patients the response to cholinesterase inhibitors is equivalent to "turning back the clock" on their disease by 6–12 months. In other words, we expect that their memory and general level of functioning

BOX 14.2 MEDICATIONS THAT MAY INTERACT WITH CHOLINESTERASE INHIBITORS

- Amiodarone (may increase cholinesterase inhibitor levels)
- Anticholinergics (may decrease cholinesterase inhibitor efficacy)
- Aspirin and aspirin combination drugs (may increase risk of gastrointestinal bleeding)
- Azole antifungals (may increase cholinesterase inhibitor levels)
- Beta blockers (may cause bradycardia and bronchospasm)
- Bupropion (may lower seizure threshold, may increase cholinesterase inhibitor levels)
- Carbamazepine (may decrease cholinesterase inhibitor levels)
- Chloramphenicol (may increase cholinesterase inhibitor levels)
- Chlorpromazine (may increase cholinesterase inhibitor levels)
- Cholinergic agents (may increase cholinergic effects and cholinergic toxicity)
- Cholinesterase inhibitors, including ophthalmic agents (may increase cholinergic effects and cholinergic toxicity)
- Cinacalcet (may increase cholinesterase inhibitor levels)
- Clarithromycins (may increase cholinesterase inhibitor levels)
- Clozapine (may decrease cholinesterase inhibitor levels)
- Conivaptan (may increase cholinesterase inhibitor levels)
- Cyclobenzaprine (may decrease cholinesterase inhibitor efficacy)
- Cyclopentolate/phenylephrine ophthalmic (may decrease efficacy of ophthalmic agent)
- Darifenacin (may decrease anticholinergic efficacy)
- Darunavir (may increase cholinesterase inhibitor levels)
- Delavirdine (may increase cholinesterase inhibitor levels)
- Dexamethasone (may decrease cholinesterase inhibitor levels)
- Diclofenac topical (may increase risk of gastrointestinal bleeding)
- Dipyridamole (may decrease cholinesterase inhibitor efficacy)
- Erythromycins (may increase cholinesterase inhibitor levels)
- Fluvoxamine (may increase cholinesterase inhibitor levels)
- Haloperidol (may increase cholinesterase inhibitor levels)
- Imatinib (may increase cholinesterase inhibitor levels)
- Inhaled anesthetics (may decrease efficacy of neuromuscular blocking effect as well as efficacy of antimyesthenic agent)
- Itraconazole (may increase cholinesterase inhibitor levels)
- Ketoconazole (may increase cholinesterase inhibitor levels)
- Lindane topical (may lower seizure threshold)
- Local anesthetics, esters (chloroprocaine, procaine) (may increase risk of local anesthetic toxicity)
- Modafinil (may decrease cholinesterase inhibitor levels)
- Nefazodone (may increase cholinesterase inhibitor levels)
- Neuromuscular blockers, non-depolarizing (may decrease non-depolarizing neuromuscular blocker efficacy)
- Nevirapine (may decrease cholinesterase inhibitor levels)
- Nilotinib (may increase cholinesterase inhibitor levels)
- Non-steroidal anti-inflammatory drugs (NSAIDs) and NSAID combinations (may increase risk of gastrointestinal bleeding)
- Olanzapine/fluoxetine (may increase cholinesterase inhibitor levels)
- Orphenadrine (may decrease cholinergic agent efficacy)
- Oxcarbazepine (may decrease cholinesterase inhibitor levels)
- Perphenazine (may increase cholinesterase inhibitor levels)
- Phenobarbital (may decrease cholinesterase inhibitor levels)
- Phenytoins (may decrease cholinesterase inhibitor levels)
- Posaconazole (may increase cholinesterase inhibitor levels)
- Primidone (may decrease cholinesterase inhibitor levels)
- Propafenone (may increase cholinesterase inhibitor levels)

Continued

BOX 14.2 MEDICATIONS THAT MAY INTERACT WITH CHOLINESTERASE INHIBITORS—Cont'd

- Propoxyphene (may increase cholinesterase inhibitor levels)
- Protease inhibitors (may increase cholinesterase inhibitor levels)
- Quinidine (may increase cholinesterase inhibitor levels)
- Ranolazine (may increase cholinesterase inhibitor levels)
- Rifabutin (may decrease cholinesterase inhibitor levels)
- Rifampins (may decrease cholinesterase inhibitor levels)
- Rifapentine (may decrease cholinesterase inhibitor levels)
- Ritonavir (may increase cholinesterase inhibitor levels)
- SSRIs 1 (2D6 inhibitors) (may increase cholinesterase inhibitor levels)
- Sodium phosphate (may lower seizure threshold)
- Solifenacin (may decrease cholinesterase inhibitor effects)
- Telithromycin (may increase cholinesterase inhibitor levels)
- Terbinafine (may increase cholinesterase inhibitor levels)
- Thioridazine (may increase cholinesterase inhibitor levels)
- Thiotepa (may increase cholinesterase inhibitor levels)
- Tigabine (may lower seizure threshold)
- Tipranavir (may increase cholinesterase inhibitor levels)
- Tramadol (may lower seizure threshold)
- Voriconazole (may increase cholinesterase inhibitor levels)

Note: This box contains some of the common and/or serious drug interactions that have been reported. It is not meant to be an exhaustive list nor a substitute for clinical judgment. When in doubt regarding a serious side-effect or interaction, discontinue the cholinesterase inhibitor and fully evaluate the patient.

Adapted from www.online.epocrates.com, Aricept, Razadyne ER, and Exelon, accessed 8/15/2009.

---

will return to where they were 6–12 months ago. For these reasons as well as the data from well-done research studies, we generally recommend a trial on one of these drugs to our patients with Alzheimer's disease.

Thus, it is clear from the preceding discussion that cholinesterase inhibitors are safe and effective in the majority of patients. But how do we know if a cholinesterase inhibitor is working in an individual patient?

IS THE MEDICATION WORKING?

One of the thorniest problems facing the practicing clinician who treats patients with Alzheimer's disease is how to judge the benefit (or lack thereof) of an anti-dementia drug in an individual patient. In our clinical research setting, each patient undergoes a comprehensive cognitive evaluation during most visits. These visits can take between 1 and 1.5 hours. By using the data from these evaluations in conjunction with interviewing the patients and caregivers we can make highly reliable judgments regarding the efficacy of the treatment. But we certainly recognize that this type of evaluation is not feasible in the context of a busy primary care or even specialty practice. The challenge then becomes to find techniques to judge the efficacy of treatment that work day-to-day in a busy practice setting.

In general, we would recommend two general strategies in addition to speaking with the patient and family for evaluating the effects on cognition of anti-dementia compounds. The first is to use a brief objective measure of cognition. The second is to use a global measure of overall functioning of the patient. As the reader may recognize, these strategies are similar to criteria used to measure drug benefit in clinical trials of anti-dementia compounds.

In terms of visit frequency, we generally see the patient 2–3 months after starting a cholinesterase inhibitor and then every 6 months thereafter.

Measuring cognition

As discussed in Chapter 2: *Evaluating the patient with memory loss* and in Appendix A: *Cognitive test and questionnaire forms, instructions, and normative data*, there are numerous brief measures of cognition which can be used to assess the efficacy of cholinesterase inhibitors. Probably the two which are most commonly used are the Mini-Mental State Examination (MMSE; Folstein et al., 1975) and the Blessed Information, Memory, and Concentration (BIMC) test (Blessed et al., 1968). The Montreal Cognitive Assessment (MoCA; www.mocatest.org) test is a newer test. Each of these can be administered in less than 10 minutes by office staff. In general, after successful treatment with cholinesterase inhibitors patients tend to improve 2 or 3 points on the MMSE and the MoCA and 3 or 4 points on the BIMC test.

Measuring general functioning

In contrast to measures of cognition, there are few measures of general functioning that are appropriate for the practicing clinician. Rather than using a specific instrument, we tend to use a structured interview that generally asks about three areas: cognition, mood and behavior, and function. The interview is typically carried out in about 10 minutes, with the patient and caregiver either together or separately (Table 14.3). At the end of the interview, we attempt to arrive at a judgment as to whether the patient shows:

- marked improvement
- moderate improvement
- mild improvement
- unchanged
- mild worsening
- moderate worsening
- marked worsening.

Box 14.3 provides some guidelines that we find helpful in determining into which of the above categories we would place a particular patient. We often find it helpful to compare the results of the current interview with the interview we conducted when we initially evaluated the patient to determine how things have changed. If our judgment is that the patient is unchanged or improved in the initial follow-up visit, we take this as evidence that the drug is having benefit—especially when this judgment is supported by the results of a brief cognitive test. (Remember that the expectation is that over a 6-month period the patient will decline.) If the patient is only mildly worse, we also typically extend treatment for another 6 months. For patients who are moderately or markedly worse, we question whether the medication is working, and we would often try another cholinesterase inhibitor.

Sudden changes

A word of caution when the patient is moderately or significantly worse. If there are sudden and rapid changes we consider the possibility of a medical or psychiatric condition that may affect cognition. The most common medical conditions include a urinary tract

Table 14.3 Brief clinical interview for follow-up visits
Instructions: Note changes in any of the following cognitive areas. If there are changes, you may find it helpful to briefly note the nature of the changes (i.e., what area improved or worsened)

	YES (a change) (better or worse?)	NO (no change)	N/S (not sure)
Forgetting information over short periods of time			
Repeating stories or questions about events of the day			
Difficulty handling financial matters (e.g, problems with checkbook or paying bills)			
Problems with judgment (e.g., poor financial decisions, difficulty making decisions)			
Confusion about the correct day, date, month or year			
Seeming bewildered or confused in a familiar setting			
Difficulty learning something new (e.g., learning to use a new appliance, gadget or computer program)			
Social withdrawal (e.g., participating less in conversations)			
Loss of interest in usual activities (e.g., hobbies)			
Difficulty with everyday activities (e.g., self-care or dressing, household tasks, finding one's way around, using appliances such as telephone or television)			

BOX 14.3 CRITERIA FOR IMPROVEMENT OR WORSENING OF GENERAL FUNCTION

- *Mild improvement:* A noticeable improvement in the patient's functioning, social interactions, or mental clarity in any aspect of performance, capabilities, tendencies, or tolerances. The change should be noticeable enough to make a difference in some aspect of day-to-day function and behavior even if it does not result in any greater independence for the patient.
- *Moderate improvement:* Similarly defined but with the additional requirement that some measure of functional independence—social, instrumental, cognitive—has been regained.
- *Marked improvement:* Carries the additional requirement that a major activity in the patient's daily routine or in mental status has been regained, in addition to regaining some measure of functional independence.
- *Mild worsening:* A noticeable decline in patient's functioning, social interactions, or mental clarity in any aspect of performance, capabilities, tendencies, or tolerances. The change should be noticeable enough to make a difference in some aspect of day-to-day function and behavior even if it does not result in any greater dependence on the part of the patient.
- *Moderate worsening:* Similarly defined but with the additional requirement that, on some measure, functional dependence has emerged.
- *Marked worsening:* Carries the additional requirement that a major activity in the patient's daily activity or mental status has been lost, in addition to loss of functional independence on some measure.

infection or pneumonia, either one of which can have dramatic deleterious effects on cognition in our experience. Strokes and other more serious conditions can of course also occur. The most common psychiatric conditions, especially early in the disease when the patient maintains insight, are depression and anxiety. In these cases, treating the medical or psychiatric condition will often positively affect cognition.

WHICH CHOLINESTERASE INHIBITOR SHOULD I PRESCRIBE?

There are currently three cholinesterase inhibitors available. How should a clinician choose? In general, this decision can be made based on four factors: efficacy, safety and tolerability, convenience for the patient/caregiver, and cost.

Efficacy and tolerability

Was Joe Louis a better boxer than Mohammed Ali? Were the 1927 Yankees better than the 1998 Yankees? These questions can lead to interesting and sometimes contentious conversation in the local sports bar and they are the stuff that computer simulations are made of. But no amount of debate, discussion or contention, and no computer program can answer these questions. There is only one way to solve the debate: the 1927 Yankees would have to play the 1998 team on the same field (artificial turf or grass), with the same baseball (live vs. dead ball era), in the same weather, with the same fans. In short, we would need to have "head-to-head" competition.

Is rivastigmine (Exelon) better than galantamine (Razadyne)? Is galantamine (Razadyne) better than donepezil (Aricept)? There are now dozens of studies on each of these drugs individually reporting efficacy and safety. And while it is tempting to compare the percentage of patients who experience side-effects on each drug or the number of points that each drug differs from placebo in each trial, these are entirely inappropriate comparisons. Although on the surface the studies appear to have similar patients, designs, and outcome measures, the only way to answer this question (as in the sports analogy) is to conduct a head-to-head comparison. That is, test multiple cholinesterase inhibitors in the same study with the same group of patients, the same experimental design, and the same outcome measures. To date only a few direct comparisons have been done.

The results of the head-to-head studies do not yield any clear choice. To date there have been a number of head-to-head trials comparing the effects of different cholinesterase inhibitors. The data from the majority of these trials are difficult to interpret because they were conducted using an "open-label design," that is, the patients knew what drugs they were taking (Wilkinson et al., 2002; Wilcock et al., 2003; Jones et al., 2004; Bullock et al., 2005).

In our experience, donepezil (Aricept) at doses of 5 and 10 mg is equally efficacious and well tolerated as galantamine (Razadyne) ER (extended release) at doses of 8 and 16 mg. Galantamine (Razadyne) ER at the 24 mg dose is probably equivalent to 15 mg (a non-standard dose) of donepezil (Aricept); in each case the efficacy is greater than the lower dose but so are the side-effects. Our clinical experience suggests that the rivastigmine (Exelon) capsule may have somewhat more side-effects than either galantamine (Razadyne) ER or donepezil (Aricept) at therapeutic doses, consistent with one of the open-label trials (Wikinson et al., 2002). However, our experience is also that the rivastigmine (Exelon) patch is both efficacious and well tolerated.

In brief, there is no reason to believe that one cholinesterase inhibitor is more or less effective than any other.

Convenience

Besides efficacy and tolerability, a third factor that can lead to favoring one cholinesterase inhibitor over another is convenience (Table 14.1). Two primary factors seem important: (1) how frequently is the drug taken and (2) how complex is the titration scheme.

Remembering to take medications is challenging for everyone. It is especially challenging for patients with memory problems. Because of this, medications that are taken less frequently may be desirable.

WHAT IS THE BEST DOSE?

In general, the higher the dose of a cholinesterase inhibitor the greater the efficacy but also the greater the likelihood of side-effects. Most studies of cholinesterase inhibitors have found that higher doses are more efficacious than lower doses. But higher doses are more likely to produce side-effects, typically loss of appetite, nausea, vomiting, and diarrhea as discussed above. So the prescribing clinician will generally attempt to achieve a balance of using the highest dose without producing side-effects.

Each of the three cholinesterase inhibitors mentioned provides instructions in the labeling to guide the clinician through a tested titration scheme (Table 14.1). Our experience suggests that these titration schemes work for most patients, who can achieve the highest dose in the absence of side-effects. In some cases, however, an even more gradual titration scheme may help some patients achieve the highest recommended dose.

For example, the common titration scheme for donepezil (Aricept) is that the patient begins with a dose of 5 mg once per day, taken in the evening. This continues for 1 month and, if it is well tolerated, the dose is increased to 10 mg, the highest recommended dose for mildly affected patients. In some cases, the patient tolerates the 5 mg dose with no side-effects, but when the dose is increased to 10 mg he or she may experience gastrointestinal distress or other side-effects. In these cases, we immediately return the patient to the 5 mg dose until the side-effects resolve. We may then attempt a slower titration schedule. For example, we may have them alternate 5 and 10 mg doses (5 mg every other day with 10 mg on the alternate days) for several weeks before increasing to 10 mg daily. In some patients we have found that this will help them tolerate the higher dose. For some patients 5 mg in the morning and 5 mg in the evening is easier than 10 mg all at once. And although not quite as good as 10 mg per day, 5 mg daily is a perfectly acceptable dose. Note that some clinicians (including us) have used donepezil off-label in a 15 mg dose. Again, the logic is that, for those who can tolerate the dose, more is better. Supporting this idea, the FDA has recently approved a 23 mg dose of donepezil for patients with moderate to severe Alzheimer's disease. Patients can be tried on this higher dose after being on the 10 mg dose for 3 months. We have less experience with this higher dose but expect greater efficacy in those patients who can tolerate it.

For galantamine we would always recommend the extended release (galantamine ER) formulation as it is both once-a-day and it is also better tolerated than the older, immediate release, galantamine. Both 16 mg and 24 mg are good therapeutic doses. The 24 mg dose may have somewhat greater efficacy but also somewhat more frequent side-effects compared with the 16 mg dose. As mentioned above, in our experience 16 mg of galantamine ER is roughly equivalent to 10 mg of donepezil (Aricept), and 24 mg of galantamine ER is roughly equivalent to 15 mg of donepezil (Aricept).

For rivastigmine (Exelon) we would always recommend the patch as it is both once-a-day and also better tolerated than the capsules. Studies have shown that 9.5 mg/24 h is a good therapeutic dose; we have also found that lower starting dose of 4.6 mg/24 h has been helpful in some patients who are particularly sensitive to cholinesterase inhibitors. The patch has one particular side-effect which is related to its being a patch: there can be skin irritation when it is removed. Although there is some debate regarding the exact cause of this irritation, in our experience it is mainly local irritation related to how the patch is pulled off. The patch should be pulled off slowly. It should NOT be pulled off quickly like a Band-Aid. The patch sticks on very tight. The strong adhesive has the advantage of allowing the patient to swim and shower with it—without it falling off. But it has the disadvantage that it must be carefully taken off, usually slowly by the caregiver using two hands, one to lift up the patch, and one to hold down the skin. Additional instructions can be found on the comprehensive package insert.

WHEN SHOULD THE MEDICATIONS BE TAKEN?

Donepezil (generic and Aricept) is taken once a day. In general, we start patients taking the drug in the evening. The rationale is that, if they experience mild gastrointestinal side-effects, they will sleep through them. But another common side-effect of donepezil (Aricept) is vivid dreams. These are not nightmares and most cases are not disturbing to patients—some patients even enjoy these dreams—but in some cases patients do complain of these dreams. In these cases we recommend that the patients take the medication in the morning and this usually alleviates the vivid dreams. For galantamine ER we usually start patients taking the drug in the morning and then switch to evening if needed to help reduce gastrointestinal side-effects. For the rivastigmine (Exelon) patch the medication is delivered continuously, such that the time of day the new patch is applied does not matter.

DOES IT HELP TO SWITCH MEDICATIONS?

One question that often comes up is whether switching from one cholinesterase inhibitor to another might be beneficial in terms of either efficacy or side-effects. Although the medications all work in the same way so that in theory there is no reason why a patient should show more benefits or side-effects on one medication than another, in practice there is some variability of response, both real and perceived. So that if shortly after starting one cholinesterase inhibitor there is not only no improvement but also no stabilization (or there is a decline), and/or there are notable side-effects, we may try another cholinesterase inhibitor. Everyone is different, and some patients do better with one medication than another. Note, however, that in our clinic switching is uncommon and we will end up doing this in fewer than one in 25 patients.

In a different scenario, sometimes after a patient has been on a cholinesterase inhibitor for a time, either the patient or the family will ask whether switching to another cholinesterase inhibitor might provide him or her with more benefit. As long as the patient had a good response initially, we would recommend that he or she continue the current medication as it is unlikely that the patient will benefit more from one cholinesterase inhibitor than another, and the new medication may not work as well as the original.

HOW DO I DISCUSS WITH THE PATIENT WHETHER THE CHOLINESTERASE INHIBITOR IS WORKING?

Determining whether an antihypertensive medication is efficacious is a straightforward process: you measure blood pressure and ask about side-effects. If the pressure is reduced and side-effects are absent or minimal, the drug is working well. Determining whether an anti-dementia compound is working is more complex for several reasons, as follows.

- As discussed above, we do not have a "blood pressure cuff" for cognition. There is no single, readily used measure that is appropriate in day-to-day practice that gives an accurate measure of changes in cognition.
- The patient may be benefiting from the anti-dementia medication even if there is no apparent symptomatic improvement. About half of our patients and their families report improved cognition with the use of cholinesterase inhibitors. But the other half report no change. No change, however, may actually be benefit in a progressive degenerative disease such as Alzheimer's. Any drug that can "turn the clock back" on this decline is beneficial. But conveying this information to patients and their families can be challenging.

When we treat patients with cholinesterase inhibitors, we try first to explain: (1) what is happening in their brain, (2) how these drugs affect the ongoing process in their brain, (3) what they can expect from these drugs, and (4) how we will measure this. The conversation might proceed as follows:

Mrs. Jones, as we have discussed, the cause of your memory and related problems is Alzheimer's disease. Alzheimer's is a brain disease. What is happening in your brain is that brain cells called neurons are slowly dying. Unlike cells in other parts of your body, brain cells do not regenerate. Once they die they are lost forever. Although the drug that you will be taking will not prevent these brain cells from dying, it can help with the symptoms of your disease—your thinking and memory—by allowing the remaining brain cells to function more efficiently. By doing this we hope that we can turn the clock back on your brain disorder. If the medication is working we will expect that your thinking and memory will return to how they were about 6–12 months ago. So we would not expect any huge changes, but we do hope to see small but noticeable and important changes. We will see you back in 2–3 months to get a sense as to how you are doing and whether the medication is working. Even if you do not notice any changes, the medication may still be working. We will talk with you and your family and we will also give you tests of memory, much like the ones you have already done in this clinic. We will decide together at that time whether to continue the medication or try another. After that we will see you about every 6 months. Many of our patients ask if we can stop the decline of Alzheimer's disease. With the medications currently available we cannot. Although we can turn the clock back on your memory loss, we cannot stop the decline that occurs over time. However, the vast majority of people do benefit from this medication, and there are new medications being developed every day, many of which do have the potential to significantly slow down or halt this disease.

We have found that, when we establish appropriate expectations at the beginning of the medication trial, patients are more likely to remain on medication for a long enough period of time to determine if it is indeed providing benefit. As discussed, using Table 14.3 and Box 14.3 for measuring the general functional outcome can be useful, along with talking with the patient, talking with family or other caregivers, and (if possible) repeating a brief cognitive test.

CHOLINESTERASE INHIBITORS IN LATE-STAGE DISEASE

Donepezil (generic and Aricept) is FDA approved to treat severe Alzheimer's disease, and in our experience all of the cholinesterase inhibitors can be helpful to preserve function in late-stage disease. For this reason, we would always continue the patient's cholinesterase inhibitor into the severe stage of Alzheimer's disease. We recommend discontinuing the cholinesterase inhibitor when the patient is no longer able to enjoy any aspect of life and the goal of treatment changes to that of trying to help the patient die with comfort and dignity. Typically this occurs after the patient has been living in a nursing home for a number of years, can no longer feed him- or herself, and no longer takes any pleasure in visits with family members. Within 2 weeks of discontinuing the cholinesterase inhibitor the patient generally shows a fairly dramatic decline in function (equivalent to about a 6- to 12-month decline), which generally hastens death.

We also recommend starting a cholinesterase inhibitor in the severe stage of the disease as long as there is function that one wishes to preserve. The one difference in starting a cholinesterase inhibitor at this stage of Alzheimer's disease is that we do not expect to see benefit or even stabilization. All the studies of patients with severe Alzheimer's disease have consistently shown less decline, rather than improvement or stabilization, with cholinesterase inhibitors compared with control.

CHOLINESTERASE INHIBITORS IN OTHER DISORDERS

Should cholinesterase inhibitors be used in disorders other than Alzheimer's disease? Other causes of dementia? Other memory disorders? There are a number of studies which have examined the use of cholinesterase inhibitors in disorders other than Alzheimer's disease, and we have had experience using cholinesterase inhibitors in these plus a few additional disorders (Box 14.4). As discussed in the relevant chapters, there are a number of well-conducted randomized double-blind placebo-controlled trials examining the use of

---

BOX 14.4 OTHER DISORDERS TO CONSIDER THE USE OF CHOLINESTERASE INHIBITORS

- Mild Cognitive Impairment (MCI)
- Dementia with Lewy bodies
- Vascular dementia
- Multiple sclerosis impairing memory
- Traumatic brain injury impairing memory
- Single strokes impairing memory
- Tumor resection impairing memory

cholinesterase inhibitors in mild cognitive impairment (e.g., Petersen et al., 2005), vascular dementia (e.g., Moretti et al., 2003), and Parkinson's disease dementia (dementia with Lewy bodies) (e.g., McKeith et al., 2000). The majority of these studies have found benefit with cholinesterase inhibitors. Further, the FDA has approved the rivastigmine (Exelon) patch for Parkinson's disease dementia. Our clinical experience in all of these disorders is similar: we believe that cholinesterase inhibitors are of benefit, with patients showing improvement of the same order of magnitude as patients with Alzheimer's disease experience. Therefore, we generally recommend or prescribe cholinesterase inhibitors for patients with mild cognitive impairment, vascular dementia, and Parkinson's disease dementia (dementia with Lewy bodies), just as we would for Alzheimer's disease.

There are a few additional disorders that we have also had positive experience with using cholinesterase inhibitors and/or there are suggestive studies (though not necessarily randomized, double-blind, and placebo-controlled). There are a number of studies which have examined either multiple sclerosis (Christodoulou et al., 2006) or traumatic brain injury (Kim et al., 2009), almost all of which found that cholinesterase inhibitors showed benefit. Our experience is similar: patients with multiple sclerosis and traumatic brain injury generally show benefit from cholinesterase inhibitors, particularly if memory and/or attention is one of the major problems for these patients. Although there are few or no studies to support it, we have also found that patients who experience memory problems due to single strokes or tumor resections may also benefit from cholinesterase inhibitors. In general, we find that as a class the cholinesterase inhibitors are medications which can improve memory, regardless of the underlying cause of the memory loss. Therefore, if there are patients who experience memory loss from other disorders (e.g., encephalitis), we would be willing to give a trial of a cholinesterase inhibitor to see if it is helpful.

Lastly, there are a few disorders in which we would not recommend cholinesterase inhibitors or we would recommend using extreme caution. Patients with frontotemporal dementias typically do not benefit from cholinesterase inhibitors. There is no biochemical deficit of acetylcholine in frontotemporal dementia, and our experience is that sometimes these patients become further agitated and/or disinhibited when given a cholinesterase inhibitor. Similarly, we would tend to avoid cholinesterase inhibitors in patients with bipolar disorder, or other tendencies toward mania. Please also see Box 14.1 for additional disorders that require caution in the use of cholinesterase inhibitors.

References

Birks, J., 2006. Cholinesterase inhibitors for Alzheimer's disease. Cochrane Database Syst. Rev. CD005593.

Blessed, G., Tomlinson, B.E., Roth, M., 1968. The association between quantitative measures of dementia and of senile change in the cerebral grey matter of elderly subjects. Br. J. Psychiatry 114, 797–811.

Bullock, R., Touchon, J., Bergman, H., et al., 2005. Rivastigmine and donepezil treatment in moderate to moderately-severe Alzheimer's disease over a 2-year period. Curr. Med. Res. Opin. 21, 1317–1327.

Christodoulou, C., Melville, P., Scherl, W.F., et al., 2006. Effects of donepezil on memory and cognition in multiple sclerosis. J. Neurol. Sci. 245, 127–136.

Cummings, J.L., 2004. Alzheimer's disease. N. Engl. J. Med. 351, 56–67.

Folstein, M.F., Folstein, S.E., McHugh, P.R., 1975. A practical method for grading the cognitive state of patients for the clinician. J. Psychiatr. Res. 12, 189–198.

Jones, R.W., Soininen, H., Hager, K., et al., 2004. A multinational, randomised, 12-week study comparing the effects of donepezil and galantamine in patients with mild to moderate Alzheimer's disease. Int. J. Geriatr. Psychiatry 19, 58–67.

Kim, Y.W., Kim, D.Y., Shin, J.C., et al., 2009. The changes of cortical metabolism associated with the clinical response to donepezil therapy in traumatic brain injury. Clin. Neuropharmacol. 32, 63–68.

McKeith, I., Del Ser, T., Spano, P., et al., 2000. Efficacy of rivastigmine in dementia with Lewy bodies: a randomised, double-blind, placebo-controlled international study. Lancet 356, 2031–2036.

Moretti, R., Torre, P., Antonello, R.M., et al., 2003. Rivastigmine in subcortical vascular dementia: a randomized, controlled, open 12-month study in 208 patients. Am. J. Alzheimers Dis. Other. Demen. 18, 265–272.

Petersen, R.C., Thomas, R.G., Grundman, M., et al., 2005. Vitamin E and donepezil for the treatment of mild cognitive impairment. N. Engl. J. Med. 352, 2379–2388.

Wilcock, G., Howe, I., Coles, H., et al., 2003. A long-term comparison of galantamine and donepezil in the treatment of Alzheimer's disease. Drugs Aging 20, 777–789.

Wilkinson, D.G., Passmore, A.P., Bullock, R., et al., 2002. A multinational, randomised, 12-week, comparative study of donepezil and rivastigmine in patients with mild to moderate Alzheimer's disease. Int. J. Clin. Pract. 56, 441–446.

15 Memantine (Namenda)

QUICK START: MEMANTINE (NAMENDA)

Mechanism of action and cognitive benefit
- Memantine (Namenda) has two mechanisms of action: (1) modulating glutamate and (2) enhancing dopamine transmission.
- It improves attention, alertness, apathy, and global functioning.

Indications and recommendations
- Memantine (Namenda) is approved for patients with moderate to severe Alzheimer's disease (MMSE < 15).
- It is prescribed twice a day, and generally titrated as follows:
  - Week 1: 5 mg QAM
  - Week 2: 5 mg BID
  - Week 3: 10 mg QAM, 5 mg QPM
  - Week 4: 10 mg BID
- Combination therapy—cholinesterase inhibitors plus memantine—gives the best short- and long-term outcomes in patients with moderate to severe Alzheimer's disease.

Common side-effects
- Common side-effects include dizziness, confusion, and drowsiness.

Judging efficacy
- Memantine (Namenda) improves attention and alertness (not memory per se).
- To determine whether the medication is working, ask the family and evaluate the patient's cognition, social engagement, and function 2 months after starting the medication.

Off-label uses
- Memantine (Namenda) is sometimes helpful in mild Alzheimer's disease when treating impaired attention, alertness, and apathy.
- Patients with vascular dementia and dementia with Lewy bodies (and Parkinson's disease dementia) also benefit from memantine (Namenda), following the same guidelines as for Alzheimer's disease.
- Patients with frontotemporal dementia sometimes benefit from memantine (Namenda).

Memantine (Namenda) was approved by the FDA for the treatment of moderate to severe Alzheimer's disease in 2003. It has become the second most widely used drug after donepezil (Aricept) to treat Alzheimer's disease. Much of what we have discussed regarding the cholinesterase inhibitors also pertains to memantine (Namenda). But, in addition to a different mechanism of action, there are also important differences between memantine (Namenda) and the cholinesterase inhibitors in terms of which patients are most likely to benefit, how the drug is administered, and its side-effect profile. We will also discuss how memantine (Namenda) can be combined with cholinesterase inhibitors.

MECHANISM OF ACTION

Memantine (Namenda) has an entirely different mechanism of action than the cholinesterase inhibitors. There are, in fact, at least two mechanisms of action for memantine (Namenda) which may be clinically relevant: modulating glutamate and enhancing dopamine transmission.

Modulating glutamate transmission

Memantine (Namenda) acts on neurons that use glutamate as a neural transmitter. Glutamate is one of a group of neural transmitters knows as *amino acid neural transmitters.* Other amino acid neural transmitters include GABA, aspartame, and others, although glutamate is the most abundant in this group. In fact, glutamate is the most abundant excitatory neural transmitter in the central nervous system, and it is present in about 40% of synapses. Like acetylcholine, glutamate is also very important in learning and memory. Numerous preclinical studies conducted in animals have shown that, when glutamate synapses are blocked, new memories cannot be formed (Wang & Morris, 2010). Additionally, there is evidence that the amnesia produced in humans from anoxia (e.g., oxygen deficiency due to cardiac arrest) is the result of the death of glutamatergic neurons.

When glutamate is released from the presynaptic neuron, it crosses the synapse and affects one or a number of different kinds of receptors on the postsynaptic neuron. One of these is the *N*-methyl-D-aspartic acid (NMDA) receptor. The NMDA receptor appears to be the crucial receptor in the formation of new memories. Memantine (Namenda) acts by regulating the NMDA receptor (Fig. 15.1).

Enhancing dopamine transmission

In addition to its effects at the NMDA receptor, there is also much evidence that memantine (Namenda) is a dopamine agonist. It stimulates dopamine receptors in vitro (Peeters et al., 2003), increases dopaminergic function in animal models (Spanagel et al., 1994), and patients with Parkinson's disease show improvement in their Parkinsonian symptoms (Merello et al., 1999). Why memantine (Namenda) has this effect is not entirely clear, but it is structurally similar to amantadine (Symmetrel), which is a known dopamine agonist used to treat patients with Parkinson's disease (Fig. 15.2).

WHICH PATIENTS SHOULD TAKE MEMANTINE (NAMENDA)?

Memantine (Namenda) has been approved in Europe for the treatment of vascular dementia since the 1980s. The initial research using memantine (Namenda) for Alzheimer's disease was begun in the mid-1990s. Unlike the cholinesterase inhibitors, which are FDA approved for patients with mild, moderate, and severe Alzheimer's disease, memantine (Namenda) is FDA approved only for patients in the moderate to severe stages of the disease (MMSE 5–14). Clinical trials in this stage of disease have shown that the magnitude of the benefit of the drug is comparable to that seen with cholinesterase inhibitors (Reisberg et al., 2003), although there have been no head-to-head studies. Memantine (Namenda) has also been shown to benefit Alzheimer's disease patients who are residing in nursing homes (Winblad & Poritis, 1999).

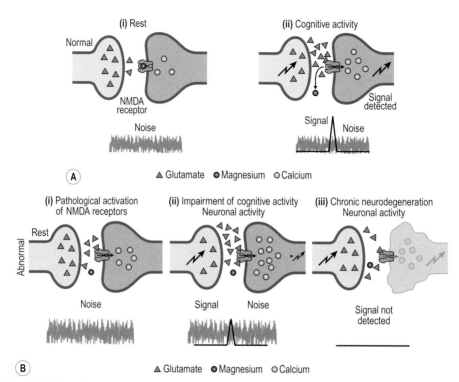

FIGURE 15.1 Possible mechanism of action of memantine (Namenda) at the NMDA receptor.

(**A**) Normal physiological function of the NMDA receptor. (i) At rest the presynaptic neuron (left) is filled with glutamate and a magnesium ion blocks the channel of the NMDA receptor on the postsynaptic neuron (right). Very few glutamate molecules are in the synaptic cleft. (ii) During cognitive activity an action potential (lightning arrow) reaches the presynaptic neuron, (1) glutamate is released from the presynaptic neuron, (2) interacts with the NMDA receptor on the postsynaptic neuron, (3) the magnesium ion pops off, (4) calcium enters the cell, and (5) an action potential (lightning arrow) is generated in the postsynaptic neuron. If we had an electrode measuring the current of the postsynaptic receptor we would find a low level of noise at rest (i), and enough of a calcium signal to rise up above the level of the noise, triggering an action potential in the postsynaptic neuron (ii). (**B**) Pathological state due to Alzheimer's disease. (i) Due to Alzheimer's disease, cells are dying, releasing their intracellular stores of glutamate, and thus too much glutamate is in the extracellular fluid. Some of this excess glutamate finds its way into the synaptic cleft and interacts with the NMDA receptor, causing the magnesium ion to pop off and calcium to trickle into the cell—even though no action potential has occurred. This trickle of calcium into the cell causes a high level of noise. (ii) Now when an action potential (lightning arrow) reaches the presynaptic neuron (left), again glutamate is released from the presynaptic neuron and interacts with the NMDA receptor of the postsynaptic neuron (right). But this time, because the magnesium ion has already popped off and calcium has been trickling into the cell, the signal cannot be detected above the high level of noise, and an action potential cannot be generated. (iii) Additionally, when calcium chronically trickles into cells it is toxic to them, killing the cells.

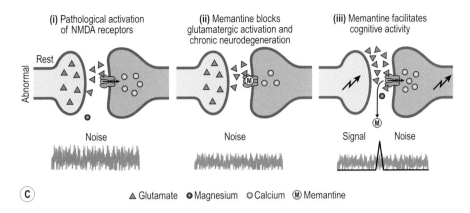

(i) Pathological activation of NMDA receptors

(ii) Memantine blocks glutamatergic activation and chronic neurodegeneration

(iii) Memantine facilitates cognitive activity

△ Glutamate ● Magnesium ○ Calcium Ⓜ Memantine

FIGURE 15.1—Cont'd

(C) Memantine restores physiological function. (i) The pathological state due to Alzheimer's disease (same as B(i)). (ii) Despite there being too much glutamate in the extracellular fluid, stimulating the NMDA receptor, memantine sits in the ion channel—like a "super" magnesium ion—stopping calcium from trickling into the cell, and reducing the noise to a normal, low level. (iii) When the action potential (lightning arrow) reaches the presynaptic neuron on the left and a large amount of glutamate is released, it again interacts with the NMDA receptor of the postsynaptic neuron. Now the memantine molecule pops off just like the magnesium ion and calcium can enter the cell, propagating the action potential (lightning arrow) in the postsynaptic neuron, and physiological function is restored (Parsons et al., 1999, 2007).

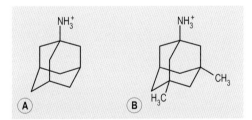

FIGURE 15.2 Chemical structure of amantadine (Symmetrel (A)) and memantine (Namenda (B)).

EFFICACY OF MEMANTINE (NAMENDA)

As is the case with the cholinesterase inhibitors, a number of randomized, double-blind studies have demonstrated that, compared with placebo, patients with moderate to severe Alzheimer's disease treated with memantine (Namenda) do better in terms of both objective cognitive tests and clinician ratings (Winblad & Poritis, 1999; Reisberg et al., 2003). Cognitively, memantine (Namenda) mainly improves attention and alertness, although memory may be improved secondarily (since memory will be improved if attention is improved). Most importantly, all the studies with memantine (Namenda) show improvements in social engagement and function.

What we hear most from families regarding patients in the moderate to severe stage of Alzheimer's disease are statements like, "he's got his spark back!," or "I've got the old Joe back," or "he's more like his old self." Other comments include the patient being more alert, talkative, engaged, outgoing, and "brighter" overall. Sometimes the results from patients in the severe stage of the disease can be quite dramatic.

One of our patients was severely impaired although still able to live at home because she was not incontinent or agitated. She went to daycare 5 days a week, and would mainly spend her time napping in a chair there. We started her on memantine and after about 4 weeks received this phone message that was saved on our voicemail:

I think the medicine is helping her, she seems a little bit more alert, she's talking a little more, and she seems to be happier. I called the daycare and they can tell a difference with her, she's not sleeping as much as she has, and she's doing more joking, and she seems to be happy. She hasn't had any side-effects from what I can see, so maybe it's a good sign...

SAFETY AND TOLERABILITY OF MEMANTINE (NAMENDA)

In general, memantine (Namenda) is a well-tolerated drug. The most common side-effects reported during the clinical trials were headache, constipation, dizziness, agitation, and confusion. None of these, however, occurred significantly more in patients treated with memantine (Namenda) than in those treated with placebo (and agitation was actually numerically less than those treated with memantine (Namenda)).

The most common side-effects that we routinely see with memantine (Namenda) are confusion and drowsiness. That confusion and drowsiness are common side-effects means that one needs to be careful in prescribing this medication, since confusion and drowsiness are common in any patient with dementia, and it can sometimes be tricky in sorting out when confusion is due to a medication side-effect and when it is simply a part of the dementia (or due to an infection, etc.). However, if you, as the clinician, always evaluate the patient after he or she has been started on the medication as described below, it should be possible to distinguish between these possibilities without too much difficulty.

One potentially interesting aspect of these side-effects is that we tend to observe them more in patients with milder disease. As discussed below, we will sometimes prescribe memantine to patients in the mild stage of Alzheimer's disease, and in our experience it is these patients who are most likely to encounter difficulties with confusion and/or drowsiness.

TITRATING MEMANTINE (NAMENDA)

Memantine (Namenda) is taken twice daily and is titrated over a 4-week period to the maximum dose of 20 mg/day (10 mg, BID) (Box 15.1). As is the case for the cholinesterase inhibitors, higher doses of Namenda are more efficacious and, in the absence of side-effects at the lower doses, the goal is to titrate patients to the highest dose. We generally provide patients with a starter sample pack (blister pack) that takes them through the 4-week titration and prescription for 10 mg BID with instructions to fill the prescription if they do not

---

BOX 15.1 MEMANTINE (NAMENDA) TITRATION

- Week 1: 5 mg QAM
- Week 2: 5 mg BID
- Week 3: 10 mg QAM, 5 mg QPM
- Week 4: 10 mg BID

---

experience side-effects during the titration period. In our experience, most patients have no difficulty with the titration. We typically revisit with them in 2 months to evaluate the medication's benefit and any side-effects, with the instructions to call us sooner if they experience dizziness, drowsiness, confusion, or other side-effects.

If they do experience side-effects, it is almost always dose-related; that is, there is usually a dose in which they were doing well, and we have now exceeded that dose. We encourage patients (with their family's help) to decrease the medication until they reach a dose which provides the desired benefits (improved attention, alertness, etc.) without side-effects.

COMBINING MEMANTINE (NAMENDA) WITH CHOLINESTERASE INHIBITORS

Because memantine (Namenda) and the cholinesterase inhibitors work on different neuro-transmitter systems, it is a reasonable hypothesis that combining the two medications would provide more benefit than either alone.

Indeed, a number of studies have shown that adding memantine (Namenda) to cholines-terase inhibitors produces additional benefit. The first of these studies was carried out in 404 patients with moderate to severe Alzheimer's disease (MMSE 5–14) who were stable on donepezil (Aricept) (Tariot et al., 2004). These patients were typically taking donepezil (Aricept) at 10 mg for an average duration of approximately 2 years. In this double-blind study, half of the patients were randomized to a group that added memantine (Namenda) to the donepezil (Aricept) and the other half added a placebo. At the end of a 24-week period, patients on the combination therapy were doing significantly better than patients taking Aricept alone. There are also data for patients taking either rivastigmine (Exelon) (Olin et al., 2010) or galantamine (Porsteinsson et al., 2008) along with memantine (Namenda).

Two retrospective studies have looked at the effects of combining memantine (Namenda) and cholinesterase inhibitors over longer periods of time. Lopez and colleagues (2009) found that time to nursing home placement was delayed by cholinesterase inhibitors alone and that this effect was significantly augmented when memantine (Namenda) was added. Interestingly (and we would argue importantly) there was no change in time to death for either cholinesterase inhibitors alone or in combination with memantine (Namenda) (Lopez et al., 2009). Atri and colleagues (2008) analyzed a large amount of retrospective data and were able to look at cognitive function and activities of daily living for up to 4 years, again finding a significant benefit of combination therapy over cholinesterase inhibitors alone in patients with very mild, mild to moderate, and moderate to severe disease. These latter data are particularly interesting because this benefit was found in patients with very mild Alzheimer's disease, although the largest effects were seen in patients with moderate to severe disease.

In general we have found that most patients tolerate the combination of a cholinesterase inhibitor and memantine (Namenda) about as well as they tolerate these medications individually. Based on the results of the studies reviewed above and on our clinical experience, we typically start our patients with Alzheimer's disease on a cholinesterase inhibitor, titrating them to their highest tolerated dose. We generally add memantine (Namenda) when patients reach the moderate stage of disease (MMSE <15), continuing the cholinesterase inhibitor. Sometimes, however, we do consider adding memantine (Namenda) in patients in the mild stage of Alzheimer's disease (see below). In these cases it is especially important to monitor for increased confusion.

MEMANTINE (NAMENDA) IN THE MILD STAGE OF ALZHEIMER'S DISEASE

Whereas the data strongly suggest that memantine (Namenda) is beneficial for the treatment of patients with Alzheimer's disease in the moderate to severe stages of the disease, the data regarding patients in earlier stages of Alzheimer's disease are equivocal with some studies showing benefit and others not. Similarly, the studies that have been conducted adding memantine (Namenda) to donepezil (Aricept) in mild Alzheimer's disease have not shown any additional benefit over taking donepezil (Aricept) alone. Based on these data, the FDA did not grant an approval of memantine for mild disease. Nevertheless, some clinicians feel that they have seen patients in earlier disease stages benefit from memantine (Namenda), and we see many patients with mild Alzheimer's disease who come to our clinic already taking this medication "off-label."

In general, we consider adding memantine (Namenda) in patients with mild Alzheimer's disease who are already taking a cholinesterase inhibitor if there are symptoms which we believe will be helped with this medication. In many patients memantine (Namenda) can provide rapid symptomatic improvement in alertness, attention, apathy, and—perhaps because of these cognitive improvements—global function. Although apathy is common, most patients with Alzheimer's disease do not have significant trouble with alertness and attention in the mild stage of the disease. However, when we do see patients with Alzheimer's disease who are having significant trouble with alertness and attention, we consider adding memantine (Namenda) even if the patients are in the mild stage of the disease. In our experience approximately half of these mild patients show symptomatic benefit with the medication. (In the other half who do not show improvement, we would generally discontinue it and try it again when the patient reaches the moderate stage of disease.)

MEMANTINE (NAMENDA) IN OTHER DEMENTIAS

Should memantine (Namenda) be used in other dementias? Several published studies address this issue. Memantine (Namenda) showed benefit in a large-scale study of patients with vascular dementia (MMSE ranging from 12 to 20) (Orgogozo et al., 2002). Improvements were seen on the MMSE, a cognitive scale (ADAS-cog), as well as a behavioral scale (Nurses' Observational Scale for Geriatric Patients). A somewhat smaller study found that memantine (Namenda) provided benefit in patients with dementia with Lewy bodies and Parkinson's disease dementia (Aarsland et al., 2009). This study found improvement in these patients cognitively in their speed on attentional tasks, and most importantly on the Clinical Global Impression of Change. Treatment in patients with frontotemporal dementia has been more mixed, with benefits found in some patients but not in others (Swanberg, 2007; Diehl-Schmid et al., 2008; Boxer et al., 2009).

Our clinic experience parallels these studies. We find that most of our patients with vascular dementia and dementia with Lewy bodies (or Parkinson's disease dementia) benefit from memantine (Namenda), particularly when they reach the moderate to severe stage of these disorders, or when they show problems with alertness, attention, or apathy. Our experience in patients with frontotemporal dementias is mixed. Some patients seem to benefit significantly, whereas other patients show no change or a decrement in function. This variability in the response to memantine (Namenda) in frontotemporal dementia may reflect differences in either clinical phenotype or in the underlying pathophysiology.

In short, we will generally try memantine in patients with vascular dementia or dementia with Lewy bodies in the same manner as if they had Alzheimer's disease. In patients with frontotemporal dementias we will often also try memantine, but explain to the family that this may or may not be helpful and could make things worse, so that we need to watch them closely to see how they do.

References

Aarsland, D., Ballard, C., Walker, Z., et al., 2009. Memantine in patients with Parkinson's disease dementia or dementia with Lewy bodies: a double-blind, placebo-controlled, multicentre trial. Lancet Neurol. 8, 613–618.

Atri, A., Shaughnessy, L.W., Locascio, J.J., et al., 2008. Long-term course and effectiveness of combination therapy in Alzheimer disease. Alzheimer Dis. Assoc. Disord. 22, 209–221.

Boxer, A.L., Lipton, A.M., Womack, K., et al., 2009. An open-label study of memantine treatment in 3 subtypes of frontotemporal lobar degeneration. Alzheimer Dis. Assoc. Disord. 23, 211–217.

Diehl-Schmid, J., Forstl, H., Perneczky, R., et al., 2008. A 6-month, open-label study of memantine in patients with frontotemporal dementia. Int. J. Geriatr. Psychiatry 23, 754–759.

Lopez, O.L., Becker, J.T., Wahed, A.S., et al., 2009. Long-term effects of the concomitant use of memantine with cholinesterase inhibition in Alzheimer disease. J. Neurol. Neurosurg. Psychiatry 80, 600–607.

Merello, M., Nouzeilles, M.I., Cammarota, A., et al., 1999. Effect of memantine (NMDA antagonist) on Parkinson's disease: a double-blind crossover randomized study. Clin. Neuropharmacol. 22, 273–276.

Olin, J.T., Bhatnagar, V., Reyes, P., et al., 2010. Safety and tolerability of rivastigmine capsule with memantine in patients with probable Alzheimer's disease: a 26-week, open-label, prospective trial (Study ENA713B US32). Int. J. Geriatr. Psychiatry 25, 419–426.

Orgogozo, J.M., Rigaud, A.S., Stoffler, A., et al., 2002. Efficacy and safety of memantine in patients with mild to moderate vascular dementia: a randomized, placebo-controlled trial (MMM 300). Stroke 33, 1834–1839.

Parsons, C.G., Danysz, W., Quack, G., 1999. Memantine is a clinically well tolerated N-methyl-D-aspartate (NMDA) receptor antagonist: a review of preclinical data. Neuropharmacology 38, 735–767.

Parsons, C.G., Stoffler, A., Danysz, W., 2007. Memantine: an NMDA receptor antagonist that improves memory by restoration of homeostasis in the glutamatergic system: too little activation is bad, too much is even worse. Neuropharmacology 53, 699–723.

Peeters, M., Maloteaux, J.M., Hermans, E., 2003. Distinct effects of amantadine and memantine on dopaminergic transmission in the rat striatum. Neurosci. Lett. 343, 205–209.

Porsteinsson, A.P., Grossberg, G.T., Mintzer, J., et al., 2008. Memantine treatment in patients with mild to moderate Alzheimer's disease already receiving a cholinesterase inhibitor: a randomized, double-blind, placebo-controlled trial. Curr. Alzheimer Res. 5, 83–89.

Reisberg, B., Doody, R., Stoffler, A., et al., 2003. Memantine in moderate-to-severe Alzheimer's disease. N. Engl. J. Med. 348, 1333–1341.

Spanagel, R., Eilbacher, B., Wilke, R., 1994. Memantine-induced dopamine release in the prefrontal cortex and striatum of the rat: a pharmacokinetic microdialysis study. Eur. J. Pharmacol. 262, 21–26.

Swanberg, M.M., 2007. Memantine for behavioral disturbances in frontotemporal dementia: a case series. Alzheimer Dis. Assoc. Disord. 21, 164–166.

Tariot, P.N., Farlow, M.R., Grossberg, G.T., et al., 2004. Memantine treatment in patients with moderate to severe Alzheimer disease already receiving donepezil: a randomized controlled trial. JAMA 291, 317–324.

Wang, S.H., Morris, R.G., 2010. Hippocampal-neocortical interactions in memory formation, consolidation, and reconsolidation. Annu. Rev. Psychol. 61, 49–79.

Winblad, B., Poritis, N., 1999. Memantine in severe dementia: results of the 9M-Best Study (Benefit and efficacy in severely demented patients during treatment with memantine). Int. J. Geriatr. Psychiatry 14, 135–146.

Vitamins, herbs, supplements, and anti-inflammatories

QUICK START: VITAMINS, HERBS, SUPPLEMENTS, AND ANTI-INFLAMMATORIES

- Vitamin E:
  - One study was positive in patients with Alzheimer's disease, but many other studies were negative.
  - We do not recommend vitamin E for our patients.
- B complex vitamins—folic acid, B6, B12:
  - There are a lot of retrospective and theoretical data to suggest that these vitamins would be helpful in Alzheimer's disease.
  - A large 18-month study showed no benefit for patients with Alzheimer's disease.
  - We do not recommend B complex vitamins for our patients.
- *Ginkgo biloba*
  - One study was positive in patients with Alzheimer's disease, but many other studies were negative.
  - We do not recommend ginkgo for our patients.
- DHA (phosphatidylcholine docosahexaenoic acid) (fish oil):
  - A large retrospective study suggested that DHA may reduce the risk of Alzheimer's disease.
  - A recently completed large, multicenter, randomized, placebo-controlled trial showed no benefit.
  - We neither encourage nor discourage DHA for our patients.
- Anti-inflammatories:
  - Several large retrospective studies suggested that non-steroidal anti-inflammatory drugs (NSAIDs) may help prevent Alzheimer's disease.
  - Several randomized controlled clinical trials for NSAIDs and cyclo-oxygenase (COX)-2 inhibitors showed no benefit related to Alzheimer's disease.
  - NSAIDs and COX-2 inhibitors have significant side-effects and risks associated with them.
  - We do not recommend NSAIDs or COX-2 inhibitors for our patients with Alzheimer's disease.

Many of our patients and their families ask us about whether they should take any one of the many supplements, herbs, vitamins, or over-the-counter medications they have seen in the supermarkets or on television infomercials. Other patients are already taking some of these additives and wonder if they are doing any good or even whether they are harmful. Because many of these compounds have demonstrated or are purported to have antioxidant effects, and because oxidative stress is thought to be harmful to brain cells, there is a rational basis for hypothesizing that these drugs could slow progression of Alzheimer's disease. We generally explain this rationale to the patient and family, but we also explain to them that, unlike medication approved by the US Food and Drug Administration (FDA), these supplements have not undergone careful evaluation, and, just like prescription medications, vitamins and supplements have benefits as well as risks and side-effects, and the decision of whether to take them should be made by weighing the relative risks and side-effects versus the benefits.

VITAMIN E

A paper published in the *New England Journal of Medicine* in 1997 reported the results of a large, double-blind, placebo-controlled, randomized trial demonstrating beneficial effects of high doses (2000 IU/day) of vitamin E in patients with mild to moderate Alzheimer's disease (Sano et al., 1997). After adjustment for unequal baseline MMSE scores by including MMSE as a covariate, vitamin E-treated patients reached milestones in Alzheimer's disease, such as loss of an important activity or placement in a nursing home, later than placebo-treated patients. Additionally, vitamin E was well tolerated and without significant reported side-effects. Based upon the results, most physicians recommended that their patients with Alzheimer's disease start taking high doses of vitamin E. Additionally, it became a widespread practice for people concerned about getting Alzheimer's disease (for example patients with mild cognitive impairment) to take vitamin E.

Although there have been no subsequent randomized studies of vitamin E in Alzheimer's disease, there have been other relevant studies with vitamin E. A randomized, double-blind, placebo-controlled study that evaluated vitamin E versus donepezil (Aricept) versus placebo in mild cognitive impairment in over 750 patients showed no benefit for vitamin E. The primary outcome measured in the study was whether individuals with mild cognitive impairment would progress to Alzheimer's disease over a 3-year period. Vitamin E showed no difference compared with placebo (Petersen et al., 2005). Other studies evaluated the cardio-vascular and/or cancer-reducing benefit of vitamin E. Not only was there no benefit found (Lee et al., 2005), but also there was the suggestion of an increased risk of heart failure in patients with diabetes or vascular disease (Yusuf et al., 2000; Lee et al., 2005; Lonn et al., 2005). Lastly, a meta-analysis of vitamin E trials reported an increase in deaths (Miller et al., 2005). (Note that this study was criticized for its methodology. See the raging debate in the Annals of Internal Medicine, July 19, 2005, Volume 143, Issue 2, which included the following critiques: vitamin E was often combined with other antioxidants in the analyzed trials; trials using the natural single isomer RRR-α-tocopherol and the synthetic racemic mixture of all seven α-tocopherol isomers were combined; trials with 10 or fewer deaths were excluded; and participants in many of the trials had serious medical illnesses including Alzheimer's disease.)

So what do we recommend to our patients? To summarize, there is only one randomized trial that showed benefit without risk in patients with Alzheimer's disease, and that trial only reached significance after a statistical adjustment for unequal baseline MMSE scores. At present, there is no evidence that vitamin E can prevent the disease in cognitively healthy patients or in those with mild cognitive impairment. Moreover, vitamin E may increase the risk of cardiac events in individuals with vascular disease or diabetes. Lastly, vitamin E may cause problems with bleeding and/or easy bruising in some individuals (Traber, 2008).

Based upon these data, regardless of whether they are cognitively healthy or they have been diagnosed with mild cognitive impairment or Alzheimer's disease, we do not recommend vitamin E supplementation for our patients, and if they are already taking vitamin E to prevent or retard Alzheimer's disease, we recommend that they discontinue it.

B COMPLEX VITAMINS: FOLIC ACID, B6, B12

On Valentine's Day in 2002, an article from the Framingham Heart Study was published in the *New England Journal of Medicine* showing that elevated plasma levels of homocysteine were a risk factor for the development of dementia and Alzheimer's disease (Seshadri et al., 2002). Later that year another study was published in the journal *Neurology* suggesting that elevated levels of homocysteine were related to cerebrovascular disease and not the plaques and tangles of Alzheimer's pathology (Miller et al., 2002). Regardless of the specific cause, some studies have also found elevated levels of homocysteine in patients with Alzheimer's disease (Religa et al., 2003), although others have not (Luchsinger et al., 2004). Like the article published in *Neurology*, many clinicians and researchers believe that the risk of dementia related to elevated levels of homocysteine is mediated through its effect on cerebrovascular disease (Sachdev et al., 2004; Scott et al., 2004; Matsui et al., 2005).

It is well known that deficiencies of folic acid or its cofactors vitamins B6 and B12 can cause an elevation of homocysteine levels. Some studies have found that low levels of these vitamins directly correlate with cognitive decline or brain pathology (Scott et al., 2004; Kado et al., 2005). Studies have also examined whether the combination of vitamins B6, B12, and folic acid could lower the levels of homocysteine in patients with Alzheimer's disease, and found that they could (Aisen et al., 2003a). Studies have also examined retrospectively whether individuals who took higher amounts of the vitamins folic acid, B6, or B12 were less likely to develop Alzheimer's disease. One study found that higher levels of folic acid intake (but not B6 or B12) did decrease the risk of later developing Alzheimer's disease (Luchsinger et al., 2008).

So can we reduce the risk of developing Alzheimer's disease or perhaps slow the progression of the disorder in those already diagnosed? One very small study reported a positive effect of folic acid supplementation in those who had mild Alzheimer's disease (Connelly et al., 2008). But most studies have found no effect. A study from Taiwan in 89 patients with mild to moderate Alzheimer's disease found that supplementation with folic acid, B6, and B12 for 26 weeks produced a reduction of homocysteine levels but no beneficial effect on cognition or function (Sun et al., 2007). And a large, multicenter study in 409 patients with mild to moderate Alzheimer's disease over 18 months from the Alzheimer's disease Cooperative Study (ADCS) group found no benefit to supplementation with folic acid, B6, and B12 (Aisen et al., 2008).

In summary, the data suggest the following. First, there is an association between elevated levels of homocysteine and Alzheimer's disease. Second, there is an association between elevated levels of homocysteine and cerebrovascular disease in patients with Alzheimer's disease. Third, there is also an association between low levels of folic acid and Alzheimer's disease. And fourth, levels of homocysteine were reduced in patients with Alzheimer's disease when they took supplementation with folic acid, B6, and B12. Unfortunately, despite all these promising preliminary data, the large 18-month trial of supplementation with folic acid, B6, and B12 showed no beneficial effect in patients with Alzheimer's disease. We therefore do not recommend supplementation with the B complex vitamins—folic acid, B6, and B12—for our patients whose vitamin B12 levels are normal.

GINKGO BILOBA

We see many patients for initial evaluation who are already taking ginkgo. Ginkgo is purported to have antioxidant properties and is also purported to enhance memory. A study of ginkgo in Alzheimer's disease patients published in the *Journal of the American Medical Association* (LeBars et al., 1997) in 1997 was portrayed by the media as showing benefit in patients with Alzheimer's disease. More careful scrutiny of the study, however, indicated minimal benefit for Alzheimer's disease patients, and not nearly what is seen with FDA-approved medications. Since then there have been other randomized trials that have not shown any benefit in Alzheimer's disease patients. Other studies have shown that there is no effect of ginkgo in reducing the development of Alzheimer's disease or dementia in those with normal cognition or mild cognitive impairment (DeKosky et al., 2008). Additionally, a placebo-controlled, double-blind, randomized trial in healthy elderly also showed no cognitive benefit for ginkgo (Solomon et al., 2002).

Ginkgo is generally a safe drug, but it can have side-effects. Most prominent is its anti-coagulant effects. This may pose a particular risk when ginkgo is taken in conjunction with aspirin or warfarin, both of which are common in the aging population we treat. Based on the results of these studies we do not recommend *Ginkgo biloba* either as a treatment or as preventative for Alzheimer's disease.

DHA (FISH OIL)

Recently, there has been considerable interest in the potential beneficial effects on cognition and the prevention of Alzheimer's disease by DHA (phosphatidylcholine docosahexaenoic acid), an omega-3 polyunsaturated fatty acid which is found in fish oil.

In one study, researchers followed 899 men and women over a 9-year period who were part of the Framingham Heart Study (Schaefer et al., 2006). During this time, 71 of these participants developed Alzheimer's disease. But people with the highest levels of DHA in their blood had a 39% lower risk of developing Alzheimer's disease. People in this study with the highest DHA levels reported that they ate two to three servings of fish per week, much more than those with lower DHA levels. Fatty fish like mackerel, lake trout, herring, sardines, albacore tuna and salmon are high in DHA. Based on this study and other results, the Alzheimer's Disease Cooperative Study (ADCS) recently completed a prospective, randomized trial to determine whether DHA can slow the progression of Alzheimer's disease. An initial report of the results (Quinn et al., 2009) showed that, compared with placebo controls, patients with mild to moderate Alzheimer's disease taking 2 g per day of DHA showed no benefit on either cognitive tests or overall functioning. Additional results should be available over the next few years.

At this time we neither recommend nor discourage our patients taking DHA or eating several servings of fish per week.

ANTI-INFLAMMATORIES

A retrospective study from the Baltimore Longitudinal Study of Aging examined 1686 older individuals regarding their risk of Alzheimer's disease in relation to their use of aspirin or other non-steroidal anti-inflammatory drugs (NSAIDs). The results showed that individuals taking NSAIDs for more than 2 years—compared with aspirin or acetaminophen—were much less likely to develop Alzheimer's disease (Rich et al., 1995; Stewart et al., 1997). Other retrospective studies provided similar results (Szekely et al., 2004). The hypothesis put forth to explain this finding was that amyloid plaques could cause local inflammation in the brain, which in turn could injure neurons. In support of this hypothesis, a number of markers of inflammation including activated microglia and astrocytes, complement components, and inflammatory cytokines are associated with Alzheimer's disease (Tuppo and Arias, 2005).

Based upon these retrospective findings of disease prevention, randomized prospective studies have evaluated the use of anti-inflammatories to treat patients who were already diagnosed with Alzheimer's disease. The Alzheimer's Disease Cooperative Study (ADCS) conducted a study in which patients were randomized to receive the cyclo-oxygenase (COX)-2 inhibitor rofecoxib (Vioxx), the non-specific NSAID naproxen (Naprosyn), or a placebo. Patients with mild to moderate disease took daily doses of the assigned drug for 1 year. The results indicated that there was no change in the rate of cognitive decline in those taking rofecoxib (Vioxx) or naproxen (Naprosyn) compared with placebo (Aisen et al., 2003b). Thus, despite these agents' possible use in the prevention of Alzheimer's disease, they are not helpful in treating the disease once it has already been diagnosed.

In brief, we do not recommend treatment with either NSAIDs or COX-2 inhibitors for our patients who already have Alzheimer's disease. The studies reviewed above do not show benefit in these patients and the side-effects and risks of these medications related to gastrointestinal bleeding and heart disease are well known. Regarding the use of these medications in patients who are at risk for, but do not yet have, Alzheimer's disease, we await the results of randomized prospective clinical trials.

References

Aisen, P.S., Egelko, S., Andrews, H., et al., 2003a. A pilot study of vitamins to lower plasma homocysteine levels in Alzheimer disease. Am. J. Geriatr. Psychiatry 11, 246–249.

Aisen, P.S., Schafer, K.A., Grundman, M., et al., 2003b. Effects of rofecoxib or naproxen vs placebo on Alzheimer disease progression: a randomized controlled trial. JAMA 289, 2819–2826.

Aisen, P.S., Schneider, L.S., Sano, M., et al., 2008. High-dose B vitamin supplementation and cognitive decline in Alzheimer disease: a randomized controlled trial. JAMA 300, 1774–1783.

Connelly, P.J., Prentice, N.P., Cousland, G., et al., 2008. A randomised double-blind placebo-controlled trial of folic acid supplementation of cholinesterase inhibitors in Alzheimer's disease. Int. J. Geriatr. Psychiatry 23, 155–160.

DeKosky, S.T., Williamson, J.D., Fitzpatrick, A.L., et al., 2008. Ginkgo biloba for prevention of dementia: a randomized controlled trial. JAMA 300, 2253–2262.

Kado, D.M., Karlamangla, A.S., Huang, M.H., et al., 2005. Homocysteine versus the vitamins folate, B6, and B12 as predictors of cognitive function and decline in older high-functioning adults: MacArthur Studies of Successful Aging. Am. J. Med. 118, 161–167.

LeBars, P.L., Katz, M.M., Berman, N., et al., 1997. A placebo-controlled, double-blind, randomized trial of an extract of Ginkgo biloba for dementia. North American EGb Study Group. JAMA 278, 1327–1332.

Lee, I.M., Cook, N.R., Gaziano, J.M., et al., 2005. Vitamin E in the primary prevention of cardiovascular disease and cancer: the Women's Health Study—a randomized controlled trial. JAMA 294, 56–65.

Lonn, E., Bosch, J., Yusuf, S., et al., 2005. Effects of long-term vitamin E supplementation on cardiovascular events and cancer: a randomized controlled trial. JAMA 293, 1338–1347.

Luchsinger, J.A., Tang, M.X., Shea, S., et al., 2004. Plasma homocysteine levels and risk of Alzheimer disease. Neurology 62, 1972–1976.

Luchsinger, J.A., Tang, M.X., Miller, J., et al., 2008. Higher folate intake is related to lower risk of Alzheimer's disease in the elderly. J. Nutr. Health Aging 12, 648–650.

Matsui, T., Nemoto, M., Maruyama, M., et al., 2005. Plasma homocysteine and risk of coexisting silent brain infarction in Alzheimer's disease. Neurodegener. Dis. 2, 299–304.

Miller III, E.R., Pastor-Barriuso, R., Dalal, D., et al., 2005. Meta-analysis: high-dosage vitamin E supplementation may increase all-cause mortality. Ann. Intern. Med. 142, 37–46.

Miller, J.W., Green, R., Mungas, D.M., et al., 2002. Homocysteine, vitamin B6, and vascular disease in AD patients. Neurology 58, 1471–1475.

Petersen, R.C., Thomas, R.G., Grundman, M., et al., 2005. Vitamin E and donepezil for the treatment of mild cognitive impairment. N. Engl. J. Med. 352, 2379–2388.

Quinn, J.F., Raman, R., Thomas, R.G., et al., 2009. A clinical trial of docosahexanoic acid (DHA) for the treatment of Alzheimer's disease, Alzheimer's Association International Conference on Alzheimer's Disease, Presentation O1-04-02, 7/12/2009.

Religa, D., Styczynska, M., Peplonska, B., et al., 2003. Homocysteine, apolipoprotein E and methylenetetrahydrofolate reductase in Alzheimer's disease and mild cognitive impairment. Dement. Geriatr. Cogn. Disord. 16, 64–70.

Rich, J.B., Rasmusson, D.X., Folstein, M.F., et al., 1995. Nonsteroidal anti-inflammatory drugs in Alzheimer's disease. Neurology 45, 51–55.

Sachdev, P., Parslow, R., Salonikas, C., et al., 2004. Homocysteine and the brain in midadult life: evidence for an increased risk of leukoaraiosis in men. Arch. Neurol. 61, 1369–1376.

Sano, M., Ernesto, C., Thomas, R.G., et al., 1997. A controlled trial of selegiline, alpha-tocopherol, or both as treatment for Alzheimer's disease. The Alzheimer's Disease Cooperative Study. N. Engl. J. Med. 336, 1216–1222.

Schaefer, E.J., Bongard, V., Beiser, A.S., et al., 2006. Plasma phosphatidylcholine docosahexaenoic acid content and risk of dementia and Alzheimer disease: the Framingham Heart Study. Arch. Neurol. 63, 1545–1550.

Scott, T.M., Tucker, K.L., Bhadelia, A., et al., 2004. Homocysteine and B vitamins relate to brain volume and white-matter changes in geriatric patients with psychiatric disorders. Am. J. Geriatr. Psychiatry 12, 631–638.

Seshadri, S., Beiser, A., Selhub, J., et al., 2002. Plasma homocysteine as a risk factor for dementia and Alzheimer's disease. N. Engl. J. Med. 346, 476–483.

Solomon, P.R., Adams, F., Silver, A., et al., 2002. Ginkgo for memory enhancement: a randomized controlled trial. JAMA 288, 835–840.

Stewart, W.F., Kawas, C., Corrada, M., et al., 1997. Risk of Alzheimer's disease and duration of NSAID use. Neurology 48, 626–632.

Sun, Y., Lu, C.J., Chien, K.L., et al., 2007. Efficacy of multivitamin supplementation containing vitamins B6 and B12 and folic acid as adjunctive treatment with a cholinesterase inhibitor in Alzheimer's disease: a 26-week, randomized, double-blind, placebo-controlled study in Taiwanese patients. Clin. Ther. 29, 2204–2214.

Szekely, C.A., Thorne, J.E., Zandi, P.P., et al., 2004. Nonsteroidal anti-inflammatory drugs for the prevention of Alzheimer's disease: a systematic review. Neuroepidemiology 23, 159–169.

Traber, M.G., 2008. Vitamin E and K interactions: a 50-year-old problem. Nutr. Rev. 66, 624–629.

Tuppo, E.E., Arias, H.R., 2005. The role of inflammation in Alzheimer's disease. Int. J. Biochem. Cell. Biol. 37, 289–305.

Yusuf, S., Dagenais, G., Pogue, J., et al., 2000. Vitamin E supplementation and cardiovascular events in high-risk patients. The Heart Outcomes Prevention Evaluation Study Investigators. N. Engl. J. Med. 342, 154–160.

Future treatments of memory loss

17

QUICK START: FUTURE TREATMENTS OF MEMORY LOSS

Symptomatic and disease-modifying treatment

- Alzheimer's disease can be treated either to improve symptoms and function or to slow disease progression.
- Symptomatic treatments work by altering neurotransmitter function.
- Most disease-modifying treatments are aimed at decreasing β-amyloid protein in the brain.
- Some disease-modifying treatments in development are directed against neurofibrillary tangle formation.

Disease-modifying treatments: amyloid plaques

- The amyloid cascade hypothesis describes how a build-up of β-amyloid can lead directly to amyloid plaques, neurofibrillary tangles, neurotransmitter disruption, and dementia.
- Approaches to decrease β-amyloid have included active immunotherapy, passive immunotherapy, and reducing the formation, accumulation, or oligomerization of β-amyloid.
- No disease-modifying treatments have yet proven efficacious.
- Many disease-modifying treatments are currently in clinical trials.
- Disease-modifying treatments may need to be started at the earliest signs of β-amyloid in the brain—perhaps years or decades prior to the onset of symptoms.

Disease-modifying treatments: neurofibrillary tangles

- As tangles are further downstream in the cascade that leads to clinical symptoms, treatments directed against tangles may be more efficacious in patients who have already developed clinical Alzheimer's disease than treatments directed against β-amyloid.
- Tangle formation may be the final common pathway in many degenerative diseases and thus treatments directed against tangles may also be efficacious against other dementias such as frontotemporal dementia and chronic traumatic encephalopathy.

Because of the rapid aging of the population and the accompanying increase in the prevalence of Alzheimer's disease, there is enormous interest from both the federal government and private industry in developing new and better treatments. In general, these treatments are aimed at two targets: treating the symptoms of Alzheimer's disease and attempting to slow the progression of the disease.

STRATEGIES TO TREAT THE SYMPTOMS OF ALZHEIMER'S DISEASE

As discussed in Chapter 13: *Goals of Treatment*, patients for whom we prescribe a cholinesterase inhibitor, memantine (Namenda), or a combination of the two often ask how these medications work and what else can be done. After explaining the mechanism of these standard, FDA approved medications, we often have a brief discussion of some of the types of treatment that are currently being developed. There are two basic reasons why we discuss future treatments. One is to give patients (and their children who are often worried about developing Alzheimer's disease when they are older) hope for the future. The second is that some patients may be interested in participating in one of the numerous clinical trials of novel medications that are being developed for Alzheimer's disease, available in most large medical centers.

Additional symptomatic treatments

One strategy to further help patients with Alzheimer's disease is to facilitate neuronal transmission, that is, communication between brain cells. The cholinesterase inhibitors and memantine (Namenda) improve the function of neurons that use acetylcholine, glutamate, and dopamine as their neurotransmitters. There are, however, other neurotransmitter systems in addition to these which can be augmented. It is now well documented that Alzheimer's disease affects many neurotransmitter systems. Table 17.1 summarizes these transmitter systems. At some point we might envision a drug cocktail that will boost the level of multiple neurotransmitter systems, thereby facilitating cognition. We are now at the beginning of this type of strategy when we combine memantine (Namenda) with a cholinesterase inhibitor. We may become sufficiently sophisticated to tailor the cocktail based on the specific symptoms that the patient is experiencing or even the patient's genotype.

There is currently considerable research ongoing aimed at developing additional symptomatic treatments. Over the past few years, clinical trials have been undertaken to determine the effects of drugs that affect transmitter systems including serotonin, norepinephrine, dopamine, somatostatin, histamine, GABA, and others, in addition to acetylcholine and glutamate.

Table 17.1 Neurotransmitters depleted in Alzheimer's disease

Transmitter system	Degree of involvement in Alzheimer's disease	Approved medications	Clinical trials ongoing?
Acetylcholine	√ √ √	donepezil (Aricept), rivastigmine (Excelon), galantamine (Razadyne)	√√√
Glutamate	√ √ √	memantine (Namenda)	√
Serotonin	√ √	---	√ √ √
Norepinephrine	√ √	---	√
Dopamine	√	memantine (Namenda)	√
GABA	√	---	√
Peptides	√	---	√

DISEASE-MODIFYING TREATMENTS

Development of symptomatic treatments notwithstanding, the major focus of new drug development for Alzheimer's disease is on disease-modifying drugs (sometimes called mechanism-based treatments). That is, drugs that address the underlying cause of the disease and in doing so prevent cell death. If this strategy is successful, then the progression of the disease could theoretically be halted. If this strategy could be combined with both early diagnosis and the use of symptomatic drugs, we could be on the horizon of successfully managing this disease.

Although the cause of Alzheimer's disease is unknown, there are a number of promising hypotheses regarding the pathogenesis of the disease, and these hypotheses have led to the development of potential disease-modifying drugs. The leading view of the cause of cell death in Alzheimer's disease is the *amyloid cascade hypothesis*.

Alzheimer's initial observations

When Alois Alzheimer had the opportunity to examine the brain of his first patient, Anna O, in 1906, he characterized the two forms of pathology that are the neuropathological hallmarks of the disease that now bears his name: senile plaques and neurofibrillary tangles.

Senile plaques appear to have a fluffy central core surrounded by thick irregular processes (Fig. 17.1). The central core is made up of a sticky protein called amyloid, and the surrounding material is a combination of dystrophic processes (axons and dendrites) and astrocytes. These plaques are primarily found in the association areas of the frontal, parietal, and temporal cortices and the piriform cortex, hippocampus, and amygdala (Fig. 2.1). Neurofibrillary tangles are intraneuronal cytoplasmic structures that are composed of paired filaments. Under the microscope they look like skeins of yarn (Fig. 17.1). These tangles appear to consist primarily of a hyperphosphorylated form of the microtubule-associated protein *tau*. Microtubules are one of three major constituents of the neuronal cytoskeleton; neurofilaments and microfilaments are the other two. All of these can be thought of as infrastructural elements of neurons that participate in functions such as axonal transport and maintenance of the structural integrity of the cell. In Alzheimer's disease, neurofibrillary tangles are present in the cortex, hippocampus, amygdala, nucleus basalis of Meynert, dorsal raphe, other brainstem nuclei, and ultimately in many other brain regions.

(See Chapter 3: *Alzheimer's disease* for additional information on senile plaques and neurofibrillary tangles.)

Baptists vs. tauists

There has been ongoing debate regarding which form of pathology, senile plaques or neurofibrillary tangles, is the primary culprit in Alzheimer's disease. The debate has become known as the "baptists" versus the "tauists." The baptists favor the view that β-amyloid protein and β-amyloid plaques are the real culprits that start an inexorable cascade that ultimately destroys neurons. They are referred to as baptists because β-amyloid protein (or plaque) can be shortened to βAP or "bap." The tauists put forth the view that neurofibrillary tangles are the primary cause of cell death. They are called tauists because of the role of *tau* in forming the tangles. Although there is great interest in both, the prevailing view is currently that

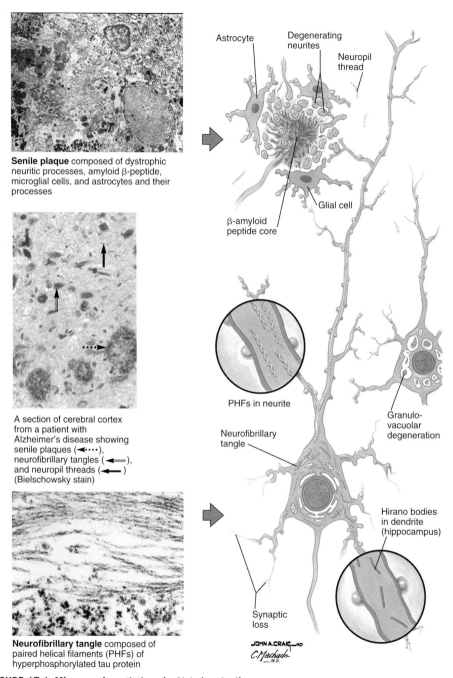

Senile plaque composed of dystrophic neuritic processes, amyloid β-peptide, microglial cells, and astrocytes and their processes

A section of cerebral cortex from a patient with Alzheimer's disease showing senile plaques (◀····), neurofibrillary tangles (◀═), and neuropil threads (◀─) (Bielschowsky stain)

Neurofibrillary tangle composed of paired helical filaments (PHFs) of hyperphosphorylated tau protein

Astrocyte

Degenerating neurites

Neuropil thread

Glial cell

β-amyloid peptide core

PHFs in neurite

Neurofibrillary tangle

Granulo-vacuolar degeneration

Hirano bodies in dendrite (hippocampus)

Synaptic loss

JOHN A.CRAIG—MD
C.Machado—M.D.

FIGURE 17.1 Microscopic pathology in Alzheimer's disease.

A color version of this figure is available online at http://www.expertconsult.com.

β-amyloid accumulation is the primary pathogenic event—the event that, if it were prevented, would prevent the death of neurons. Because of this view, the central focus of disease-modifying treatments in current development is on attacking β-amyloid and β-amyloid plaques. These treatments have become know as *"plaque busters."*

The amyloid cascade hypothesis

The amyloid cascade hypothesis starts with the premise that the primary culprit in the pathogenesis of Alzheimer's disease is the accumulation of toxic forms of amyloid. It then follows that the focus of treatment of disease-modifying drugs is either to affect amyloid directly (the "plaque busters") or to affect the downstream consequences of amyloid accumulation, such as reducing inflammation, oxidative stress, and neurofibrillary tangle formation.

Figure 3.10 summarizes the amyloid cascade hypothesis (Hardy & Selkoe, 2002; Solomon & Budson, 2003; Haass & Selkoe, 2007). As Figure 3.10 shows, the initial assumption is that different gene defects can lead, either directly or indirectly, to an increase in toxic forms of β-amyloid. This increase may either be due to either overproduction of or failure to clear these toxic forms of amyloid. Gradual accumulation of aggregated β-amyloid protein leads to a multistep cascade that includes inflammation, neuritic and synaptic changes, neurofibrillary tangles, neurotransmitter loss, and gliosis, and ultimately results in dementia.

β-amyloid is a small piece of a much larger protein called the amyloid precursor protein (APP). The APP is a transmembrane protein that, when activated, is cut into smaller segments which operate either inside or outside the neuron. There are several ways that the APP can be cut, one of which leads to the production of β-amyloid (Figs 17.2 and 3.11).

There is considerable evidence to support the amyloid cascade hypothesis, for example:

- In a few hundred extended families worldwide, researchers have discovered mutations in genes that virtually guarantee an individual will develop Alzheimer's disease at a young age. Each of these abnormal genes increases β-amyloid production (those in the APP, presenilin 1, or presenilin 2).
- All Alzheimer's disease patients have amyloid plaque counts that far exceed those found in normal aging.
- Down's syndrome patients, who invariably develop Alzheimer's disease pathology by age 50, produce too much β-amyloid protein from birth (presumably because they have a third copy of the gene coding for the APP, found on chromosome 21).
- β-amyloid fibrils damage neurons in culture and activate brain inflammatory cells (microglia).

Despite this evidence, the amyloid cascade hypothesis is only a hypothesis, and as with all hypotheses there are unanswered questions. Nevertheless, the amyloid cascade hypothesis continues to be the most widely accepted view of the pathogenesis of Alzheimer's disease and as such amyloid is a major therapeutic target. Considerable research is now ongoing in an attempt to develop drugs that will intervene in this cascade and in doing so slow (or even stop) the progression of the disease. Some of these drugs act to directly modulate β-amyloid while others are aimed at the downstream effects of β-amyloid plaque such as inflammation.

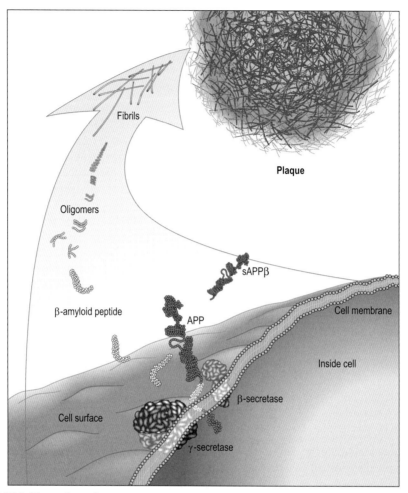

FIGURE 17.2 Plaque formation.

(From: NIA/NIH, 2008. Alzheimer's disease: unraveling the mystery. NIH Publication 08-3782, p. 23.)

Amyloid-directed treatments

There are three major ongoing approaches to intervening in the amyloid cascade (Figs 3.10, 3.11, 17.2, 17.3). The first, secretase inhibitors, involves blocking the formation of β-amyloid by interfering with the enzymes that cleave the amyloid precursor protein in a manner that yields the toxic form of β-amyloid. The second approach, anti-aggregants, is aimed at preventing the aggregation of single strands of β-amyloid (monomers) into units containing multiple strands (oligomers) of the toxic molecule. There is some evidence that, although monomers are not neurotoxic, as few as two aggregated strands (dimers) may be (Haass & Selkoe, 2007). The third strategy, vaccines, involves removing the neuronal plaques, which consist of an aggregated β-amyloid core surrounded by parts of dying neurons.

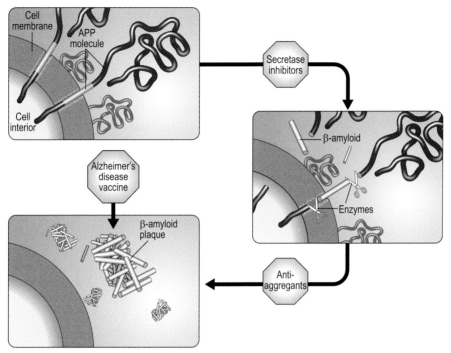

FIGURE 17.3 Possible points of intervention for anti-amyloid treatments.

Active immunotherapy

Also known as the Alzheimer's disease active vaccine, the basic strategy here is to mobilize the immune system to produce antibodies to recognize and attack β-amyloid. The role of these antibodies is to remove existing plaque and to block the formation of subsequent plaques. To accomplish this goal patients are injected with a fragment of the β-amyloid protein.

Initial studies in mice that were genetically engineered to produce pathological forms of β-amyloid (and experienced difficulty in maze learning and other learning and memory tasks) benefited from β-amyloid vaccination. Vaccinated mice had both fewer plaques and relatively enhanced learning and memory compared with non-vaccinated mice.

The first large-scale clinical trial in humans conducted by Elan Pharmaceuticals was with the entire 42 amino acid β-amyloid protein (compound AN1792) or a placebo infused into volunteers (Gilman et al., 2005). The trial received enormous publicity and was enrolled quickly with 300 volunteers with Alzheimer's disease. The trial, however, was stopped prematurely because of side-effects. The goal of AN1792 infusions was to produce an immune response to β-amyloid, but approximately 6% of patients in the trial experienced an inflammatory response (i.e., encephalitis). On the positive side, many of the patients in the study have been followed since their vaccinations in 1999. Several cases have come to autopsy and the results indicated substantially less plaque in the brain of patients from the study who received active vaccine as opposed to placebo (Fig 17.4) (Nicoll et al., 2003; Holmes et al., 2008). Additionally, some of these patients received follow-up at 1 and 4.5 years after vaccination.

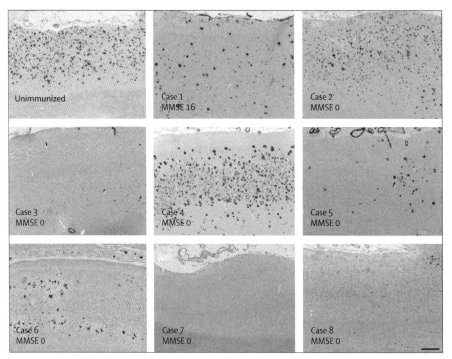

FIGURE 17.4 Histological patterns of Aβ in the temporal lobe neocortex after immunization with AN1792.

An unimmunized control (top left) has a high density of plaques. **Cases 1–8** are all patients who were immunized with Aβ42. **Case 1** died 4 months after the first immunization dose and showed an early stage of Aβ removal. **Cases 2–8** survived 20–64 months after the first immunization dose. **Case 2** did not develop anti-Aβ antibodies and showed no evidence of plaque clearance. **Cases 3–6** showed an intermediate range of plaque clearance. **Cases 7** and **8** showed very extensive (**case 8**) to nearly complete (**case 7**) removal of Aβ plaques throughout the cerebral cortex. All the long-term survivors (i.e., **cases 2–8**) continued to have progressive dementia with cognitive function declining to an unrecordable level (i.e., MMSE=0) before death. Scale bar=0.5 mm. A color version of this figure is available online at http://www.expertconsult.com.

From Holmes, C., Boche, D., Wilkinson, D., et al., 2008. Long-term effects of Abeta42 immunisation in Alzheimer's disease: follow-up of a randomised, placebo-controlled phase I trial. Lancet, 372, 216-223.

At 1 year, vaccinated antibody responders (those with increased titers) did better on a cognitive test battery. A subset of these patients were again evaluated 4.5 years after their initial vaccination. These 17 patients all continued to show increased titers of antibody against β-amyloid compared with placebo controls. Additionally, compared with placebo controls, the vaccinated patients showed significantly less functional decline on measures of activities of daily living and dependence on a caregiver. These patients also did not show any additional episodes of brain inflammation (encephalitis) (Vellas et al., 2009).

In 2009 Wyeth Pharmaceuticals initiated a phase II study with an active vaccine (ACC-001). This vaccine differs from Elan's AN1792 in that it consists of a fragment of the 42 amino acid β-amyloid protein. This modification was made in the hope of eliminating the inflammatory response seen with AN1792. There are currently several ongoing clinical trials with ACC-001. There are also a number of other active vaccines currently in development, but no data from human clinical trials are as yet available.

Passive immunotherapy

The basic strategy here is to administer laboratory-produced antibodies to β-amyloid. The idea is that this Alzheimer's disease passive vaccine might be safer because antibodies are produced in a laboratory and passively administered instead of mobilizing the body's immune system. To accomplish this antibodies are produced in mice. They are then "humanized" to be suitable for humans and ultimately infused in patients. Laboratory-produced antibodies can be given like any other drug in fixed doses, and unlike an active vaccine do not persist in the body after the dosing stops.

Several companies are developing passive anti-β-amyloid antibodies. A joint effort between Elan and Wyeth pharmaceuticals completed a phase II study testing multiple doses of anti-β-amyloid antibodies (bapinuezumab) in approximately 240 patients with Alzheimer's disease (Salloway et al., 2009). In this study patients were given either the anti-β-amyloid antibodies or a placebo for an 18-month period. During this time, they periodically underwent cognitive testing and volumetric MRI to determine whether brain cells were being preserved. The purpose of this study was to evaluate the safety of bapinuezumab. The safety results showed that the primary side-effect was vasogenic edema. Vasogenic edema is a condition in which fluid accumulates in the brain because of an increase in vessel permeability due to the inflammatory process. In this study vasogenic edema occurred in about 5% of patients. Almost all of these patients were taking the highest dose of bapinuezumab. Based on these phase II data, the phase III studies were designed to include only the lower doses of the vaccine. In almost all cases the vasogenic edema resolved without treatment, and in most cases it did not produce symptoms but rather was detected on the routine MRIs. Two large-scale (2000 patients each) phase III clinical trials are currently enrolling and data should be available some time in 2011–2012. Bapineuzumab is now being developed by Janssen Alzheimer's Immunotherapy.

A second passive vaccine developed by Lilly (solenuzumab) also recently reported safety results from a phase II study that indicated no significant side-effects. A large-scale trial (1000 patients) is ongoing. Data should be available in 2012.

Many other companies, including Pfizer, Genentech, Merck, and GlaxoSmithKline (and as many as a dozen others), have passive vaccines in various stages of clinical development.

Blocking the formation of β-amyloid

Recall that β-amyloid is cleaved from the larger amyloid precursor protein (APP) (Figs 3.11 and 17.2). The cleaving is accomplished in a two-step process by enzymes called secretases. APP is one of many proteins that is associated with the neuronal cell membrane. As it is being produced in the cell it penetrates through the cell membrane and eventually resides inside, through, and outside the neuron. There are three enzymes that cut or cleave APP and, depending upon which enzyme is involved and where the cleaving occurs, APP can follow one of two pathways.

In normal processing, the amyloid precursor protein (695–770 amino acids long) is first cleaved by α-secretase and then by γ-secretase to form harmless soluble fragments called sAPP α. sAPP α has beneficial properties related to neuronal growth and survival. In abnormal processing, however, the amyloid precursor protein is first cut by β-secretase and then by γ-secretase to form the toxic β-amyloid proteins (42 amino acids sometimes known as $A\beta_{1-42}$) that self-aggregate to first form oligomers and then fibrils and then plaques. The plaques are clearly toxic to neurons, but now there is evidence that even oligomers may be toxic (Haass & Selkoe, 2007; Moreno et al., 2009).

Changing the behavior of either β-secretase or γ-secretase could reduce or prevent the formation of harmful β-amyloid. Drugs that can block or alter the clipping action of these secretases are called *secretase inhibitors*. There are a number of secretase inhibitors in development, but recent results from a γ-secretase inhibitor (Lilly, LY450139, semagacestat) has led to questions regarding this approach. Preliminary results from two large-scale (more than 2600 patients) ongoing phase III trials demonstrated that the drug not only failed to slow cognitive decline in people with mild to moderate Alzheimer disease, but that it actually made them worse. Based upon this, both trials were immediately halted. Why a γ-secretase inhibitor would disrupt cognition in patients with Alzheimer's disease is unclear, but it may have to do with Notch, a crucial signaling molecule that regulates the fate of a wide variety of cell types. The current view is that it may be necessary to develop Notch-sparing modulation of γ-secretase activity.

A related approach to blocking the formation of amyloid used by Myriad Pharmaceuticals with its compound Flurizan (R-flurbiprofen) is to alter the way secretases work in order to encourage the amyloid precursor protein to cut into fragments other than the toxic β-amyloid protein; that is, to encourage the formation of less toxic forms of $A\beta1$–42 such as $A\beta1$–38 or $A\beta1$–39. Unfortunately, a large clinical trial showed no benefit of this novel drug in patients with mild to moderate Alzheimer's disease (Imbimbo, 2009). The drug has been withdrawn from development.

Blocking accumulation of β-amyloid

Because β-amyloid exists in many forms in the human brain, one important question becomes which form is most toxic. As Figures 17.2 and 3.11 show, when β-amyloid is initially cleaved it forms single pieces or monomers. The monomers are soluble and may not yet be toxic. The monomers are then thought to combine into clusters to form β-amyloid oligomers, and finally the oligomers form insoluble fibrils also known as β-sheets. This process is collectively known as aggregation. These β-sheets further accumulate and become deposited as plaques. It is not clear how long this entire process takes, but some researchers hypothesize that it occurs over many years.

The importance of fully understanding this amyloid cascade is that it provides the opportunity to develop interventions. When researchers initially hypothesized that the β-amyloid did not become toxic until the stage of insoluble beta sheets, they proposed that interventions that blocked this stage could be therapeutic. The more recent view as mentioned above, however, is that β-amyloid may be toxic as early as formation of oligomers and perhaps as early as a cluster of two monomers (dimers) (Haass & Selkoe, 2007).

The first anti-aggregation drug to be tested in patients was Alzhemed (3-amino-1-propanosulfonic acid, 3APS), which is in development by the Canadian pharmaceutical company Neurochem. Alzhemed binds to soluble β-amyloid and in doing so is hypothesized to block the chain of events leading to the formation of toxic beta sheets. Studies in cell culture and in animals lent support to this hypothesis.

In a phase II clinical trial (Aisen et al., 2006), 58 patients with Alzheimer's disease were randomized to receive either placebo or one of three doses of Alzhemed over a 3-month double-blind period. The results of the study indicated that the drug was generally safe and well tolerated. Analyses of cerebrospinal fluid (CSF) also showed that there was a reduction of β-amyloid. Unfortunately, neither this phase II nor two large phase III studies showed any efficacy of Alzhemed in reducing cognitive decline in patients with Alzheimer's disease.

A more recent approach to blocking aggregation of β-amyloid monomers involves treatment with the compound ELND-005 (scyllo-inositol, AZD-103, Elan Pharmaceuticals/ Transition Therapeutics). The hypothesized mechanism of action of this compound is to both block accumulation of Aβ oligomers and prevent Aβ oligomer formation. A recently completed phase II study revealed that the drug did not significantly improve cognition or function in participants with mild to moderate Alzheimer's disease; however, the compound had an effect on CSF Aβ, perhaps suggesting that the compound affected underlying pathology. Based on these data, Elan/Transition have announced that they plan to conduct a phase III trial.

Another approach to preventing the aggregation of amyloid involves clearing less harmful forms of amyloid before they aggregate. One theoretical method to accomplish this is through the use of cholesterol-lowering drugs. As we discussed in Chapter 3: *Alzheimer's disease*, certain forms of the cholesterol-carrying protein apolipoprotein E (APOE) can increase the risk of Alzheimer's disease, while other forms (alleles) lower the risk. One view of why this occurs involves the effects of various alleles of APOE on clearing β-amyloid. The hypothesis is that the risk-inducing allele, E4, is not able to clear β-amyloid as well as the more common E3 allele, whereas the protective allele, E2, facilitates clearance even better than E3.

Retrospective studies showed that individuals who took the statin cholesterol-lowering drugs, typically for hypercholesterolemia, had a significantly lower risk of having Alzheimer's disease than those who did not (Wolozin et al., 2004). However, data from a completed 72-week randomized trial failed to show any difference between patients with mild to modererate Alzheimer's disease taking donepezil (Aricept) plus artorvostatin (Lipitor) and those taking donepezil plus a placebo (see Sparks, 2009).

Downstream approaches

According to the amyloid cascade hypothesis, amyloid plaques lead to neuronal death through a variety of mechanisms including inflammation and oxidative stress. If this is the case, then anti-inflammatories and antioxidants could prevent neuronal death. See Chapter 16: *Vitamins, herbs, supplements, and anti-inflammatories* for a discussion of some of the available anti-inflammatories and antioxidants. But to summarize briefly, there is currently no evidence that any of these treatments provide benefit and we do not recommend them to our patients.

Targeting the neurofibrillary tangle: tau and neurofibrillary degeneration

So far, we have been discussing emerging therapies that target β-amyloid, but as mentioned above there is also a school of thought, the *tauists*, that argues therapeutic approaches for disease progression should target the neurofibrillary tangle. Neurofibrillary lesions, made up from aggregated hyperphosphorylated forms of the microtubule-associated protein tau, represent the second defining form of pathology in Alzheimer's disease (Fig. 17.5).

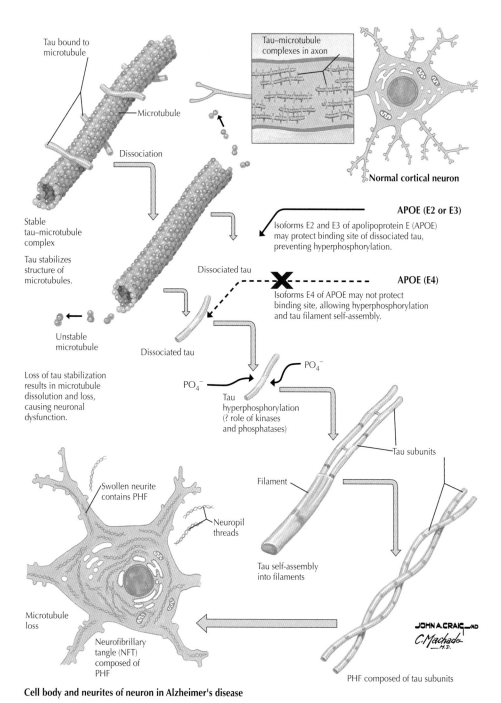

Tau bound to microtubule

Tau–microtubule complexes in axon

Microtubule

Dissociation

Normal cortical neuron

Stable tau–microtubule complex

Tau stabilizes structure of microtubules.

APOE (E2 or E3)

Isoforms E2 and E3 of apolipoprotein E (APOE) may protect binding site of dissociated tau, preventing hyperphosphorylation.

Dissociated tau

APOE (E4)

Isoforms E4 of APOE may not protect binding site, allowing hyperphosphorylation and tau filament self-assembly.

Unstable microtubule

Dissociated tau

PO_4^-

PO_4^-

Loss of tau stabilization results in microtubule dissolution and loss, causing neuronal dysfunction.

Tau hyperphosphorylation (? role of kinases and phosphatases)

Tau subunits

Swollen neurite contains PHF

Neuropil threads

Filament

Tau self-assembly into filaments

Microtubule loss

Neurofibrillary tangle (NFT) composed of PHF

JOHN A. CRAIG—AD
C. Machado—M.D.

PHF composed of tau subunits

Cell body and neurites of neuron in Alzheimer's disease

FIGURE 17.5 Tangle formation in Alzheimer's disease.

A color version of this figure is available online at http://www.expertconsult.com.

The primary role of tau is to stabilize microtubules in the neuron, much like railroad ties stabilize the rails of the track. These microtubules normally serve in axonal transport of cellular nutrients and precursors of neural transmitters. When abnormal phosphorylation occurs, the microtubule network breaks down, there is a disruption of axonal transport, and eventually there is neurodegeneration (Mandelkow & Mandelkow, 1998). Additionally, there is evidence that certain forms of tau may have direct neurotoxic properties (Klafki et al., 2006).

Although the preponderance of evidence is that the senile plaque is the primary culprit in Alzheimer's disease and that the neurofibrillary tangle is part of the chain (the amyloid cascade) that eventually leads to neuronal degeneration and dementia, there is also evidence that, at least for some causes of dementia, the neurofibrillary tangle may be the primary cause.

A familial form of frontal lobe dementia, known as familial frontal lobe dementia with parkinsonism (FDP-17), has been linked to chromosome 17 (see Chapter 7: *Frontotemporal dementia*). In this form of dementia, dysregulation of tau alone can cause neurodegeneration. As discussed in the next section on the pathophysiology of chronic traumatic encephalopathy, it is possible that, once tangle formation begins, the tangles can progress on their own.

Because of the potential role of tau in neurodegeneration, a number of therapeutic strategies are now being pursued that influence the regulation of tau. The basic strategy is to block the abnormal hyperphosphorylation of tau and, in doing so, to stop the formation of neurofibrillary tangles and the destabilization of neurons (Klafki et al., 2006).

The TauRx compound LMTB is hypothesized to inhibit tau protein aggregation and thus block formation of tangles (www.taurx.com). Preliminary phase II data presented at the International Conference on Alzheimer's Disease in 2009 suggested that disease progression was slowed in a double-blind placebo-controlled trial and, based upon these data, phase III trials are now planned. Additionally, because the drug is aimed at the neurofibrillary tangle, it may also be evaluated in frontotemporal dementia (Chapter 7) and progressive supranuclear palsy (Chapter 8), as these and other disorders involve tau pathology in the absence of amyloid plaques.

LESSONS FROM FAILED TRIALS AND CHRONIC TRAUMATIC ENCEPHALOPATHY

To date, there are now at least three different drugs that have shown evidence at reducing β-amyloid or its aggregation but have not shown efficacy in stopping or significantly slowing dementia (Flurizan, Alzhemed, and AN1792). The questions thus naturally arise: Is the amyloid cascade hypothesis wrong? Is β-amyloid incidental to Alzheimer's disease? At present, the answers to these important questions are unknown.

One clue, however, to the relationship between β-amyloid, tangle formation, and dementia comes from our current understanding of chronic traumatic encephalopathy (CTE; McKee et al., 2009). Chronic traumatic encephalopathy is a condition that has existed for more than 80 years. It was formerly known as dementia pugilistica because it was initially described in boxers who received multiple blows to the head and later developed dementia (DeKosky et al., 2010). More recently, chronic traumatic encephalopathy is being discovered in other athletes and particularly professional football players. In each case, it is thought to be brought about by repetitive head trauma (McKee et al., 2009).

As discussed in Chapter 12: *Other disorders*, once the trauma damages the brain sufficiently for tangle formation to get started in chronic traumatic encephalopathy, the evidence suggests that tangles progress on their own. What is particularly notable is that often the brain trauma occurred years or decades prior to the onset of the dementia. This fact raises the possibility that not only does it take decades for dementia to develop after the start of β-amyloid collecting in the brain, but that once tangle formation is underway it may continue on its own at that point regardless of whether β-amyloid is present or not. If this suggestion is correct, it would mean that β-amyloid may be the prime mover in the cause of Alzheimer's disease, but that treatments directed against β-amyloid must be initiated prior to the development of dementia—and probably prior to the development of any cognitive impairment. Future studies will determine whether this interesting hypothesis is correct.

THE FUTURE OF ALZHEIMER'S DISEASE THERAPY

Alzheimer's disease is a devastating neurodegenerative disease for patients, their families, and society. The difficulty of managing this disease for all concerned will grow dramatically over the next 30–40 years, as the number of cases increases four- to five-fold. As with all major illnesses, early detection and treatment will be critical factors in the successful management of Alzheimer's disease. We have suggested that there are three major areas in which substantial progress needs to be made in order to successfully treat Alzheimer's disease: (1) early detection and diagnosis, (2) further development of symptomatic medications, and related treatment and care, and (3) development of disease-modifying medications (Solomon & Budson, 2003; Gold & Budson, 2008; Solomon & Murphy, 2008). We can only hope that the progress in the next 20 years will eclipse the progress of these past productive 20 years.

References

Aisen, P.S., Saumier, D., Briand, R., et al., 2006. A phase II study targeting amyloid-beta with 3APS in mild-to-moderate Alzheimer disease. Neurology 67, 1757–1763.

DeKosky, S.T., Ikonomovic, M.D., Gandy, S., 2010. Traumatic brain injury: football, warfare, and long-term effects. N. Engl. J. Med. 363, 1293–1296.

Gilman, S., Koller, M., Black, R.S., et al., 2005. Clinical effects of Abeta immunization (AN1792) in patients with Alzheimer's disease in an interrupted trial. Neurology 64, 1553–1562.

Gold, C.A., Budson, A.E., 2008. Memory loss in Alzheimer's disease: implications for development of therapeutics. Expert Rev. Neurother. 8, 1879–1891.

Haass, C., Selkoe, D.J., 2007. Soluble protein oligomers in neurodegeneration: lessons from the Alzheimer's amyloid beta-peptide. Nat. Rev. Mol. Cell. Biol. 8, 101–112.

Hardy, J., Selkoe, D.J., 2002. The amyloid hypothesis of Alzheimer's disease: progress and problems on the road to therapeutics. Science 297, 353–356.

Holmes, C., Boche, D., Wilkinson, D., et al., 2008. Long-term effects of Abeta42 immunisation in Alzheimer's disease: follow-up of a randomised, placebo-controlled phase I trial. Lancet 372, 216–223.

Imbimbo, B.P., 2009. Why did tarenflurbil fail in Alzheimer's disease? J. Alzheimers Dis. 17, 757–760.

Klafki, H.W., Staufenbiel, M., Kornhuber, J., et al., 2006. Therapeutic approaches to Alzheimer's disease. Brain 129, 2840–2855.

Mandelkow, E.M., Mandelkow, E., 1998. Tau in Alzheimer's disease. Trends Cell. Biol. 8, 425–427.

McKee, A.C., Cantu, R.C., Nowinski, C.J., et al., 2009. Chronic traumatic encephalopathy in athletes: progressive tauopathy after repetitive head injury. J. Neuropathol. Exp. Neurol. 68, 709–735.

Moreno, H., Yu, E., Pigino, G., et al., 2009. Synaptic transmission block by presynaptic injection of oligomeric amyloid beta. Proc. Natl Acad. Sci. U.S.A. 106, 5901–5906.

Nicoll, J.A., Wilkinson, D., Holmes, C., et al., 2003. Neuropathology of human Alzheimer disease after immunization with amyloid-beta peptide: a case report. Nat. Med. 9, 448–452.

Salloway, S., Sperling, R., Gilman, S., et al., 2009. A phase 2 multiple ascending dose trial of bapineuzumab in mild to moderate Alzheimer disease. Neurology 73, 2061–2070.

Solomon, P.R., Budson, A.L., 2003. Alzheimer's disease. Clinical Symposia: Dannemiller Memorial Educational Foundation (formerly Ciba Symposium) 54 (1), 1–44.

Solomon, P.R., Murphy, C.M., 2008. Early diagnosis and treatment of Alzheimer's disease. Expert Rev. Neurother. 8 (5), 769–780.

Sparks, L., 2009. Statins and cognitive function. J. Neurol. Neurosurg. Psychiatry 80, 1–2.

Vellas, B., Black, R., Thal, L.J., et al., 2009. Long-term follow-up of patients immunized with AN1792: reduced functional decline in antibody responders. Curr. Alzheimer Res. 6, 144–151.

Wolozin, B., Brown III, J., Theisler, C., et al., 2004. The cellular biochemistry of cholesterol and statins: insights into the pathophysiology and therapy of Alzheimer's disease. CNS Drug. Rev. 10, 127–146.

18 Non-pharmacological treatment of memory loss

> ## QUICK START: NON-PHARMACOLOGICAL TREATMENT OF MEMORY LOSS
>
> - Non-pharmacological treatments to help memory loss can improve function equal to or greater than medication.
> - External memory aids such as calendars, lists, and white-boards can be helpful in keeping patients functional.
> - It is important to keep the memory aid in the same place.
> - Learning habits (using procedural memory) allow patients with even moderate Alzheimer's disease to improve their function.
> - Pictures are easier to remember for patients with Alzheimer's disease.
> - The Mediterranean diet or diets high in resveratrol (red grapes, red wine, and blueberries) or antioxidants have been suggested to reduce memory loss, although their value is currently uncertain.
> - Social and cognitively stimulating activities, as found in an enriched environment, have been shown to improve function.
> - Aerobic exercise can stimulate the development of new neurons in the hippocampus and improve cognition, in addition to its effects on cardiovascular health and mood.

Pharmacological treatment of memory loss, present or future, can only help so much when dealing with Alzheimer's and other diseases affecting memory. Non-pharmacological treatments are invaluable, and can often help daily function as much as, if not more than, medications (Burgener et al., 2009). An entire book could be written on this important subject. In this chapter we briefly touch on a number of relevant topics.

EXTERNAL MEMORY AIDS

Almost all of us use external devices to augment our memory. These include traditional simple items, such as a list, calendar, Filofax or organizer, as well as more sophisticated electronic devices including cell phone, BlackBerry, or iPad to store names, addresses, phone numbers, appointments, and other information. Prior to their illness, most patients with memory problems also used such devices to a greater or lesser extent. Not surprisingly, patients who always depended upon external devices are, in general, able to continue using them early on in the disorder to compensate for their declining memory. Patients who, by contrast, always depended upon their memory to keep themselves organized tend to suffer more swift and severe functional impairment as their memory declines, because they do not automatically reach for external devices to compensate for their impaired memory. As the illness progresses, however, almost all patients would benefit from additional use of external devices to compensate for their memory problems. What follows are some of the simple ways that a number of our patients have found functional improvement in the face of memory impairment.

Calendar

Knowing the day, date, month, season, and year are important basic components of knowledge that most of us take for granted. Such knowledge is important insofar as we have appointments, meetings, lunch dates, or television shows that we want to keep, participate in, or watch. Losing track of this information is one of the first things that occurs when memory becomes impaired.

There are, of course, many different types of calendars that can be used. Early in the disease course (e.g., in mild cognitive impairment or very mild Alzheimer's disease) any of these would be fine, as a certain amount of new learning is possible. However, the best approach—and the only approach that works as the disease progresses—is to use a calendar system that can easily become a habit to the patient (Box 18.1).

In general we recommend a large desk or wall calendar that always stays in one place. In this way it will not become lost, and the patient with memory loss will be able to get into the habit of going there to look at it. It is important that the previous days are "crossed off," so that the patient will automatically know what the current date is.

BOX 18.1 THE IMPORTANCE OF HABIT

Using a system that can become a habit is critically important when teaching a patient with memory loss new skills. Habits do not depend upon the episodic memory system—the memory system that is affected by Alzheimer's disease and other disorders of memory. Habits depend upon a different kind of memory, procedural memory. Procedural memory is the type of memory we use when riding a bike, touch typing, playing the violin, and dialing a phone number that we have done hundreds of times without thinking about it. It is due to procedural memory that, when we are not paying attention to where we are driving, we may make turns toward a familiar location—but not necessarily the one we had intended to go to! Procedural memory is quite well preserved in Alzheimer's disease and other memory disorders until quite late in the disease. This preservation of procedural memory allows us to teach the patient with Alzheimer's disease new functional skills even when their episodic memory is devastated. See Appendix C: *Our current understanding of memory* for more on the different types of memory systems in the brain.

Teaching by doing is the key to learning with procedural memory. Think again about learning to ride a bike: it is not learning verbally with words. Has anyone ever asked you for a phone number and you've had to say, "Hold on, let me dial it?" You have to dial it because that number is stored in your procedural memory, not your episodic memory.

Here is an example. The wife of a patient with mild Alzheimer's disease has just bought a new wall calendar that she is keeping all of their appointments on. Although they had not previously used a wall calendar, she is very pleased with her new system, which works very well for her. She reports to us, however, that it is not working for her husband. He is continually asking her what they are doing for the day, and although she has told him a thousand times to go look at the calendar, he never does this on his own, although he will go to it after she tells him to.

We then explained to her that she needs to actually lead him to the calendar each time he asks what they are doing for the day, so that "his feet can learn where to go." At first it seems like no progress is being made. But over the course of a few weeks of her leading him to the calendar every time he asks, he begins to go to look at the calendar automatically.

Special places

In the same way that the patient with memory loss can get into the habit of going to look at the calendar, so can the patient get into the habit of going to other places as well. For example, shoes can be kept in a special place in the front hall so that there is never a search for them. Shopping lists can be kept on the left side of the refrigerator. Microwave dinners can be kept on the right-hand side of the freezer. Clothes for the next day can be laid out on a certain chair such that the patient never needs to ask what they should wear for the day. And even the order of the clothes, laid out in the same way each day, helps the patient to get dressed properly (e.g., underpants first, then pants).

At a more general level we discourage caregivers from rearranging closets or the kitchen drawers or any other organizational system with which the patient is familiar. We have even heard reports from caregivers that rearranging furniture can be a disorienting experience for the patient. Alzheimer's patients can continue to function in longstanding environments because they can rely upon their intact remote memories.

Bulletin and white-boards

Just like the calendar and special places to keep shoes, clothes, and shopping lists, bulletin boards and white-boards mounted in a special place can provide a way to help the patient with memory loss know what is ongoing.

Let's return to the patient and his wife described in Box 18.1. Several years have passed, and he is more impaired, now in the moderate stage of Alzheimer's disease. He is too impaired to read. And the calendar is now too complicated for him to figure out, even with the dates crossed off. But with the help of their daughter, they have found a new system that works. In place of the calendar, in the same spot in which it had hung, they have a magnetic board. Here they put up pictures that let the patient know what is going on that day (Box 18.2). Using the camera on her cell phone, the daughter has taken pictures of many of the common friends and family members that they see, common places they visit, such as the post-office, bank, grocery store, and a favorite restaurant, as well as activities such as walking and gardening. Each morning his wife puts up the people, places, and activities that they will be seeing, visiting, and doing that day. She tells us that she isn't sure that he can remember the things on the board for more than a minute or two, but now he simply goes and looks—sometimes 10 or 20 times in an hour—rather than asking her every time.

SPECIFIC DIETS?

Are there specific diets that will either improve memory loss due to Alzheimer's disease or prevent Alzheimer's disease? This is a question that we often hear from our patients and caregivers. The short answer is that there is no firm evidence to suggest that there is any special diet that is helpful in treating or preventing Alzheimer's disease. One study found that older adults were less likely to develop Alzheimer's disease if they ate more salad, nuts, fish, tomatoes, poultry, vegetables (in particular the cabbage and broccoli family of vegetables), fruits, and dark green leafy vegetables, and less high-fat dairy products, red meat, organ meat, and butter (Gu et al., 2010). Some advocate for foods that are high in resveratrol, which can be found in foods such as red grapes, red wine, and blueberries (Albani et al., 2010). Others advocate for a Mediterranean diet (Berr et al., 2009; Scarmeas et al., 2009a; Scarmeas et al., 2009b). And some recommend diets high in antioxidants or

---

BOX 18.2 POWER OF PICTURES

It is said that a picture is worth a thousand words (Fig. 18.1). For patients with Alzheimer's disease, this is certainly true. Some of our research, in fact, has shown that, although memory is enhanced by pictures relative to words for young adults, this effect of pictures is greater for healthy older adults, greater still for patients with mild cognitive impairment, and is the greatest for patients with Alzheimer's disease (Ally et al., 2009). This enhancement of memory for pictures versus words in Alzheimer's disease is likely attributable to a number of things. We all tend to pay more attention to pictures. Pictures are more distinctive and therefore easier to remember. When we see a picture we may store the information twice: once as an image and once as its meaning. And patients with Alzheimer's disease develop difficulty processing written words as the disease progresses.

   The simple take home message is this: using pictures is one way to help the patient with Alzheimer's disease remember information. So instead of simply telling the patient that his granddaughter will be visiting today, show him her picture.

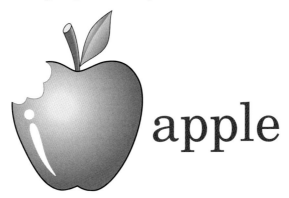

FIGURE 18.1 A picture is worth a thousand words

---

calorie restriction (Burgener et al., 2008). At the present time we consider all of these diets to be promising, but not proven. So, if your patients enjoy having a bowl of blueberries for breakfast, and drinking a glass of Chianti with their antipasti for dinner, by all means encourage them to continue—it can only help. We would not, however, recommend at this time that patients change their diets to something they do not like with the hope that it will help memory loss or prevent Alzheimer's disease.

SOCIAL AND COGNITIVELY STIMULATING ACTIVITIES

A 79-year-old patient with mild Alzheimer's disease, socially isolated and living alone, comes to see us with her daughter in the clinic. She is forgetting to take her medications, and only thinks about eating when she is reminded. She scores 21 out of 30 on the Mini-Mental State Examination (MMSE). She is clearly failing at home, and the decision is made to move her to assisted living. After several weeks of acclimating in the facility, a seemingly miraculous change comes about. She is the "life" of her unit, has many friends, and now appears to have little or no difficulty in navigating her routines. In fact, she seems *better* than when she entered the facility over a month ago. A routine follow-up of her MMSE confirms this: she now scores 25 out of 30!

The scenario outlined above is very common. Why it occurs is not exactly clear. Certainly some of the change may be attributable to improvements in mood, apathy, or both. We know, however, that there are other positive psychological and neurophysiological changes that occur (Nithianantharajah & Hannan, 2009). Whatever the mechanism, when patients move from an isolated to an enriched environment, we typically see clinically relevant improvements in function.

Even if there is no change in living, it has also been proven that leisure activities, particularly those that are socially and cognitively stimulating, can be helpful in slowing memory loss, preventing Alzheimer's disease, reducing neuropsychiatric symptoms, and improving function (Boyke et al., 2008; Akbaraly et al., 2009; Leung et al., 2010).

AEROBIC EXERCISE

Probably the most important non-pharmacological activity to retard memory loss, reduce the risk of Alzheimer's disease, and actually improve memory is to participate in aerobic exercise (Scarmeas et al., 2009a). It has been known for many years that in rodents aerobic exercise leads to hippocampal neurogenesis—new brain cells growing in the hippocampus. More recently, evidence has been found in older adults as well that aerobic exercise can increase brain volume (Colcombe et al., 2006; Gordon et al., 2008). Most importantly, exercise has been shown to improve cognitive function (Weuve et al., 2004). And this benefit of exercise is in addition to the benefits to cardiovascular health and mood. Thus, we advocate for all of our patients to participate in aerobic exercise, such as walking or swimming. And because the studies in rodents show a linear relationship between the amount of exercise and the increase in hippocampal neurogenesis, we tell our patients and families that some exercise is good, and more is better. (See Galvan & Bredesen (2007) for a review of neurogenesis in the adult human brain and the implications for Alzheimer's disease.)

References

Akbaraly, T.N., Portet, F., Fustinoni, S., et al., 2009. Leisure activities and the risk of dementia in the elderly: results from the Three-City Study. Neurology 73, 854–861.

Albani, D., Polito, L., Forloni, G., 2010. Sirtuins as novel targets for Alzheimer's disease and other neurodegenerative disorders: experimental and genetic evidence. J. Alzheimers Dis. 19, 11–26.

Ally, B.A., Gold, C.A., Budson, A.E., 2009. The picture superiority effect in patients with Alzheimer's disease and mild cognitive impairment. Neuropsychologia 47, 595–598.

Berr, C., Portet, F., Carriere, I., et al., 2009. Olive oil and cognition: results from the Three-City Study. Dement. Geriatr. Cogn. Disord. 28, 357–364.

Boyke, J., Driemeyer, J., Gaser, C., et al., 2008. Training-induced brain structure changes in the elderly. J. Neurosci. 28, 7031–7035.

Burgener, S.C., Buettner, L., Coen, B.K., et al., 2008. Evidence supporting nutritional interventions for persons in early stage Alzheimer's disease (AD). J. Nutr. Health Aging 12, 18–21.

Burgener, S.C., Buettner, L.L., Beattie, E., et al., 2009. Effectiveness of community-based, nonpharmacological interventions for early-stage dementia: conclusions and recommendations. J. Gerontol. Nurs. 35, 50–57.

Colcombe, S.J., Erickson, K.I., Scalf, P.E., et al., 2006. Aerobic exercise training increases brain volume in aging humans. J. Gerontol. A. Biol. Sci. Med. Sci. 61, 1166–1170.

Galvan, V., Bredesen, D.E., 2007. Neurogenesis in the adult brain: implications for Alzheimer's disease. CNS Neurol. Disord. Drug Targets 6, 303–310.

Gordon, B.A., Rykhlevskaia, E.I., Brumback, C.R., et al., 2008. Neuroanatomical correlates of aging, cardiopulmonary fitness level, and education. Psychophysiology 45, 825–838.

Gu, Y., Nieves, J.W., Stern, Y., et al., 2010. Food combination and Alzheimer disease risk: a protective diet. Arch. Neurol. 67, 699–706.

Leung, G.T., Fung, A.W., Tam, C.W., et al., 2010. Examining the association between participation in late-life leisure activities and cognitive function in community-dwelling elderly Chinese in Hong Kong. Int. Psychogeriatr. 22, 2–13.

Nithianantharajah, J., Hannan, A.J., 2009. The neurobiology of brain and cognitive reserve: mental and physical activity as modulators of brain disorders. Prog. Neurobiol. 89, 369–382.

Scarmeas, N., Luchsinger, J.A., Schupf, N., et al., 2009a. Physical activity, diet, and risk of Alzheimer disease. JAMA 302, 627–637.

Scarmeas, N., Stern, Y., Mayeux, R., et al., 2009b. Mediterranean diet and mild cognitive impairment. Arch. Neurol. 66, 216–225.

Weuve, J., Kang, J.H., Manson, J.E., et al., 2004. Physical activity, including walking, and cognitive function in older women. JAMA 292, 1454–1461.

CHAPTER

19   Evaluating the behavioral and psychological symptoms of dementia

---

QUICK START: EVALUATING THE BEHAVIORAL AND PSYCHOLOGICAL SYMPTOMS OF DEMENTIA

The behavioral and psychological symptoms of dementia	• The behavioral and psychological symptoms of dementia are usually the most difficult for patients and caregivers to manage.
	• Symptoms usually assessed on the basis of interviews with patients and relatives include anxiety, depression, hallucinations, and delusions.
	• Symptoms usually identified on the basis of observation of patient behavior include aggression, screaming, restlessness, agitation, wandering, culturally inappropriate behaviors, sexual disinhibition, hoarding, cursing, and shadowing.
Benefits of treatment	• Improves quality of life for patients and caregivers.
	• Reduces caregiver stress.
	• Reduces the likelihood of institutionalization.
	• Decreases the patient's dependence upon the caregiver.
	• May improve cognition and function.
Evaluating behavioral and psychological symptoms of dementia	• It is important for the clinician to evaluate:
	• Apathy
	• Mood
	– Depression
	– Anxiety
	• Psychosis
	– Agitation
	– Disinhibition
	– Hallucinations
	– Delusions.
Formulating a treatment plan	• Caring for and educating the caregiver (Chapter 20)
	• Non-pharmacological treatment of the patient (Chapter 21)
	• Pharmacological treatment of the patient (Chapter 22)

Patient EB is an 84-year-old woman who is living with her two nieces. She moved to the United States at age 22, never married, and worked in the fashion industry in New York, retiring at age 65. She has memory problems (denies having conversations, constantly repeats questions), problems with executive functioning (she has great difficulty managing her finances and has inappropriately given away money), and visuospatial functioning (she can become lost walking in her neighborhood). She also entirely denies any cognitive deficits and does not understand why she needs to live with her nieces. She is agitated and this agitation is expressed by constantly berating her nieces, denying her problems, and attempting to wander in the neighborhood. Her nieces are extremely frustrated in attempting to care for her. We diagnosed her with Alzheimer's disease and then had a discussion with the patient and her nieces regarding treatments.

Recall the case of EB from Chapter 13. Until now we have been discussing treatments for the cognitive aspects of Alzheimer's disease. But, as case EB demonstrates, changes in cognition and the problems that this causes are only part of the problem in Alzheimer's disease (as well as other dementing illnesses). There are accompanying behavioral symptoms, as well, which have significant management consequences. To wit, we have learned from our families that, in many respects, the stresses and demands of caring for a patient with behavioral problems is often the primary challenge. As one caregiver succinctly characterized the challenges in dealing with the behavioral and psychological symptoms of dementia:

> *When my wife would forget to buy my favorite foods at the supermarket I was upset, but when she started screaming at me to get out of our bed because she did not sleep with strangers, I knew the disease had reached a whole different level.*

There has been considerable effort in recent years to develop both behavioral and pharmacological treatments for what has become known as "the behavioral and psychological signs and symptoms of dementia" (Finkel et al., 1996). Clinicians now realize that caring for these symptoms is a central part of caring for the patient with Alzheimer's disease and other dementias (Table 19.1).

WHAT CONSTITUTES BEHAVIORAL AND PSYCHOLOGICAL SYMPTOMS OF DEMENTIA?

There are many symptoms that can be classified in the category of behavioral and psychological symptoms of dementia, and considerable effort has been devoted to arriving at a classification scheme. One such scheme that was presented at the first consensus conference for these symptoms in 1996 (Finkel et al., 1996) suggests that two general categories of symptoms can be evaluated:

- Symptoms usually assessed on the basis of interviews with patients and relatives. These symptoms include anxiety, depressive mood, hallucinations, and delusions.
- Symptoms usually identified on the basis of observation of patient behavior including aggression, screaming, restlessness, agitation, wandering, culturally inappropriate behaviors, sexual disinhibition, hoarding, cursing, and shadowing.

Table 19.1 Dementias and selected neurodegenerative disorders that commonly manifest behavioral and psychological symptoms

Behavioral/ psychological symptom	Dementia
Apathy	• Alzheimer's disease • Vascular dementia • Frontotemporal dementia • Dementia with Lewy bodies • Corticobasal degeneration
Depression	• Alzheimer's disease • Parkinson's disease • Vascular dementia • Corticobasal degeneration • Dementia with Lewy bodies
Hallucinations	• Dementia with Lewy bodies • Parkinson's disease (following treatment with dopaminergic agonists) • Vascular dementia (if infarcts involve the visual system)
Delusions	• Alzheimer's disease • Dementia with Lewy bodies • Parkinson's disease (following treatment with dopaminergic agonists)
Agitation/aggression	• Alzheimer's disease • Dementia with Lewy bodies • Frontotemporal dementia
Disinhibition	• Frontotemporal dementia

After Cummings, J.L., 2003. The Neuropsychiatry of Alzheimer's Disease and Related Dementias. Martin Dunitz Ltd, London, Ch. 2, p. 32.

THE BENEFITS OF TREATING BEHAVIORAL AND PSYCHOLOGICAL SYMPTOMS OF DEMENTIA

Treating these symptoms has many potential benefits for patients and caregivers. Both patients and caregivers report experiencing considerable distress when patients experience these symptoms. As noted above, it has been our experience that little is more distressing to caregivers than these symptoms. Treating these symptoms can help reduce stress in the family setting. By reducing stress, treating behavioral and psychological symptoms of dementia can improve the quality of life for patients and caregivers and may reduce the risk of institutionalization. Additionally, treating these symptoms may improve cognition and functional ability and decrease the patient's dependence on the caregiver.

MEASURING BEHAVIORAL AND PSYCHOLOGICAL SYMPTOMS OF DEMENTIA

There are now a variety of methods of measuring behavioral and psychological symptoms of dementia, ranging from informant interviews to validated scales. Some scales focus on a single symptom (e.g., depression) whereas others rate multiple symptoms. The Geriatric Depression Scale (Yesavage et al., 1983) and the Cornell Scale for Depression (Alexopoulos et al., 1988) are commonly used to rate depression, and the Cohen-Mansfield Agitation Inventory is widely used to measure agitation (Cohen-Mansfield, 1986). The BEHAVE-Alzheimer's disease (Reisberg et al., 1987) is an example of a multisymptom rating scale, as is the widely used Neuropsychiatric Inventory (Cummings et al., 1994).

The Neuropsychiatric Inventory is designed to provide a multidimensional profile of the behavioral and psychological symptoms that accompany dementia (Cummings et al., 1994). It is predicated on three assumptions that have been supported by research findings:

- As cognition worsens, behavioral changes become more likely.
- Multiple, simultaneous symptoms are the rule in patients with Alzheimer's disease (Fig. 19.1). For example, patients commonly exhibit agitation, psychosis, and depression.
- Once symptoms occur, they tend to persist.

The behavioral and psychological symptoms that are included in the Neuropsychiatric Inventory provide both a summary of what clinicians might expect to encounter and a framework for measuring/evaluating these symptoms (Table 19.2).

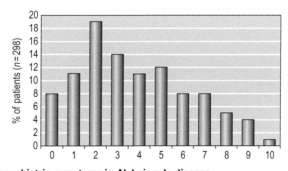

FIGURE 19.1 Neuropsychiatric symptoms in Alzheimer's disease.

Percentage of patients with Alzheimer's disease who exhibited 0, 1, 2, 3, etc., neuropsychiatric symptoms elicited with the 10-item Neuropsychiatric Inventory. Note that 92% showed at least one symptom, and 51% had four or more symptoms.

After Cummings, J.L., 2003. The Neuropsychiatry of Alzheimer's Disease and Related Dementias. Martin Dunitz Ltd, London, Ch. 1, p. 7.

Table 19.2 Neuropsychiatric screening questions

Behavioral/ psychological symptom	Probe from the Neuropsychiatric Inventory
Delusions	Does the patient have beliefs that you know are not true (for example, insisting that people are trying to harm him/her or steal from him/her)? Has he/she said that family members are not who they say they are or that the house is not their home? I'm not asking about mere suspiciousness; I am interested if the patient is *convinced* that these things are happening to him/her.
Hallucinations	Does the patient have hallucinations, such as seeing false visions or hearing imaginary voices? Does he/she seem to see, hear or experience things that are not present? By this question, we do not mean just mistaken beliefs such as stating that someone who has died is still alive; rather, we are asking if the patient actually has abnormal experiences of sounds or visions.
Agitation/ aggression	Does the patient have periods when he/she refuses to cooperate or won't let people help him/her? Is he/she hard to handle?
Depression	Does the patient seem sad or depressed? Does he/she say that he/she feels sad or depressed?
Anxiety	Is the patient very nervous, worried, or frightened for no apparent reason? Does he/she seem very tense or fidgety? Is the patient afraid to be apart from you?
Elation/euphoria	Does the patient seem too cheerful or too happy for no reason? I don't mean the normal happiness that comes from seeing friends, receiving presents, or spending time with family members. I am asking if the patient has a persistent and *abnormally* good mood or finds humor where others do not.
Apathy/indifference	Has the patient lost interest in the world around him/her? Has he/she lost interest in doing things or does he/she lack motivation for starting new activities? Is he/she more difficult to engage in conversation or in doing chores? Is the patient apathetic or indifferent?
Disinhibition	Does the patient seem to act impulsively without thinking? Does he/she do or say things that are not usually done or said in public? Does he/she do things that are embarrassing to you or others?
Irritability	Does the patient get irritated and easily disturbed? Are his/her moods very changeable? Is he/she abnormally impatient? We do not mean frustration over memory loss or inability to perform usual tasks; we are interested to know if the patient has *abnormal* irritability, impatience, or rapid emotional changes different from his/her usual self.
Aberrant motor behavior	Does the patient pace, do things over and over such as opening closets or drawers, or repeatedly pick at things or wind string or threads?
Sleep and night-time behavior disorders	Does the patient have difficulty sleeping? (Do not count as present if the patient simply gets up once or twice per night only to go to the bathroom and falls back asleep immediately.) Is he/she up at night? Does he/she wander at night, get dressed in the middle of the night, or disturb your sleep?
Appetite and eating disorders	Has he/she had any change in appetite, weight, or eating habits? (Count as NA if the patient is incapacitated or has to be fed.) Has there been any change in the type of food he/she prefers?

EVALUATING BEHAVIORAL AND PSYCHOLOGICAL SYMPTOMS OF DEMENTIA: PRAGMATIC GUIDELINES FOR THE CLINICIAN

An important part of any diagnostic and treatment plan of the demented patient is evaluating behavioral and psychological symptoms. In general, we have found that discussing three areas with the patient and caregiver in the course of either the initial or a follow-up interview will generally provide information regarding these symptoms.

We generally probe:

- apathy
- mood (anxiety, depression)
- psychosis (hallucinations, delusions, agitation, disinhibition).

The clinician may wish to address these areas using the screening questions from the Neuropsychiatric Inventory (Table 19.2).

Apathy

Apathy is among the most common and earliest symptoms of Alzheimer's disease (Mega et al., 1996; Fig. 19.2)

- *Probe:* lack of interest in usual activities, pursuits, and hobbies.
- *Probe:* loss of interest in social engagements including meeting friends or engaging with family members.
- *Probe:* loss of emotional engagement including reduced affect and intimacy.

Mood (anxiety and depression)

- *Probe:* patients must exhibit either a depressed mood or a decreased positive affect or pleasure
- *Probe:* has there been anxiety, nervousness, or tension?
- *Probe:* has there been increased irritability?
- *Probe:* has the patient had manifestations of sadness, helplessness, or hopelessness?

Note: Depression and anxiety occur in greater than 50% of patients with Alzheimer's disease.

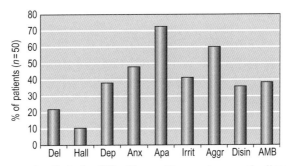

FIGURE 19.2 Percentage of patients (*n*=50) with specific symptoms on the Neuropsychiatric Inventory.

Del, delusions; Hall, hallucinations; Dep, depression; Anx, anxiety; Apa, apathy; Irrit, irritability; Aggr, aggression/agitation; Disin, disinhibition; AMB, aberrant motor behavior.

After Cummings, J.L., 2003. The Neuropsychiatry of Alzheimer's Disease and Related Dementias. Martin Dunitz Ltd, London, Ch. 1, p. 7.

Psychosis (hallucinations, delusions, agitation, disinhibition)

Agitation

Note – Agitation is among the most common symptoms of Alzheimer's disease, occurring in about 70% of patients at some point in the course of the disease.

- *Probe:* has the patient exhibited aggressive, disruptive, and resistive behaviors such as threats, hitting, shouting, or cursing?
- *Probe:* has the patient exhibited less severe behaviors including pacing and frequent repetition of questions?

Disinhibition

Note – Disinhibition is characterized by inappropriate social and interpersonal interactions. This is not typical in Alzheimer's disease, but may occur and can be prominent in frontotemporal dementia.

- *Probe:* has the patient exhibited impulsive behavior including tactless and lewd comments?
- *Probe:* has the patient disregarded usual social conventions, for example inappropriately touching someone?
- *Probe:* has the patient exhibited behaviors that have been embarrassing to their family?

Hallucinations and delusions

Note – The combined prevalence of hallucinations and delusions is 40–65% in Alzheimer's disease patients.

- *Probe:* presence of hallucinations or delusions that occur after the onset of dementia symptoms?

Note: Hallucinations or delusions must have been present at least intermittently for 1 month or longer, must not be due to delirium, and must be severe enough to disrupt patient function.

Note – Visual hallucinations that occur as presenting or early symptoms of a dementia syndrome are suggestive of dementia with Lewy bodies.

FORMULATING A TREATMENT PLAN FOR BEHAVIORAL AND PSYCHOLOGICAL SYMPTOMS: PRAGMATIC GUIDELINES FOR THE CLINICIAN

In our experience, treatment of behavioral and psychological symptoms can be approached in three ways.

- caring for and educating the caregiver
- non-pharmacological treatment of the patient
- pharmacological treatment of the patient.

These approaches are by no means mutually exclusive; it is best, in fact, when approaches are used together. For example, non-pharmacological (e.g., behavioral treatments) are typically instituted by the caregiver based on a plan from the education provided by the clinician. Similarly, in many cases, combinations of pharmacological and non-pharmacological interventions produce the best outcome. In the following chapters we will provide specific pharmacological and non-pharmacological strategies for different behavioral and psychological symptoms. Before doing so, however, it may be useful to provide a general discussion of caring and educating the caregiver. We will consider caring for the caregiver in Chapter 20, non-pharmacological treatments for the patient in Chapter 21, and pharmacological treatments in Chapter 22.

References

Alexopoulos, G.S., Abrams, R.C., Young, R.C., et al., 1988. Cornell Scale for Depression in Dementia. Biol. Psychiatry 23, 271–284.

Cohen-Mansfield, J., 1986. Agitated behaviors in the elderly. II. Preliminary results in the cognitively deteriorated. J. Am. Geriatr. Soc. 34, 722–727.

Cummings, J.L., Mega, M., Gray, K., et al., 1994. The Neuropsychiatric Inventory: comprehensive assessment of psychopathology in dementia. Neurology 44, 2308–2314.

Finkel, S.I., Costa e Silva, G., Cohen, et al., 1996. Behavioral and psychological signs and symptoms of dementia: a consensus statement on current knowledge and implications for research and treatment. Int. Psychogeriatr. 8 (Suppl. 3), 497–500.

Mega, M.S., Cummings, J.L., Fiorello, T., et al., 1996. The spectrum of behavioral changes in Alzheimer's disease. Neurology 46, 130–135.

Reisberg, B., Borenstein, J., Salob, S.P., et al., 1987. Behavioral symptoms in Alzheimer's disease: phenomenology and treatment. J. Clin. Psychiatry 48 (Suppl.), 9–15.

Yesavage, J.A., Brink, T.L., Rose, T.L., et al., 1983. Development and validation of a geriatric depression screening scale: a preliminary report. J. Psychiatr. Res. 17, 37–49.

20 Caring for and educating the caregiver

QUICK START: CARING FOR AND EDUCATING THE CAREGIVER

- Alzheimer's is a disease that affects the entire family.
- Approximately 70% of patients with Alzheimer's disease are cared for at home by a family member.
- Supporting the caregiver is vitally important.
  - Listen to the caregiver
  - Educate the caregiver
  - Make sure the caregiver is taking care of his or her own health
    - Does the caregiver have a primary care physician?
    - Would the caregiver benefit from referral to a psychotherapist?
- Helpful books for caregivers include:
  - *The Alzheimer's Action Plan* (Doraiswamy & Gwyther, 2008)
  - *The 36-Hour Day* (Mace & Rabins, 2006)
  - *Learning to Speak Alzheimer's* (Coste, 2003).
- Three predictable transition points where the caregiver needs help:
  - Coping with the diagnosis
    - Understanding the nature of the disease
    - Understanding the stage of disease
    - Prognosis: What is the disease progression?
    - Familial/genetic implications?
    - Treatment options
    - Is there resistance to the diagnosis?
    - Financial and legal planning
  - Disease progression
    - Accepting outside help, e.g., home health aide, homemaker, social worker
    - Alzheimer's Association has many resources (www.alz.org)
    - Support groups can provide caregivers with great benefit
  - Late-stage decisions
    - The decision to seek 24-hour care is not a selfish decision but one that is almost always in the best interest of the patient
    - There is no absolute right or wrong time to make this move
    - Because the decision to institute 24-hour care can come about with little warning, a plan should be in place

Continued

Memory Loss: A Practical Guide for Clinicians.

QUICK START: CARING FOR AND EDUCATING THE CAREGIVER—Cont'd

- Relinquishing primary caregiving does not mean the caregiver will not be involved
- We encourage caregivers to begin to consider how they will fill the void when they are no longer spending considerable time caregiving.

See also Chapter 23: *Life adjustments,* for additional discussion of these important topics.

Alzheimer's is a disease that has effects on many more individuals than just those with the dementia. The effect of the disease on families and other caregivers is staggering.

- Approximately 70% of patients with Alzheimer's disease are cared for at home, typically by a family member.
- Caregivers spend an average of 863 hours per year (16.6 hours per week) providing direct care—an impressive figure when compared with the average of 1800 hours per year that Americans work at their full-time job (US Department of Labor, www.dol.gov/dol/topic/statistics, accessed 2009).
- In 2008, 9.8 million American family members and other unpaid caregivers provided 8.4 billion hours of unpaid care, an economic contribution valued at over $89 billion dollars annually (Alzheimer's Association, 2010).
- Over half of the $100 billion spent annually on Alzheimer's disease-related services are attributed to the treatment of caregivers, who are at increased risk for medical and psychiatric illness.

To help the families of our newly diagnosed patients we often recommend that they read a book for caregivers such as *Learning to Speak Alzheimer's* (Coste, 2003), *The 36-Hour Day* (Mace & Rabins, 2006), or *The Alzheimer's Action Plan* (Doraiswamy & Gwyther, 2008). In *The 36-Hour Day*, a classic now in its fourth edition, the authors, Nancy Mace, a social worker, and Peter Rabins, a psychiatrist, take a pragmatic approach to many of the problems faced by Alzheimer's disease patients and their families. In *The Alzheimer's Action Plan*, Murali Doraiswamy, a psychiatrist, and Lisa Gwyther, a social worker, take a very pragmatic approach to diagnosis, treatment, and caregiving. In all of these books, there are topics that range from diagnosis, to medical care, to dealing with problems of mood and behavior. Introducing these books also allows us to discuss with the caregiver our understanding of what is perhaps one of the most difficult jobs: caring for the Alzheimer's disease patient. (In some respects the title, *The 36-Hour Day,* tells all.) Our goal in this conversation is fourfold:

1. To let the caregiver know that we fully understand the difficult job they are undertaking.
2. To help them understand that Alzheimer's is a disease that affects the whole family.
3. To introduce the concept that this disease is best treated as a partnership between the patient, the caregiver, and the clinician.
4. To let them know that the treatment of this disease involves treating, supporting, and educating the caregiver along with the patient. We often tell caregivers:

Once the diagnosis and treatment plan is in place, it is likely that our staff and we will spend more time with you than with the patient. This is because we recognize that the single most important aspect of how the patient does throughout the disease is how the caregiver does.

We encourage and try to help everyone become a "4-star caregiver." Having said this, we also recognize that some individuals are more suited to be caregivers than others. This is never presented as a criticism, but simply that each individual has their own strengths and weaknesses. Later in this chapter we will discuss strategies for recognizing and handling this situation. If we as clinicians have learned one thing in the more that 20 years we have been caring for Alzheimer's disease patients and their families, it is to do our best not to be judgmental.

As is common in the typical medical model, caregivers often feel that, although they are provided with adequate information and support when the diagnosis is given, support in the subsequent care may be lacking (Laakkonen et al., 2008). In our roles as health professionals we work to try to help the patient and caregiver throughout the entire disease process.

CARING FOR THE CAREGIVER

Caregivers, simply by virtue of being caregivers, are at increased risk for a variety of medical and psychological problems (Box 20.1). Caregivers have many more illnesses than non-caregiving older adults (Baumgarten et al., 1994, 1997; Schulz et al., 1995; Crespo et al., 2005; Ferrara et al., 2008). These are primarily stress-related illnesses such as headache and chronic fatigue. They are also susceptible to psychological illnesses, particularly anxiety and depression. Anger is also commonly reported in Alzheimer's disease caregivers. Caregivers frequently indicate that they feel captive, burdened, and distressed. There are several things the treating clinician can do to help, but often the most important and helpful is simply acknowledging that the caregiver may be experiencing these emotions.

- Referral to psychological services may be appropriate. When possible, we will take part in the initial visit between the caregiver and the therapist.
- Being sure that the caregiver has a primary care physician. We have been struck by the number of caregivers who are so busy taking care of the patient that they neglect their own health. They frequently either ignore or try to self-treat their own medical illnesses.

THREE PREDICTABLE TRANSITION POINTS WHERE THE CAREGIVER NEEDS HELP

In our experience there are three points in the course of caring for the Alzheimer's disease patient that pose particular difficulty for the caregiver: (1) diagnosis, (2) disease progression—the onset of increasingly debilitating declines in function and/or the onset of the behavioral and psychological symptoms, and (3) the transition to 24-hour care.

BOX 20.1 LISTENING TO THE CAREGIVER

In the course of a follow-up visit simply asking the question of the caregiver, "How are you doing?" and listening to their response may be the single most important part of the visit. Although we often cannot solve the problems they are facing, letting them know we are aware and concerned can do a world of good.

Coping with the diagnosis

The diagnosis of any major illness, including Alzheimer's disease, poses challenges for both the patient and family (Box 20.2). Among the issues that need to be discussed during the visit when the diagnosis is made include:

The nature of the disease

We discuss Alzheimer's disease as a brain disease in which cells in the brain are slowly, but surely, dying. As these cells die, abilities are lost. Most families and patients resonate to this discussion because they have recognized the progressive nature of their cognitive decline, and because they are fearful that Alzheimer's disease "means they are crazy," something of which they are both fearful and embarrassed. Explaining that Alzheimer's disease is a medical disorder and specifically a brain disease can thus be helpful.

We also explain that the brain not only enables cognition and memory but it also regulates personality and behavior. This fact means that, as the disease progresses, behavior and personality will change—sometimes only subtly, sometimes dramatically. So, for example, when the wife finds that her husband with Alzheimer's disease is acting in an irritable, aggressive, or inappropriate manner, it does not mean that he is being "a jerk." It means that the disease has affected his personality and behavior.

Stage of disease

It is important to present Alzheimer's as a long-lasting disease (an average of 8–12 years) that is very different in different stages. We usually discuss three stages—early, middle, and late—noting that about 3–4 years are spent in each (Table 20.1).

BOX 20.2 ISSUES TO BE DISCUSSED WITH THE CAREGIVER WHEN THE DIAGNOSIS IS DISCLOSED

- The nature of the disease
  - Brain cells are dying, causing a decline in cognition and memory
  - Changes also occur in personality and behavior
- There are different stages of Alzheimer's disease, each with their own challenges
- The disease progresses over time
- As in most other major illnesses, family members are at higher risk of developing the disease
- There are a number of treatment options available
- Financial and legal planning will be needed at some time

Table 20.1 Three stages of Alzheimer's disease

Stage	Mini-Mental State Examination range	Description
I (Early)	>18	Subtle changes in cognition; patient can often live alone with supervision that must increase as the patient progresses throughout this stage
II (Middle)	10–18	Patient now needs supervision/help with most activities. Living alone is now impossible.
III (Late)	<10	24-hour care is present or imminent

We then discuss with the patient and caregiver which stage the patient falls into, and the level of care that is likely to be necessary in each stage.

Progression

Patients typically want to know how quickly the disease will progress. We begin by noting that progression is quite variable in Alzheimer's disease. We also indicate that making predictions beyond the next year is difficult (an analogy that helps is to point out that they would have little faith in a weather forecast that predicted more than a week in advance). With this in mind, we discuss the changes in activities and living situation that we might foresee in the next year.

Genetic implications

Most families ask about this early on. At initial diagnosis we usually briefly state that like any other major illness, if a first-degree relative has the disease, family members are at greater risk. Later, we may discuss more fully what is known about the genetic risks. Of course, in the rare cases of autosomal dominant familial disease, we have a different discussion.

Treatment

Patients and families are always anxious to discuss treatment options. Please see Section III: *Treatment of Memory Loss* (Chapters 13–18).

Resistance to diagnosis

Resistance can come from the patient (most common), the caregiver/family, or both. Resistance from the patient usually goes hand-in-hand with resistance to being at the evaluation and often manifests as "there is nothing wrong with my memory." It is our experience that there is little the clinician can do at that point to persuade the patient that there is a problem. The goal in this situation is not to argue the point, but to convince him or her to begin treatment. Over time, as a relationship begins to form between the clinician, patient, and caregiver, we usually find that the patient's resistance softens. Resistance from the caregiver usually reflects underlying discomfort with the diagnosis, typically because of fear. There may be fear over the loss of the loved one, fear of being left alone (emotionally and physically), or fear of a prolonged illness that they have observed in another family member. Occasionally caregivers are reluctant to accept a diagnosis for which there is no biomarker. In these cases we offer to refer the patient and caregiver for a second opinion. It is our view that we cannot successfully treat the patient if the patient, caregiver, or both are not accepting of the diagnosis. See Carpenter & Dave (2004) for a review on the important topic of disclosing the diagnosis.

Financial and legal planning

We feel that a lengthy discussion of financial and legal ramifications of the disease at the first or second visit is perhaps too much for a family to deal with and digest. But planting the seed that these are important issues can be helpful. We then go over these points again at a later visit, typically by encouraging caregivers to discuss these issues with their family lawyer and/ or financial planner.

Disease progression

It can be surmised from the complexity described already, that, in many respects, Alzheimer's disease is not a single uniform illness. As the disease progresses, the symptoms of the patient and consequent demands on the caregiver can change significantly. At a recent talk we gave to a group of caregivers, one of the caregivers noted the following:

> *The most difficult part of being a caregiver is dealing with the progressive nature of the disease. Just when I think I have the situation in control, just when I think the programs and structure I have created are working, something changes and it is back to the drawing board.*

This caregiver, of course, is referring to both declines in cognition and/or the onset of behavioral and psychological symptoms. In these instances, families need help in accepting the changes and implementing strategies to cope.

Accepting outside help

Many caregivers are reluctant to accept any outside help. This may stem from the caregiver's belief that caring for their spouse or parent is their job, or from not wanting "strangers" in their home. It also may stem from the patient's reluctance to having anyone other than the caregiver help them. This situation can be potentially disastrous because it greatly exacerbates caregiver stress, leading to the exact situation that the clinician and both the patient and caregiver are trying to avoid: a debilitated caregiver leading to a crisis which requires immediate large amounts of outside help or earlier 24-hour care than would otherwise be necessary. Further complicating the situation is that individuals under stress are poor decision-makers.

We have found several approaches help in defusing the situation of the caregiver who refuses outside help:

- A discussion with the caregiver that they are the single most important factor in the prognosis for the patient and it is therefore essential that they remain healthy. An important part of remaining healthy is to reduce stress. Accepting outside help is an important part of stress reduction.
- Enlisting the services of a social worker, elder care services, or the Alzheimer's Association (www.alz.org) can be helpful.
- Encouraging the caregiver to attend a support group to learn how other caregivers handle stressful situations can be very beneficial.
- Asking the caregiver to consider counseling.

Late-stage decisions

Almost inevitably, patients with Alzheimer's disease will reach a point when a single caregiver can no longer adequately care for them. At this time caregivers must seek placement in a facility where caregiving is a shared responsibility. This usually means placement in an assisted living or a nursing home facility. In a small minority of cases, families attempt to arrange for round-the-clock help to come into the home. While on the surface this seems like a desirable plan, we have rarely seen it accomplished successfully. There are unfortunately a number of challenging obstacles that make this a difficult path. To begin, round-the-clock care is very expensive; by estimates of some of the families we have worked with who have done this successfully, round-the-clock care can cost up to $100,000 annually. Few families have these resources. Even when financial resources are available, it is difficult to find skilled and reliable caregivers. As we point out to families who propose this, "Whenever a caregiver does not show up, you are the backup."

In some cases, as the disease progresses, there is a stepwise transition from living at home, to assisted living, to nursing homes. In all cases these transitions are difficult for the caregiver—sometimes more so than for the patient. For our patients, whom we follow on a regular basis, we will often initiate the conversation in anticipation of these transitions.

The decision to move a loved one from the home is always a very difficult and emotionally laden decision (Lieberman & Fisher, 2001). It is important to start to plant the seed early that a move from the home will be necessary at some time, and to continue that discussion as the disease progresses. When we recognize that the caregiver can no longer successfully care for the patient at home we continue this conversation with a discussion that includes the following points that may ease the transition for the caregiver:

- *The decision to seek 24-hour care is not a selfish decision but one that is almost always in the best interest of the patient.* We usually begin by praising the caregiver's efforts to date, and reviewing all the wonderful things they have done over the past year (caregivers rarely get such outside praise). We then discuss how inevitably, in all cases of Alzheimer's disease, there comes a time that no single person can care for the patient. Moreover, attempting to do so may actually not be in the best interest of the patient. This leads to a discussion of the concept of "caregiving shared by professionals," and a discussion of ways in which this can be accomplished, including help in the home through homemakers and home health aides, adult day care, assisted living, and nursing homes.

- *There is no absolute right or wrong time to make this move.* We emphasize that all caregivers and patients are different and that the time to implement a move to assisted living or nursing home is when the caregiver—with guidance from the clinician—thinks it is appropriate and will be best for both patient and caregiver together. We also take this as an opportunity to tell the caregiver that, in our experience, the time for the move may come on suddenly.

- *Because the decision to institute 24-hour care can come about with little warning, a plan should be in place.* Because the time to start 24-hour care often comes at a time of crisis, we urge caregivers to begin to visit facilities during the middle stage of the disease (MMSE 10–17) in order to identify a facility in which they would feel comfortable having their loved one. When they find a facility, we urge them to complete the necessary paperwork to the degree that they can, so that, when the time comes, they can initiate placement with just a phone call. We also explain that there may be a delay until a place in the facility becomes available.

- *Relinquishing primary caregiving does not mean they will not be involved.* We let caregivers know that, once the move is made, how much or little they are involved in care will be up to them, again indicating that there is no right amount, but rather it is an individual decision.

- *We encourage them to begin to consider how they will fill the void when they are no longer spending considerable time caregiving.* We encourage them to consider the things they liked to do before they became a caregiver. Work (paid or volunteer), travel, hobbies, and time with family and friends should all be considered.

References

Alzheimer's Association, 2010. 2010 Alzheimer's disease facts and figures. Alzheimers Dement. 6, 158–194.

Baumgarten, M., Hanley, J.A., Infante-Rivard, C., et al., 1994. Health of family members caring for elderly persons with dementia. A longitudinal study. Ann. Intern. Med. 120, 126–132.

Baumgarten, M., Battista, R.N., Infante-Rivard, C., et al., 1997. Use of physician services among family caregivers of elderly persons with dementia. J. Clin. Epidemiol. 50, 1265–1272.

Carpenter, B., Dave, J., 2004. Disclosing a dementia diagnosis: a review of opinion and practice, and a proposed research agenda. Gerontologist 44, 149–158.

Coste, J.K., 2003. Learning to Speak Alzheimer's: a Groundbreaking Approach for Everyone Dealing with the Disease. Houghton Mifflin, Boston.

Crespo, M., Lopez, J., Zarit, S.H., 2005. Depression and anxiety in primary caregivers: a comparative study of caregivers of demented and nondemented older persons. Int. J. Geriatr. Psychiatry 20, 591–592.

Doraiswamy, M., Gwyther, L.P., 2008. The Alzheimer's Action Plan. St Martin's Press, New York.

Ferrara, M., Langiano, E., Di Brango, T., et al., 2008. Prevalence of stress, anxiety and depression in with Alzheimer caregivers. Health Qual. Life Outcomes 6, 93.

Laakkonen, M.L., Raivio, M.M., Eloniemi-Sulkava, U., et al., 2008. How do elderly spouse care givers of people with Alzheimer disease experience the disclosure of dementia diagnosis and subsequent care? J. Med. Ethics 34, 427–430.

Lieberman, M.A., Fisher, L., 2001. The effects of nursing home placement on family caregivers of patients with Alzheimer's disease. Gerontologist 41, 819–826.

Mace, N.L., Rabins, P.V., 2006. The 36-Hour Day: A Family Guide to Caring for People with Alzheimer Disease, Other Dementias, and Memory Loss in Later Life. Johns Hopkins University Press, Baltimore.

Schulz, R., O'Brien, A.T., Bookwala, J., et al., 1995. Psychiatric and physical morbidity effects of dementia caregiving: prevalence, correlates, and causes. Gerontologist 35, 771–791.

21 Non-pharmacological treatment of the behavioral and psychological symptoms of dementia

---

QUICK START: NON-PHARMACOLOGICAL TREATMENT OF BEHAVIORAL AND PSYCHOLOGICAL SYMPTOMS OF DEMENTIA

Important principles for treating behavioral and psychological symptoms of dementia—the 3 R's:

- Reassure
  - Let patients know that they will be cared for and their wishes will be respected.
- Reconsider
  - Consider how things look from the patient's point of view.
- Redirect
  - Do not confront patients when they are wrong, frustrating, or delusional
  - Distract them by moving to a different activity or topic of conversation.

General behavioral strategies for managing behavioral and psychological symptoms of dementia

- Manage the environment
  - Keep routines and other things as constant as possible
  - Use pictures liberally in signs and other written communication
  - Use night-lights and other lighting at night.
- Keep the patient safe
  - Alzheimer's Association/Medic Alert "Safe Return" bracelet
  - GPS tracking system for the watch or car
  - Locks on doors, gates, and cabinets
  - Disconnect the stove
  - Remove or lock up weapons and power tools.
- Redirect the patient
  - Change the topic of conversation
  - Participate in safe and familiar activities
    - Listen to old music
    - Watch old movies
    - Look at photo albums
    - Discuss past events
    - Fold laundry
  - Walk or drive with the patient.
- Care for the caregiver (see also Chapter 20)
  - Support groups
  - Counseling/therapy—individual and family

Continued

QUICK START: NON-PHARMACOLOGICAL TREATMENT OF BEHAVIORAL AND PSYCHOLOGICAL SYMPTOMS OF DEMENTIA—Cont'd

- Educational activities
- Respite care
- Online chat rooms, blogs, and message boards.

Dealing with specific behavioral and psychological symptoms of dementia

- Apathy
  - Involve the patient in preferred activities
  - Simplify the activities if needed
  - Do not trade apathy for agitation.
- Depression
  - Avoid asking the patient to "snap out of it"
  - Encourage social interaction
  - Seek counseling/therapy.
- Psychosis: delusions and hallucinations
  - Delusions are common
    - Stealing possessions
    - Infidelity
    - House is not their home
    - Spouse is not their spouse
  - Hallucinations
    - Visual hallucinations are common early in dementia with Lewy bodies
    - Hallucinations occur in other dementias in the middle or late stages
    - Some hallucinations require medical investigation
  - Behavioral interventions
    - React calmly
    - Help the caregiver to understand the patient's experience
    - Avoid denying the patient's experience or confronting the patient regarding the experience.

When caregivers report behavioral and psychological symptoms we begin with an evaluation of the nature of the symptoms, level of distress they are causing the patient, and level of distress they are causing the caregiver. Based upon this evaluation, the initial decision is made whether or not to treat the symptoms. For example, a commonly reported repetitive hallucination is one of a child playing in a corner. In some instances, this hallucination may have a delusional quality, that is, the patient believes it is really happening; in other instances, the patient may realize at some level that it is not real. In either case most patients are not disturbed by this hallucination nor are caregivers. In these situations we will typically not suggest any treatment. In contrast, if the repetitive hallucination is of a man breaking into the house it may be terrifying for the patient and upsetting for the caregiver, and therefore warrants treatment.

In most cases we first try to treat behavioral and psychological symptoms of dementia using behavioral (non-pharmacological) techniques. If this approach is not successful we then move on to supplementation with drugs (see Chapter 22: *Pharmacological treatment of the behavioral and psychological symptoms of dementia*).

Before discussing techniques for the treatment of specific behavioral and psychological symptoms, we would like to discuss some general principles.

SOME GENERAL PRINCIPLES FOR TREATING BEHAVIORAL AND PSYCHOLOGICAL SYMPTOMS IN DEMENTIA: THE 3 R'S

Caregivers often experience difficulty when attempting to determine if, when, and how to intervene when behavioral and psychological symptoms occur. They struggle between trying to accommodate two basic needs that are often in conflict:

1. the need for the patient to be safe, and
2. the need for the patient to be content (happy).

For example, at some point patients will need to stop driving to prevent significant risk of endangering themselves and others. However, patients are often reluctant to do so, and even a discussion of the possibility of not driving can lead to stress and agitation. It is clear that such a situation needs intervention.

One general approach to managing behavioral and psychological symptoms of dementia has become commonly known as the 3 R's: reassure, reconsider, redirect.

Reassure

One reason the person may be unwilling to give up a particular activity, driving for example, is that he or she is fearful of the loss of the ability to do the things they find necessary (going to the supermarket) or enjoyable (visiting a friend). In any discussion where a loss of an important activity may be involved, it is important for the caregiver to reassure the patient that there will be alternative ways in which the patient can continue doing what they need and like to do (Box 21.1).

Reconsider

Ask, "How do things look from the patient's point of view?"

In many cases simply trying to understand how the patient with diminished cognitive capacity might perceive the situation can be used to remediate the behavioral problem (Box 21.2).

BOX 21.1 REASSURING THE VETERAN DRIVER

One of the most contentious discussions we have ever had about driving was with a patient who was a World War II veteran. Despite several minor accidents, becoming so lost he had to be brought home by the police, and losing his car in a parking lot, he would not even entertain the possibility of not driving. His family could not even broach the subject with him without significant agitation including yelling and throwing objects. The family asked for our help, and, after several frustrating meetings, we made no progress. We finally decided to ask him to keep a daily log of where he drove. He was willing to do this task, and what emerged was that there was one place he went to nearly every day: the American Legion Post that was only a few miles from his home, but too far to walk. Other use of the car was sporadic. When we discussed with him a plan for getting him to the American Legion Post on a daily basis, his resistance to quitting driving disappeared.

What the family and we did here was to let the patient know (reassure him) that he was in a loving environment where people cared for him, respected his needs, and would do what was necessary to meet these needs.

BOX 21.2 RECONSIDERING THE TOUCHY PATIENT

Several years ago we encountered a patient who was exhibiting inappropriate sexual behavior toward a female caregiver who visited to help with his care three times a week. His wife was quite upset when the patient would inappropriately touch the caregiver during the course of the day. The patient's wife was also surprised because this type of behavior was entirely uncharacteristic for the patient. After considerable discussion with the patient and caregiver, we all came to realize that the genesis of this troublesome behavior was that one of the responsibilities of the caregiver was to help the patient bathe. The patient interpreted touching during bathing as sexual touching and thus in his view his touching the caregiver during the day was reciprocal and entirely appropriate. We rearranged the bathing schedule so that he was no longer bathed by a woman.

Redirect

Perhaps the single most important piece of advice we can provide to a caregiver is not to be confrontational (Box 21.3). And while this advice is easy to give, in many cases it may not be so easy to follow.

BOX 21.3 REDIRECTING THE GOURMET COOK

We follow a patient who was once an excellent cook, but now has great difficulty in the kitchen. As such, her husband, the primary caregiver, has taken over the duties in the kitchen. While he has become a competent cook, his main challenge is now to keep his wife out of the kitchen. The patient understandably continues to want to be engaged in activities in which she was once quite accomplished. The problem is that she would often cause difficult and potentially dangerous situations, such as putting a metal bowl in the microwave or putting a dish towel on the burner. These difficulties led to many confrontations and arguments. Her husband solved this problem by getting the patient her own oven—in this case a toy oven—and giving her a specific job during meal preparation that she cheerfully carries out.

Interacting with a demented patient—even when the patient is a spouse or parent—can be quite frustrating for the caregiver. The caregiver needs to strike a balance between what the patient wants to do and what is safe. When these conflict, there can be frustration and agitation for both patient and caregiver.

In general, we advise caregivers to carefully pick their battles. When a patient asks a caregiver for the 10th time in 15 minutes where they are going for lunch that day, it is tempting—and probably cathartic—for the caregiver to say, "Don't ask me again! I have already told you the answer 10 times in the last 15 minutes!" Unfortunately, this response will likely lead to the patient experiencing either anger and agitation or sadness and depression. A better solution is to redirect the patient to another activity that they can accomplish independently and that will distract them from focusing on lunch. In the case above, the astute caregiver took a situation that was potentially confrontational and turned it into a positive activity.

Of course, there are instances in which the caregiver must intervene more directly. These are generally cases in which safety is an imminent issue. For example, when a patient who is known to become lost in the neighborhood and cannot safely cross streets is walking out the front door, a direct approach may be necessary.

Other general strategies for dealing with behavioral and psychological symptoms in dementia using behavioral techniques are summarized in Box 21.4.

BOX 21.4 GENERAL BEHAVIORAL STRATEGIES FOR MANAGING BEHAVIORAL AND PSYCHOLOGICAL SYMPTOMS IN DEMENTIA

Manage the environment

As dementia progresses, patients become more confused and disoriented. A highly structured and consistent environment, both in terms of the physical environment and temporal routine, can be helpful. (See External memory aids in Chapter 18 for elaboration and additional suggestions.)

- Keep the daily routine as constant as possible
- Keep a calendar of daily events in a prominent place that the patient will check frequently
- Try not to rearrange the contents of cabinets, drawers, or even the location of furniture
- Use signs to direct and identify places in the home, such as the bathroom
- In signs and written communication, use pictures, rather than words, whenever possible
- Use night-lights and other lighting at night

Keep the patient safe

- Obtain an Alzheimer's Association/Medic Alert "Safe Return" bracelet for the patient (www.alz.org/safereturn)
- If the patient goes out independently, consider a GPS tracking system, often as part of a watch or attached to the car (http://www.alz.org/comfortzone)
- If the person wanders, also consider locks on doors and gates
- Disconnect the stove from the power or gas
- Use "child-proof" locks on cabinets that house knives and dangerous chemicals
- Remove or lock up power tools and weapons

Redirect the patient

- Change the topic of conversation
- Listen to familiar music, e.g., show tunes
- Watch DVDs of old and familiar movies
- Look at family albums and discuss *past* events
- Walk or drive with the patient
- Perform safe and routine activities, such as folding laundry

Care for the caregiver

- Support groups
- Counseling/therapy—individual and family
- Educational activities
- Respite care
- Online chat rooms, blogs, and message boards (http://www.alz.org/living_with_alzheimers_message_boards_lwa.asp)

DEALING WITH SPECIFIC BEHAVIORAL AND PSYCHOLOGICAL SYMPTOMS OF DEMENTIA: BEHAVIORAL TECHNIQUES

Apathy

One of the most common complaints that we hear from caregivers is that the patient does not want to do anything. The caregivers comment that patients often just want to sit in their chairs, often falling asleep. They further comment that it is difficult to keep them busy and to find appropriate activities to do with them.

As discussed earlier, apathy is perhaps the most common behavioral symptom in Alzheimer's disease. It is not clear why Alzheimer's disease patients become apathetic.

In the most global, biological sense, it is likely due to the effects the disease has on specific brain areas. There is evidence from imaging studies that Alzheimer's disease patients with apathy have more frontal white matter hyperintensities on MRI (Starkstein et al., 2009), decreased gray matter volume in the anterior cingulate and frontal cortex bilaterally, as well as the head of the left caudate and bilateral putamen (Bruen et al., 2008), and decreased metabolic activity in bilateral anterior cingulate extending inferiorly into the medial orbitofrontal region, as well as the bilateral medial thalamus (Marshall et al., 2007). A psychological explanation of why patients with Alzheimer's disease are apathetic is that it is their way of coping with a world that is complex and confusing to them. To cope, they simply withdraw.

It is tempting to consider apathy as a form of depression, but the two are separable. Although apathy and depression commonly co-occur, there can be apathy without depression and depression without apathy (Lerner et al., 2007; Nakaaki et al., 2008; Tagariello et al., 2009). It is also tempting not to bother treating apathy because it is certainly easier to care for apathetic patients than those who are agitated and upset. It is, however, vitally important to treat the apathetic patient.

Behavioral treatments for apathy

Some strategies to suggest for caregivers to help with the apathetic patient include:

- try to get the patient involved in activities they once enjoyed
- simplify and organize what you ask the patient to do (Box 21.5)
- don't trade apathy for agitation (Box 21.6).

BOX 21.5 A PLAN FOR THE GARDEN

One of our caregivers tried to get her husband up from his chair (where he would sit most of the day and not interact with anyone) and go out to their garden, a garden they planted and cared for together for many years. She would take him outside and suggest several things that he might do, including planting, weeding, and watering. Within a few minutes she would find him back in his chair, much to the frustration of the caregiver. We realized that part of the problem was that the patient had lost the ability to organize and sequence the necessary gardening steps. We suggested that the caregiver try to find time to go out to the garden to work with him and then plan, organize, and supervise a very single specific task for him, such as weeding a small part of the garden that she would delineate with some string. The reports back from the garden were that this worked well and we even reaped the fruits in the form of wonderful tomatoes.

BOX 21.6 THE PUZZLER: APATHETIC OR AGITATED?

One of our patients was an avid crossword puzzler. But he stopped doing these puzzles and became quite withdrawn and apathetic. His wife read that keeping the mind active could slow the progression of Alzheimer's disease and so she began to insist that he not sit around all day and that he complete crossword puzzles. This insistence led to significant agitation. He would uncharacteristically throw the puzzles, break his pencil, and scream at his wife. His wife had traded one manifestation of behavioral and psychological symptoms in dementia for another. We suggested that perhaps a simpler form of word game might be more successful. She substituted "word search" (a puzzle in which the person finds words in mixes of letters and circles them) for the crossword puzzle with great success.

Depression

Although we know that many patients with Alzheimer's disease also show symptoms of depression, the relationship between Alzheimer's disease and depression is complex and controversial (for review see Panza et al., 2010). There are well-done studies to suggest the following:

- a history of depression earlier in life is a risk factor for Alzheimer's disease
- symptoms of depression are common in the few years preceding the diagnosis of Alzheimer's disease, prompting some researchers to hypothesize that it is an early symptom of Alzheimer's disease, especially in individuals with no lifetime history of depression
- depression is common early in the course of Alzheimer's disease and the incidence increases as the disease progresses until all insight is lost.

Because both Alzheimer's disease and depression can produce memory dysfunction (see Chapter 12: *Other disorders*), we often see patients referred by their primary care providers who are already treated with an antidepressant. In some cases (but rarely in our experience) treating the depression eliminates the cognitive deficits. Much more commonly, the referred patient is experiencing both Alzheimer's disease and depression, and both are contributing to their cognitive deficits, and both need to be treated. To help sort out the contribution of the depression, when we evaluate these patients we ask ourselves two questions:

1. If the depression completely resolved tomorrow, would this individual's memory problems also be resolved?
2. Is the current level of depression sufficient to account for the current level of cognitive deficits?

In almost all cases, the answer to both questions is no.

Behavioral treatments for depression

Some strategies and tips to suggest for caregivers to help with the depressed patient include the following.

- Avoid asking the patient to "snap out of it"
  - This type of message conveys that the caregiver does not understand what the depressed individual is experiencing, which may lead to frustration and may exacerbate the depression.
- Encourage social interaction
  - This may best be accomplished in small groups, e.g., dinner at home with one or two close friends.
  - When the interactions are in larger groups, which can be confusing to patients, encourage the patient to talk just with one or two people there.
- Seek counseling/therapy
  - Psychotherapy is most likely to be successful in patients who have relatively mild disease, so that they can understand and remember what has transpired in the session.
  - It is important to refer to a therapist who has knowledge of and experience with Alzheimer's disease

Psychosis: delusions and hallucinations

Delusions are very common in all dementias, but particularly in patients with Alzheimer's disease (perhaps related to their memory impairment). Delusions are false beliefs, and in dementia often take on a paranoid flavor. Hallucinations also occur in dementia, particularly in patients with dementia with Lewy bodies but also in patients with Alzheimer's disease in the middle stage of the disease and beyond (roughly MMSE <16). In dementia with Lewy bodies the hallucinations occur as an early symptom and are almost always visual; in Alzheimer's disease the hallucinations can be in any sensory modality: visual, auditory, tactile, or olfactory. Hallucinations may or may not have a delusional quality. For example, a patient may report seeing children playing in the yard and be able to describe them in great detail. Yet, when questioned, they realize that the children are not really there. In contrast another patient may have the same report, but have the firm belief (from which they will not be dissuaded) that the children are real; these hallucinations have a delusional quality.

A father and son were looking at the moon. The father told his son there were two moons. The son replied, you must be seeing double. No, said the father, if I were seeing double, there would be four.

People with memory problems can become suspicious to the point of paranoia. This suspiciousness can range from a mild annoyance to the patient and family, e.g., "the cleaning person is stealing my loose change," to events that produce palpable fear and lead to destructive behaviors, e.g., "the mailman, delivery person, etc., is coming to take me from my home or to steal my furniture," leading to locking doors, resisting all help and visitors, and perhaps calling the police. More mild delusions can often be ignored, but the disruptive or dangerous delusions need to be treated (Box 21.7).

BOX 21.7 SITTING WITH A SHOTGUN

We had a patient in the middle stages of dementia who believed that anyone coming to his door (e.g., the mailman, the UPS delivery person) was there to take him from his home and take all his possessions. Initially, he simply commented upon this. But, as he became more confused and forgetful, he began to perseverate on this idea. One morning his brother came to visit, as he often did, and found the door locked. He knocked but there was no answer. When he looked in the window, he saw his brother sitting with a shotgun (that we later determined was loaded) in his lap.

It was clear that it was now time to treat these paranoid delusions.

Delusions

Delusions in Alzheimer's disease and other dementias can vary, but certain delusions seem to prevail, including the following.

- A relative or neighbor is stealing the patient's possessions
  - This often stems from patients misplacing or even hiding items, and when they cannot find them they assume others have stolen them.
  - This delusion can often lead to contention and distress when the patient confronts the family member or neighbor.
- Delusion of infidelity.
  - These delusions can be especially troublesome when the patient accuses his or her spouse of many years of an extramarital relationship and asks the spouse to leave the home.

- Their house is not their home
  - This delusion can lead to very agitated behavior in which the person constantly states that they want to go home, even when they are at home.
  - This delusion frequently occurs because the patient remembers an earlier home (often the home of their childhood), and thinks that they live there.
- Their spouse is not their spouse
  - This delusion is obviously very distressing to the spouse, making it that much more difficult to care for the patient.
  - Often the patient will be remembering a past time, either expecting the spouse to look 40 years younger or expecting their previous husband or wife.

We would, however, offer one caution when evaluating delusions, whether of infidelity, stealing, or other matters (Box 21.8). Delusions are important to treat because they can lead to agitation, aggression, anxiety, and purposeless behavior. They are frequently stressful to the patient and the caregiver.

BOX 21.8 JUST BECAUSE YOU'RE PARANOID DOESN'T MEAN THEY AREN'T OUT TO GET YOU

We followed a patient who had been married to his wife for 48 years. In talking with him at one visit, he confided to me (P.R.S.) that he felt his wife was having an affair with a younger man in Boston. He told me that on several recent occasions his wife had left him with a caregiver and gone to Boston for several days. He also was sure that this person was calling his wife at home. We discussed this at some length and it was clear that this was understandably extremely troublesome to him. He had not discussed this with his wife. I asked if I might first talk to his wife about this and perhaps then we could all discuss his feelings. He agreed. I then talked with his wife and told her that I thought her husband was having delusions and conveyed the conversation that the patient and I had. I then noticed a "deer in the headlights" look come over her face and I immediately knew her husband was not having a delusion. The patient's wife then told me that his beliefs were true and we discussed how we might manage this difficult situation.

Another of our patients was living alone in his own home. He was in the early stages of Alzheimer's disease (MMSE 24) and his daughter was his primary caregiver. They spoke on the phone daily and she saw him about once a week. He also was receiving help from three young women who lived next door to him. He had good retirement benefits and social security, yet he reported that he never had any money. His daughter found that his bank account was dwindling and no one could understand how he was spending the money. The patient felt that someone in the bank must be stealing his money. What we eventually learned was that the "helpful neighbors" were not only helping him get to the supermarket and drug store, but also to the cash machine, several times a week. Our patient did not recall these episodes.

The lesson we learned from these episodes was that some stories—even though they seem unlikely and fit the pattern of delusions seen in Alzheimer's disease—are actually true.

Hallucinations

A person with a dementing illness may hear, see, smell, or feel stimuli that are not present (Box 21.9). Visual hallucinations are often an early symptom of dementia with Lewy bodies. In Alzheimer's disease hallucinations generally occur in the middle stages of the disease and beyond (MMSE <16). As in the case of delusions, they can range from being entertaining to the patient—seeing children playing in the back yard—to being

---

> **BOX 21.9 BUGS**
>
> One hallucination deserves particular mention: that of feeling bugs crawling on one's arm. This hallucination is not uncommon, and can result from a number of causes. It may be due to medication toxicity or another medical problem, particularly one that causes itching (e.g., morphine use, renal failure). It may also be from ordinary causes of itching, such as poison ivy or even simply dry skin. The first sign of this hallucination may be raw skin on the patient's arm from "scratching the bugs." This hallucination, almost always very disturbing to the patient and caregiver, warrants medical investigation and treatment.

terrifying—seeing snakes in the bed. As with delusions, the amount of distress that the delusions cause the patient determines the nature of the treatment.

Behavioral treatments for hallucinations and delusions

Some strategies and tips to suggest for caregivers to help with patients with hallucinations and delusions include the following.

- React calmly
  - The initial occurrence of an hallucination or delusion can be disconcerting and frightening to the patient and/or family. The tendency is to treat the situation as an emergency. An emergency attitude and action can be alarming to the patient as well and may contribute to agitation, further complicating an already difficult situation.
  - As long as the hallucination or delusion is not posing a danger to the patient or others, the caregiver can simply reassure the patient and seek a medical evaluation and assistance in the usual way.
  - In many cases the combination of reassurance that this symptom is typical of the disease and a discussion of strategies to manage the symptom will handle the situation.
- Help the caregiver understand the patient's experience
  - Perhaps the most difficult aspect of hallucinations and delusions for the caregiver to embrace is that the experience for the patient is as real as any experience that the caregiver is having.
  - We often ask our caregivers, "If I tried to convince you that the chair sitting in the corner was not there, would you believe me?"
  - Once the caregiver appreciates what the patient is experiencing, discussing management strategies becomes easier.
- Avoid denying the patient's experience or confronting the patient regarding the experience (Box 21.10).
  - Although we do not recommend denying the experience, neither do we recommend endorsing it.
  - A simple statement, such as "I understand that you believe people are stealing from you, but I think your wallet is simply misplaced," may be helpful.
  - Redirecting the patient to other topics is usually the best approach.

BOX 21.10 SITTING IN THE LIVING ROOM

A mid-stage Alzheimer's disease patient (MMSE 17) visited with her daughter and told us about seeing her dead husband sitting on the living room couch on several occasions. Although the patient was remarkably calm about the events, her daughter was not. Her daughter corrected the patient, reminded her that her husband was dead, and an argument between mother and daughter ensued.

Because the experience is real for the patient, denial, confrontation, and getting upset on the part of the daughter only served to agitate the patient. Although we did not recommend endorsing this hallucination, we suggested that she simply state to her mother: "I understand that you saw dad, but I did not. I am sure this is frightening for you." We then recommended that she change the conversation and exit the situation.

References

Bruen, P.D., McGeown, W.J., Shanks, M.F., et al., 2008. Neuroanatomical correlates of neuropsychiatric symptoms in Alzheimer's disease. Brain 131, 2455–2463.

Lerner, A.J., Strauss, M., Sami, S.A., 2007. Recognizing apathy in Alzheimer's disease. Geriatrics 62, 14–17.

Marshall, G.A., Monserratt, L., Harwood, D., et al., 2007. Positron emission tomography metabolic correlates of apathy in Alzheimer disease. Arch. Neurol. 64, 1015–1020.

Nakaaki, S., Murata, Y., Sato, J., et al., 2008. Association between apathy/depression and executive function in patients with Alzheimer's disease. Int. Psychogeriatr. 20, 964–975.

Panza, F., Frisardi, V., Capurso, C., et al., 2010. Late-life depression, mild cognitive impairment, and dementia: possible continuum? Am. J. Geriatr. Psychiatry 18, 98–116.

Starkstein, S.E., Mizrahi, R., Capizzano, A.A., et al., 2009. Neuroimaging correlates of apathy and depression in Alzheimer's disease. J. Neuropsychiatry Clin. Neurosci. 21, 259–265.

Tagariello, P., Girardi, P., Amore, M., 2009. Depression and apathy in dementia: same syndrome or different constructs? A critical review. Arch. Gerontol. Geriatr. 49, 246–249.

Pharmacological treatment of the behavioral and psychological symptoms of dementia

QUICK START: PHARMACOLOGICAL TREATMENT OF BEHAVIORAL AND PSYCHOLOGICAL SYMPTOMS OF DEMENTIA

- Pharmacological treatment of behavioral and psychological symptoms of dementia should only be undertaken when one of the following situations is present:
  - The symptoms are causing distress to the patient or caregiver
  - The symptoms are dangerous to the patient or others
  - There is a specific condition for which there is a known treatment that is both efficacious and safe.
- Medications to treat cognition, cholinesterase inhibitors and memantine (Namenda), are helpful in treating the behavioral and psychological symptoms of dementia, and in general should be used first.
- Medical illnesses should always be looked for and treated.
- General principles of pharmacotherapy for behavioral and psychological symptoms of dementia:
  - Accurately diagnose the underlying dementia
  - Identify and measure specific target symptoms
  - Start low, go slow—but go
  - Instruct the caregiver and patient both verbally and in writing
  - Remove unneeded medications
  - Change only one medication at a time.
- Pharmacotherapy for depression
  - SSRIs are first-line therapy
  - Bupropion (Wellbutrin) and venlafaxine (Effexor) can also be used.
- Pharmacotherapy for anxiety
  - SSRIs are first-line therapy
  - Atypical antipsychotics can be used with caution.
- Pharmacotherapy for insomnia
  - Address sleep hygiene issues
  - Try non-pharmacological treatment
  - Treat any underlying sleep disorder

Continued

QUICK START: PHARMACOLOGICAL TREATMENT OF BEHAVIORAL AND PSYCHOLOGICAL SYMPTOMS OF DEMENTIA—Cont'd

- Treat any underlying depression or anxiety
- Can try a small dose of a long-acting stimulant medication to keep patient awake and alert during the day (see text)
- Can try a small dose of a sedative if necessary (see text).
- Pharmacotherapy for psychosis
  - Accurately diagnose the cause of the dementia.
  - Atypical antipsychotics are the preferred treatment.
- Pharmacotherapy for agitation
  - Characterize and diagnose the nature of the agitation and any underlying or comorbid condition(s) present.
  - If depression or anxiety is present, start with an SSRI.
  - If psychosis (hallucinations or delusions) is present, start with an atypical antipsychotic.
  - If no specific cause for the agitation can be determined, start with an atypical antipsychotic if rapid treatment is necessary; start with an SSRI if treatment may be initiated more slowly.
- Behavioral and psychiatric crises
  - Psychiatric hospitalizations allow medications to quickly be withdrawn and added in a safe setting.
- Use of SSRIs in dementia
  - SSRIs are generally well tolerated.
  - SSRIs can help with depression, anxiety, and agitation
  - We generally use a low dose of:
    – Sertraline (Zoloft) target 75–150 mg QD; general range for dementia 50–200 mg
    – Citalopram (Celexa) target 20 mg QD; general range for dementia 10–40 mg
    – Escitalopram (Lexapro) target 10 mg QD; general range for dementia 5–20 mg
  - Main side-effects: gastrointestinal upset and sexual dysfunction.
- Use of atypical antipsychotics in dementia
  - Atypical antipsychotics may: impair cognition, be sedating, cause Parkinsonism, lead to falls, cause hyperglycemia, increase the risk of heart disease and strokes, lower the seizure threshold, and cause dystonias and tardive dyskinesia
  - After informed consent, atypical antipsychotics should be used for as brief a period as possible, when the patient is in a situation in which he or she can be regularly observed
  - We generally use:
    - Risperidone (Risperdal); range for dementia 0.25–1 mg QD-BID
      Little sedation, recommended for daytime use
    - Quetiapine (Seroquel); range for dementia 12.5–200 mg QD-BID
      Sedating, recommended for use at bedtime
      Less likely than others to cause or worsen Parkinsonism; recommended for patients with dementia with Lewy bodies
    - Aripiprazole (Abilify); range for dementia 2.5–5 mg QD-BID
      Very little sedation, recommended for daytime use
      Least effect on carbohydrate metabolism.
- Please see text for additional discussion of atypical antipsychotics prior to use.

Note that the medications discussed in this chapter are powerful drugs with dangerous side-effects and adverse reactions and are not approved by the US Food and Drug Administration for use in patients with dementia. See CAUTION in text.

In some cases non-pharmacological treatment of the behavioral and psychological symptoms of dementia is not sufficient. In these instances the judicious use of appropriate medications can be beneficial. Our rule of thumb in introducing pharmacological treatment for the behavioral and psychological symptoms of dementia is that we only do so when one of the following situations is present:

- the symptoms are causing distress to the patient or caregiver
- the symptoms are dangerous to the patient or others
- there is a specific condition for which there is a known treatment that is both efficacious and safe.

> CAUTION: Note that the medications discussed in this chapter are powerful drugs with dangerous side-effects and adverse reactions and are not approved by the US Food and Drug Administration (FDA) for use in patients with dementia. All recommendations in this chapter are based upon the combination of published research studies, clinical experience, and use in non-demented patients. The physician (or other provider) must use appropriate clinical judgment as to whether the potential benefit of prescribing one of these medications "off-label" outweighs the risks to the patient. In addition to reviewing side-effects and adverse reactions, the physician (or other provider) must review the FDA-approved package insert, including black box warnings, contraindications and cautions, drug interactions, and safety and monitoring, before prescribing. The authors take no responsibility in the prescribing of one or more of these medications by the physician (or other provider) to his or her patients.

In general, pharmacotherapy for patients with behavioral and psychological symptoms of dementia falls into three general categories.

1. *Drugs to treat cognition.* Treating the underlying dementing disorder may also treat behavioral and psychological symptoms of dementia. Treatment with cholinesterase inhibitors and memantine (Namenda) has been shown to decrease the symptoms in patients with Alzheimer's disease, dementia with Lewy bodies, and vascular dementia (for review, see Cummings et al., 2008; see also Box 22.1). Note, however, that in some patients with frontotemporal dementia cholinesterase inhibitors will sometimes worsen the behavioral and psychological symptoms of dementia.

BOX 22.1 INCREASING MEMORY CAN REDUCE DELUSIONS

Consider three of the most common delusions in dementia:

- Possessions are being stolen
- House is not their home
- Spouse is not their spouse

These delusions are all caused in part by impaired memory. The patient who thinks people are stealing her jewelry typically put it away for safe-keeping, then forgot that she moved it (and where she put it). The patient who does not believe that his house is his home is usually remembering an earlier home—most often the home of his childhood—and thinks that is where he still lives, and perhaps that his mother is waiting for him! The patient who does not believe that her husband is her spouse is likely remembering when the husband looked younger (or perhaps is remembering a previous husband). Because memory dysfunction contributes to these delusions, it should not be surprising that improving patients' memories can reduce or eliminate these types of delusions. For this reason, when we believe that the patient's delusions are caused by memory problems, we always start by making sure that the memory medication—that is, the cholinesterase inhibitor—is maximized.

2. *Drugs to treat comorbid illnesses.* Although it may seem obvious, it is well worth reiterating that patients with dementing disorders often have comorbid illnesses that, although not the cause of their dementia, may be contributing to their poor cognition and their behavioral and psychological symptoms. For example, whenever we detect a change in cognition over a matter of days in one of our patients we always suspect an infection (such as a urinary tract infection or pneumonia) or another medical cause. Treating the medical illness should correct the sudden deterioration in behavior and cognition.

3. *Drugs to treat specific symptoms of behavioral and psychological symptoms of dementia.* Depression, anxiety, insomnia, hallucinations, delusions, and agitation are all common in dementing illnesses. These conditions also all have specific pharmacological treatment that can be helpful when implemented skillfully and judiciously.

GENERAL PRINCIPLES OF PHARMACOTHERAPY FOR BEHAVIORAL AND PSYCHOLOGICAL SYMPTOMS OF DEMENTIA

- *Accurately diagnose the underlying dementia.* Treatment of behavioral and psychological symptoms of dementia will vary depending upon the underlying dementing disorder. For example, as we saw in Chapter 5: *Dementia with Lewy bodies (including Parkinson's disease dementia),* although patients with dementia with Lewy bodies experience visual hallucinations, one must be very cautious in treating them because many antipsychotic drugs exacerbate their Parkinsonian symptoms. Knowing that the patient has dementia with Lewy bodies will lead to the use of quetiapine (Seroquel) as first-line therapy, rather than risperidone (Risperdal), since the former is less likely to exacerbate their Parkinsonism (Box 22.2).

- *Identify and measure specific target symptoms.* The clinician and caregiver should identify specific symptoms and behaviors that they wish to reduce, such as depression, wandering, or aggression. Each symptom should be measured at baseline such that, when a treatment is prescribed, the treatment effect on that symptom can be quantified. One common way to measure these symptoms and behaviors is to count how many times specific events occur in a period of time. (For example, the patient attempted to wander out of the house six times over a 2-week period, or ask the caregiver if this is happening multiple times a day, once a day, several times a week, once a week or once a month.)

- *Start low, go slow—but go.* Older adults are often more sensitive to medications. As such, doses in older individuals should start at one-third to one-half the standard adult dose. Titrations should be slower than in younger adults. Importantly, however, the drugs should be titrated until the desired response is achieved or until intolerable side-effects emerge. We have too often seen patients treated for long periods on sub-therapeutic doses of drugs that are not having the desired effect. In many cases, when the doses were increased to therapeutic levels, the patients did better.

- *Instruct the caregiver and patient both verbally and in writing.* We have been surprised how often we will have a conversation with a patient and caregiver regarding medications only to realize they misunderstood what we said when we revisit the topic later. Because of the frequency of misunderstanding, we now provide information regarding medications both verbally and in clear, written directions. These instructions include how and when to take the medication, what side-effects may occur and how to manage them, and what to do if they run out of medication. (See Box 22.3 for examples.)

BOX 22.2 USE OF ATYPICAL ANTIPSYCHOTICS IN DEMENTIA

- Atypical antipsychotics may: impair cognition, be sedating, cause Parkinsonism, lead to falls, cause hyperglycemia, increase the risk of heart disease and strokes, lower the seizure threshold, and cause dystonias and tardive dyskinesia.
- Atypical antipsychotics should be used for as brief a period as possible, and only when the patient is in a situation in which he or she can be regularly observed.
- Complications often occur with the use of atypical antipsychotics in patients with dementia; this possibility of complications should be discussed with the patient and caregiver, and consent for the use of these medications should be obtained and documented in the medical record.
- There are a number of atypical antipsychotics to choose from. The ones typically used in dementia are (target dose is always the lowest effective dose):
  - Risperidone (Risperdal); range for dementia 0.25–1 mg QD-BID. Available in tablets and also 1 mg/ml solution. One of the less sedating atypical antipsychotics, ideal for use during the day when a daytime medication is needed. Also useful in liquid form when pills cannot be swallowed. Can cause prolactinemia and exacerbate osteoporosis.
  - Quetiapine (Seroquel); range for dementia 12.5–200 mg QD-BID. Somewhat sedating, recommended for use at bedtime although can be used during the day in small doses. Less likely than others to cause or worsen Parkinsonism; ideal for patients with dementia with Lewy bodies.
  - Aripiprazole (Abilify); range for dementia 2.5–5 mg QD-BID. One of the least sedating atypical antipsychotics. Least effect on carbohydrate metabolism.
  - Ziprasidone (Geodon); intramuscular (IM) range for dementia: 20 mg IM QD-TID. Particularly useful when an intramuscular medication is needed. Switch to PO as soon as possible.
  - Olanzapine (Zyprexa); range for dementia 1.25–10 mg QD.
- If one atypical antipsychotic is not effective, others may be.
- Atypical antipsychotics should be used with caution in patients with dementia.

- *Remove unneeded medications.* It is both essential and difficult to obtain an accurate list of medications in our patients with dementia. In an informal survey that we completed several years ago, we found that our average patient reported taking eight medications (range 0–20+). In many cases neither the patients nor their caregivers knew who prescribed a number of their medications or what they were for. The typical scenario was that multiple providers added medications, but medications were rarely removed. A number of the commonly prescribed medications have potential cognitive side-effects or drug interactions, including anticholinergic medications, antihistamines, and others. (See Box 22.4 and Box 12.3: *Common classes or properties of medications causing cognitive dysfunction,* and Box 14.2: *Medications that may interact with cholinesterase inhibitors.*) We often begin by working with the patient's primary care provider to try to simplify their medication regime.
- *Change only one medication at a time.* This very obvious point is often overlooked. If more than one medication is changed at once it is generally impossible to determine the cause of either beneficial or detrimental cognitive effects. We therefore recommend changing only one medication at a time.

PHARMACOTHERAPY FOR DEPRESSION

There are few things in our society today that are as depressing and anxiety provoking as realizing that one has Alzheimer's disease, and that one is going to literally "lose one's mind." Although it rarely meets the diagnostic criteria for major depression, a significant

BOX 22.3 EXAMPLES OF MEDICATION INSTRUCTIONS FOR PATIENTS

Directions for Aricept (donepezil) sample kit
- Take one pill (white, 5 mg tablet) daily, in the evening for 4 weeks
- Then begin the yellow, 10 mg tablets, daily, in the evening for 1 week
- Possible side-effects include:
  - Vivid dreams
  - Stomach upset
  - Bloating
  - Nausea and vomiting

Directions for Lexapro (escitolopram oxalate)
- Take one pill daily every day with or without food
- Possible side-effects include:
  - Nausea
  - Insomnia
  - Sexual side-effects
  - Drowsiness
  - Increased sweating
  - Fatigue

Directions for Exelon patch (rivastigmine transdermal system)
- Cut the pouch along the dotted line and remove the patch
- Peel off the protective layer
- Put the sticky side of the patch on the upper or lower back, upper arm or chest
- Peel off the second side of the protective layer
- Press the patch firmly in place with the hand to make sure the edges stick well
  - The patch should be replaced by a new one after 24 hours
  - The application site of the Exelon patch should be changed every day, not using the same spot for at least 14 days
- Possible side-effects include:
  - Nausea
  - Vomiting
  - Diarrhea
  - Decreased appetite
  - Weight loss

BOX 22.4 THE INCONTINENCE MEDICATIONS

The incontinence medications deserve special mention. Virtually all of the medications used to control incontinence, such as hyoscyamine and oxybutynin, are anticholinergic not as a side-effect, but as their primary mode of action.

- Should these medications be discontinued in a patient with dementia who is on a cholinesterase inhibitor? The simple answer requires one question:
- Is the medication working to control the patient's incontinence such that he or she does not need to wear Depends (or similar absorbent underwear)?
  - If the answer is "yes," the medication would appear to be working and should be continued, despite any possible worsening of cognition. The reason being is that incontinence, being distressing, inconvenient, and burdensome for caregivers, is one of the major causes of patients being placed in long-term care facilities. It is therefore worth enduring cognitive side-effects if incontinence can be eliminated.
  - If the answer is "no"—as it often is—then the medication is unlikely to be doing anything to improve the patient's quality of life and should most likely be discontinued.

BOX 22.5 USE OF SELECTIVE SEROTONIN REUPTAKE INHIBITORS (SSRIs) IN DEMENTIA

- SSRIs are generally well tolerated in patients with cognitive impairment and dementia.
- SSRIs are only minimally anticholinergic, are relatively non-sedating, and are therefore unlikely to worsen cognition.
- Several SSRIs (including sertraline (Zoloft), citalopram (Celexa), and escitalopram (Lexapro)) are anxiolytics as well as antidepressants.
- We generally use a low dose of:
  - Sertraline (Zoloft) target 75–150 mg QD; general range for dementia 50–200 mg
  - Citalopram (Celexa) target 20 mg QD; general range for dementia 10–40 mg
  - Escitalopram (Lexapro) target 10 mg QD; general range for dementia 5–20 mg.
- Fluoxitine (Prozac) can have activating properties and may be beneficial when apathy is present. However, it takes twice as long to be effective (6–8 weeks versus 2–3 weeks for the others) and may interact with warfarin (Coumadin).
- As in other populations, if one SSRI is not effective, others may be.
- Main side-effects: gastrointestinal upset and sexual dysfunction.
- Note that paroxetine (Paxil) may be problematic in the elderly owing to both the common side-effect of hyponatremia and the rapid onset of withdrawal symptoms if a dose is forgotten.

---

degree of depression often occurs in patients before, during, and throughout the course of Alzheimer's disease. Depression is common in Alzheimer's disease and mild cognitive impairment, occurring in about half of the patients (Di Iulio et al., 2010). Although treatment of depression in the demented patient will not resolve the cognitive deficits, successful treatment will help the mood of the patient and in doing so will improve the patient's cognition, daily function, and overall well-being (Cummings et al., 2006).

Some general guidelines for managing depression pharmacologically:

- Selective serotonin reuptake inhibitors (SSRIs) are generally first-line therapy. See Box 22.5.
- Other antidepressant classes that may be beneficial for depression:
  - bupropion (Wellbutrin) has activating properties and can also be helpful when apathy is present; may lower the seizure threshold, particularly in doses above 300 mg per day
  - serotonin–norepinephrine reuptake inhibitors, such as venlafaxine (Effexor), are efficacious in some patients.
- Antidepressants to avoid include:
  - tricyclic antidepressants because of anticholinergic effects
  - mirtazepine (Remeron) because of anticholinergic effects
  - monoamine oxidase inhibitors because of the likelihood of dietary indiscretions in the cognitively impaired patient.

PHARMACOTHERAPY FOR ANXIETY

As mentioned above, having the slightest bit of insight into knowing that one has Alzheimer's disease is quite anxiety provoking, in addition to being depressing. Consistent with this notion, one study suggested that approximately half of patients with Alzheimer's disease (48%) showed evidence of anxiety (Mega et al., 1996). Anxiety in Alzheimer's disease may improve with cholinesterase inhibitor therapy (Mega et al., 1999), so a cholinesterase inhibitor should always be tried first (see Chapter 14: *Cholinesterase inhibitors*). As in depression, however, the mainstay of pharmacotherapy for anxiety in dementia is the SSRIs, notably sertraline (Zoloft), citalopram (Celexa), and escitalopram (Lexapro) (Box 22.5).

If the SSRIs are not effective in alleviating the anxiety, the class of medications which is typically tried next is the atypical antipsychotics. Although not as well tolerated as SSRIs, the atypical antipsychotics are helpful and sometimes necessary. Atypical antipsychotics may impair cognition and lead to sedation, falls, and cardiovascular disease. These second-line treatments should be used for as brief a period as possible, and in a situation in which the patient is regularly observed (Box 22.2).

Benzodiazepines are rarely used for anxiety in the cognitively impaired patient because they often impair cognition, lead to dependence, and have rebound effects.

PHARMACOTHERAPY FOR INSOMNIA

Pharmacological treatment for insomnia and other sleep disturbances in dementia depends upon the underlying cause. When we hear that the patient has trouble sleeping we always begin by going through the patient's day. A typical day reported by a caregiver might sound like this narrative:

> I have to wake him up around 8 a.m. so that I can get him on the van to the day care at 9 a.m. He stays at the day care until 2.30, returning home at 3 p.m. They tell me that he sleeps in the chair half of the time at day care. When he is home he generally watches TV, but he has trouble following what is going on, and so he generally naps from about 3.30 to 5.30 p.m., when I wake him up for dinner. We eat from 5.30 to 6 p.m., and then watch the news on the couch, followed by Jeopardy and Wheel of Fortune till 8 p.m. Sometimes he falls asleep during this time as well. I start getting him ready for bed at 8, and he is generally asleep by 9 p.m. I then find him wandering around the house between 3 and 6 a.m. I will put him back to sleep by 6 a.m. if he hasn't gone back to sleep already...

This patient sleeps from 6–8 a.m. (2 hours), half the time at day care (half of 9.30 a.m.–2.30 p.m. or 2.5 hours), 3.30–5.50 p.m. (2 hours), and half the time from 6–8 p.m. (1 hour). So by the time he goes to sleep at 9 p.m., starting at 6 a.m. he has already slept an average of 7.5 hours. If he then sleeps from 9 p.m. to 3 a.m. he has slept an additional 6 hours and a total of 13.5 hours. It is no wonder at all that he is awake and wandering around the house from 3 to 6 a.m.!

The patient in the example above has poor sleep hygiene; he may or may not have other sleep problems as well. Nearly half of older adults experience difficulty in initiating and maintaining sleep (Roepke & Ancoli-Israel, 2010). In normal aging there is an increase in sleep problems, including:

- restless legs syndrome; prevalence in the elderly of 8–20%
- periodic limb movements of sleep; prevalence in the elderly of up to 45%
- sleep disordered breathing; prevalence in the elderly of 45–62%
- rapid eye movement (REM) sleep behavior disorder; increased in the elderly—prevalence unclear.

In dementia, including Alzheimer's disease and dementia with Lewy bodies, these sleep disturbances are even more common (Gabelle & Dauvilliers, 2010), and there is commonly disrupted circadian rhythm (Neikrug & Ancoli-Israel, 2010). Specific sleep disturbances should be diagnosed and treated appropriately, keeping in mind that many sleep disturbances may be side-effects of medications.

Sleep problems may also be caused by depression and/or anxiety. Because depression and anxiety are common in dementia, they are also commonly causes of sleep disturbances in these patients.

The treatment for poor sleep hygiene (as in our patient above) is to limit naps during the day and thereby consolidate sleep at night. One or at the most two naps per day of 30–60 minutes each should be the maximum if the patient is expected to sleep at night.

Sometimes we will use a small dose of a stimulant medication to help the patient stay awake during the day (Box 22.6). A small dose of a stimulant medication also has the benefit of increasing alertness and attention, which may in turn improve thinking and memory. There are many that can be used. The two we most commonly use are long-acting methylphenidate (Ritalin and other brand names) and modafinil (Provigil). Note that in dementia we generally prescribe a single dose of a long-acting medication and do not increase it; in our experience if it will work for this purpose it works at a low dose, and higher doses increase side-effects and adverse reactions without an increase in efficacy. If the low dose seems to be helpful without side-effects we continue the stimulant; if it is unhelpful or causing side-effects we discontinue it.

What about sedatives to help the patient go to sleep? We would first note that, in the example above, having a patient take a "sleeping pill" at 9 p.m. is unlikely to help him stay asleep at 3 a.m.; most of its effects will have worn off by then. Sedatives at night may also lead to nocturnal incontinence if the patient is too sedated to get out of bed to use the bathroom. If the patient does get out of bed to use the bathroom, sedatives make it more likely that he will fall with potential injury occurring.

With these caveats in mind, sometimes a small dose of a sedative medication can be helpful in allowing the patient (and caregiver) to get a restful night's sleep, particularly if the main problem is difficulty falling asleep. Again we try to think about what is the underlying cause of the patient's difficulty sleeping (Box 22.7).

BOX 22.6 USE OF STIMULANT MEDICATION IN DEMENTIA

- Methylphenidate ER (Ritalin ER) 20 mg QAM
- Modafinil (Provigil) 100 mg QAM

Side-effects and adverse reactions can include dependency, abuse, confusion, psychosis, mania, agitation, aggression, arrhythmias, hypertension, myocardial infarction, stroke, sudden death, seizures, and hypersensitivity reaction including Stevens–Johnson syndrome.

PHARMACOTHERAPY FOR PSYCHOSIS

Psychosis, hallucinations, and delusions are common in the later stages of Alzheimer's disease. Visual hallucinations are also a presenting symptom of dementia with Lewy bodies, and delusions are very common in frontotemporal dementias. According to some studies,

---

BOX 22.7 STRATEGIES FOR TREATING INSOMNIA IN DEMENTIA

- Are there problems with sleep hygiene?
  - Regulate times of sleep and wake, limiting naps to no more than 1 hour per day
  - Can try a dose of melatonin 3–6 mg 1 hour prior to bed.
- Can non-pharmacological treatment help?
  - Limit naps as above.
  - Limit caffeine, tobacco, and alcohol after lunch
  - Try a glass of warm milk, soft music, soothing sounds, or a gentle back rub.
- Is there an underlying primary sleep problem?
  - Work-up and treat primary sleep problems when suspected.
- Is the problem due to underlying depression?
  - Can try a small dose of trazodone, 25–50 mg QHS, to help with insomnia and possibly treat the underlying depression (though it is not a very effective antidepressant). Side-effects in the elderly patient can include orthostatic hypotension and falls
  - Can also treat with an SSRI during the day, although note that SSRIs can worsen certain sleep disorders, such as periodic limb movements of sleep (Box 22.5).
- Is the problem due to underlying anxiety?
  - Can try a small dose of zolpidem (Ambien) 5–10 mg QHS or a small dose of a benzodiazepine.
- Is the problem due to underlying psychotic symptoms, such as delusions or hallucinations?
  - Can try a small dose of an atypical antipsychotic, typically starting with quetiapine (Seroquel) because it tends to be sedating (a good thing here) (Box 22.2).

---

hallucinations and delusions are the most common form of behavioral and psychological symptoms of dementia. See Chapters 20: *Caring for and educating the caregiver* and 21: *Non-pharmacological treatment of behavioral and psychological symptoms of dementia* for additional discussion of psychotic symptoms in dementia.

Hallucinations and delusions can manifest in a variety of ways, including agitation, anxiety, or repetitive, purposeless behavior. In general, as discussed above, we treat hallucinations and delusions only when they are troublesome to the patient.

Some general guidelines for managing hallucinations and delusions pharmacologically include:

- accurate diagnosis of the underlying dementia is crucial before determining how to treat the symptoms
- psychotic symptoms should be sufficient to disrupt the patient's functioning.
- the psychotic symptoms should be present for at least 1 month and should not be due to delirium or a pre-existing psychotic disorder or substance abuse problem
- the goal of treatment is not to eliminate the psychotic symptoms, but to reduce distress and improve function
- atypical antipsychotics are generally preferred (Box 22.2).

PHARMACOTHERAPY FOR AGITATION

Agitation is characterized by resistive verbally and sometimes physically aggressive behavior. Agitation is common in Alzheimer's disease, occurring in up to 70% of cases, and is probably even more common in some other dementias, such as frontotemporal dementia.

BOX 22.8 GENERAL GUIDELINES FOR PHARMACOLOGICAL MANAGEMENT OF AGITATION

- Characterize and diagnose the underlying condition(s) present.
- Characterize, diagnose, and treat any comorbid conditions, even if they are not thought to be contributing to the agitation.
- Characterize the nature of the agitation:
  - If depression or anxiety is present, start with an SSRI (Box 22.5)
    - Substitution of another SSRI may be appropriate
    - If sleep disturbance occurs trazodone may be added (see Pharmacotherapy for insomnia, above)
  - If psychosis (hallucinations or delusions) is present, start with an atypical antipsychotic (Box 22.2)
  - If no specific cause for the agitation can be determined, does it need to be treated quickly?
    - If the agitation needs to be treated rapidly because of danger to self or others, or difficulty providing care, start with an atypical antipsychotic (Box 22.2)
    - If the agitation can be treated more slowly, start with an SSRI (Box 22.5).

It can range from mild symptoms, such as repeating requests and demands ("When will I get dinner"), to outbursts characterized by punching, kicking, screaming, and running. It is often troublesome to both the patient and caregiver, and sometimes can only be managed by pharmacological intervention (Box 22.8).

Agitation often comes in the form of aggressive and uncooperative behavior coupled with or perhaps due to other symptoms of behavioral and psychological symptoms of dementia such as hallucinations, delusions, depression, or anxiety. It is important for clinicians to be aware that agitation is a very general term and can represent a number of different behaviors and be related to multiple underlying conditions. Characterization of how the agitation is manifesting and what underlying disorder is present is most likely to lead to successful treatment. For example, the individual with underlying psychosis may do best on an atypical antipsychotic. A patient with underlying depression may respond to an SSRI. (Note that, although valproic acid (Depakote) and other anticonvulsants are sometimes used, there are currently no data supporting their use nor do we do recommend using anticonvulsants in this setting.)

BEHAVIORAL AND PSYCHIATRIC CRISES

Despite the best efforts of caregivers and clinicians, the behavioral and psychological symptoms of dementia lead to crises in many patients. Sometimes these crises can be managed in the home, but often management in an acute psychiatric setting is necessary. Because crises are by their nature difficult to predict, we recommend to clinicians that they become familiar with the different acute psychiatric facility options available in their communities such that, when the crises invariably occur, they are ready to deal with them quickly and effectively. If we believe that there is a chance that a psychiatric hospitalization may be necessary for one of our patients, we try to let the family know ahead of time whenever possible. We stress that a short-term psychiatric hospitalization can be quite helpful, allowing medications to be withdrawn or added in a safe setting and enabling changes to occur much more quickly and easily than could be accomplished at home. We reassure the family of the high likelihood of the patient then being able to return home in a more stable clinical condition.

References

Cummings, J.L., McRae, T., Zhang, R., 2006. Effects of donepezil on neuropsychiatric symptoms in patients with dementia and severe behavioral disorders. Am. J. Geriatr. Psychiatry 14, 605–612.

Cummings, J.L., Mackell, J., Kaufer, D., 2008. Behavioral effects of current Alzheimer's disease treatments: a descriptive review. Alzheimers Dement. 4, 49–60.

Di Iulio, F., Palmer, K., Blundo, C., et al., 2010. Occurrence of neuropsychiatric symptoms and psychiatric disorders in mild Alzheimer's disease and mild cognitive impairment subtypes. Int. Psychogeriatr. 22, 629–640.

Gabelle, A., Dauvilliers, Y., 2010. Editorial: sleep and dementia. J. Nutr. Health Aging 14, 201–202.

Mega, M.S., Cummings, J.L., Fiorello, T., et al., 1996. The spectrum of behavioral changes in Alzheimer's disease. Neurology 46, 130–135.

Mega, M.S., Masterman, D.M., O'Connor, S.M., et al., 1999. The spectrum of behavioral responses to cholinesterase inhibitor therapy in Alzheimer disease. Arch. Neurol. 56, 1388–1393.

Neikrug, A.B., Ancoli-Israel, S., 2010. Sleep disturbances in nursing homes. J. Nutr. Health Aging 14, 207–211.

Roepke, S.K., Ancoli-Israel, S., 2010. Sleep disorders in the elderly. Indian J. Med. Res. 131, 302–310.

CHAPTER

Life adjustments

23

QUICK START: LIFE ADJUSTMENTS

Issues in mild cognitive impairment and Alzheimer's disease in the very mild and mild stages

- Patients with mild cognitive impairment and very mild Alzheimer's disease may be able to drive
  - A family member should ride in the passenger seat while the patient is driving once a month to help assure that the patient is driving safely
  - Driving should stop either when the patient reaches the mild stage of Alzheimer's disease or when the family member is uncomfortable riding in the car
  - When the patient does not want to stop driving, a formal driving evaluation is available at most rehabilitation hospitals.
- Patients with mild cognitive impairment and Alzheimer's disease at any stage need to have their financial affairs supervised
  - Family members or legal representatives should monitor all financial matters
  - The patient should be protected from telemarketers and other unscrupulous individuals soliciting monies and investment
  - Independent financial investing should cease immediately
- Patients with mild cognitive impairment and both very mild and mild Alzheimer's disease may be able to continue working
  - Working is healthy from the patient's perspective
  - The patient will need to be in a supervised setting
  - The job should entail no risks or dangers to the patient as well as relevant co-workers, customers, or consumers if problems in job performance were to occur.

Issues in Alzheimer's disease in the moderate and severe stages

- In general, patients with moderate to severe Alzheimer's disease should not be left alone.
- Home health aides and homemakers can provide assistance to patients and respite to caregivers
  - Home health aides help with the patient's personal needs, such as bathing
  - Homemakers help with household chores, such as cooking and laundry.
- Day programs provide a healthy routine for the patient and respite for the caregiver
  - Start at least 2 days per week; increase as needed
  - Call it a "club."
- Assisted living is ideal for patients who need more care than can be provided in the home when there is not a ready caregiver available. There are a large variety of assisted living facilities:
  - Some are almost independent living facilities
  - Some are almost nursing homes
  - And some are in-between.
- Unfortunately, most insurance does not pay for assisted living facilities.

Continued

Memory Loss: A Practical Guide for Clinicians.

> **QUICK START: LIFE ADJUSTMENTS—Cont'd**
>
> - Long-term care is necessary for almost all patients with dementia at some point in their illness
>   - Encourage families to plan ahead
>   - The family should look for a facility that they like and is close to home
>   - Units that specialize in dementia care are ideal, if available.
>
> See also Chapter 20: *Caring for and educating the caregiver*, for additional discussion of many of these important topics.

MILD COGNITIVE IMPAIRMENT AND ALZHEIMER'S DISEASE IN THE VERY MILD AND MILD STAGES

Driving

Driving is one of the most difficult issues that arises and will need to be addressed with almost every patient with dementia. How do we know if the patient in our office is safe to drive? In 2000 the American Academy of Neurology published a practice parameter paper based upon a meta-analysis of the available literature. The main finding was that patients with very mild Alzheimer's disease have motor vehicle accident rates similar to 16- to 19-year-old drivers. Since we allow 16- to 19-year-olds to drive, the conclusion was (and we agree) that it is reasonable for patients with very mild Alzheimer's disease to be allowed to drive as well (Dubinsky et al., 2000). (See Chapter 3: *Alzheimer's disease* for details on distinguishing the very mild from the mild stage of Alzheimer's disease.)

However, even if it is safe for patients with very mild Alzheimer's disease to drive in general, how do we know if it is safe for the particular very mild patient sitting in our office to drive? In 2010 the American Academy of Neurology published an update to their practice parameter paper which helped to identify additional risk factors for unsafe driving (Iverson et al., 2010) (see Fig. 23.1).

This updated practice parameter is helpful, but, even if it is safe for the patient to drive today, what about next week or next month? If it is determined that the patient with very mild Alzheimer's disease is safe to drive, we recommend that each month a family member ride as the front-seat passenger with the patient driving along their regular routes. For the most part, as long as the family member feels comfortable riding in the car with the patient driving, then we feel comfortable for the patient to continue driving. Driving should stop when either the family member no longer feels comfortable riding in the car or the patient progresses from the very mild to the mild stage of Alzheimer's disease.

If there is a controversy between the patient and his or her family, we recommend a formal driving evaluation, which can be done at most rehabilitation hospitals. These evaluations are (unfortunately) unlikely to be covered by insurance, and cost several hundred dollars. But they are much less expensive than a single accident.

Paying bills, credit and ATM cards, and investing

Having difficulties paying bills is often one of the first signs of memory loss. Some patients will forget to pay their bills, leading to loss of important services such as heat, electricity, and telephone. Other patients will pay bills twice. Some patients will have both problems.

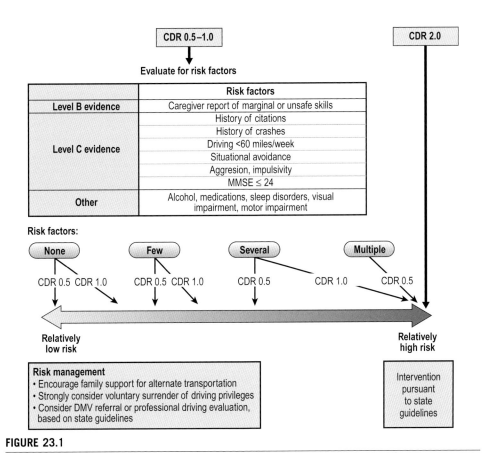

FIGURE 23.1

Possible algorithm for evaluating driving competence and risk management in patients with dementia
From Iverson, D.J., Gronseth, G.S., Reger, M.A., et al., 2010. Practice parameter update: evaluation and management
of driving risk in dementia. Report of the Quality Standards Subcommittee of the American Academy of Neurology.
Neurology 74, 1316–1324.

If a patient with mild cognitive impairment or very mild Alzheimer's disease is continuing to pay the household bills and do other banking duties, we recommend that their work be reviewed with a family member at least monthly to assure that no problems are developing.

In our society it is easy to have rapid access to large amounts of money or purchasing power using automatic teller machines (ATM) and/or credit cards. By the time the patient is in the mild stage of Alzheimer's disease it is usually prudent to remove access to these cards. As described in Chapter 21: *Non-pharmacological treatment of behavioral and psychological symptoms of dementia*, patients with ready access to cash can be easily exploited. Solicitations from unscrupulous individuals frequently appear in the mail and on the phone. We also know of several patients who, after their car was taken away to prevent them from unsafe driving, promptly went out and purchased another one, putting the down-payment on their credit card!

Even the most healthy and intelligent individual will sometimes make bad investments leading to significant financial losses. Investing is a complicated art, and depends upon being aware of the latest information along with good judgment and reasoning abilities (and of course a bit of luck). Given the complexity of investing, it is not surprising that many patients who eventually develop Alzheimer's disease or another dementia will have made poor investments in the years prior to their diagnosis. The tragedy is that sometimes life-long savings or retirement funds are lost within a short period of time. We recommend that a patient diagnosed with mild cognitive impairment or any type of dementia immediately relinquish any form of investing (Triebel et al., 2009).

Working

Should a patient with mild cognitive impairment work? As awareness of memory loss grows, and as more adults work into their 70s and 80s, there are more and more individuals who are working at the time of their diagnosis of mild cognitive impairment (and, more occasionally, very mild Alzheimer's disease). Whether individuals with mild cognitive impairment and very mild Alzheimer's disease should continue working depends upon the individual, their job, and how long they have been doing the work. If the individual has been doing the job for many years, it is likely that many of the manual and cognitive skills have already been consolidated in memory, and can therefore be maintained for a period of time (see Appendix C: *Our current understanding of memory*).

From the patient's perspective, working is almost always a good thing: working typically provides a healthy routine, intellectual stimulation, socialization, and other helpful qualities such as maintaining feelings of self-worth and avoiding depression. From the employer's and society's perspective, it depends upon whether the patient's cognitive impairment disrupts the performance of the job and/or whether there are risks or dangers involved.

For example, an individual with mild cognitive impairment could continue to work on an assembly line in which their task is procedural in nature (not requiring memory, judgment, or reasoning), is relatively circumscribed, and the person at the next stage of the assembly line will be aware of any errors made. Another example of an appropriate job to continue includes making hand-made crafts such as pottery or articles of clothing; again the work depends largely on procedural memory (not affected by mild Alzheimer's disease; see Appendix C), and the quality of the work will generally be readily apparent.

Inappropriate jobs to continue include those that involve supervision at almost any level, from watching children at a daycare center to managing a business. Other inappropriate jobs to continue include those that involve memory, judgment, and reasoning that affects people's lives at any level, such as a clinical or legal professional. Sales jobs may be appropriate if the work is circumscribed, the patient is already quite experienced, and the supervision of the patient is appropriate. For example, one of our patients was able to continue his job and be productive as a florist well into the mild stage of Alzheimer's disease.

ALZHEIMER'S DISEASE IN THE MODERATE TO SEVERE STAGES
Home alone

One way to define the moderate stage of Alzheimer's disease is when the patient is no longer able to stay home alone for more than an hour or two. As discussed in more detail in Chapter 3: *Alzheimer's disease*, problems in the moderate stage of Alzheimer's disease include severe memory difficulties, poor problem-solving, wandering, and often the start of problems of incontinence and needing help with hygiene. Not surprisingly, patients in the moderate stage of Alzheimer's disease begin to get into trouble when left alone. Even patients without incontinence who do not wander may leave the stove on. And those who do not leave the stove on may fall prey to a telemarketer or accidentally lock themselves out of the house. We therefore strongly encourage families to have round-the-clock supervision available for patients in the moderate stage of dementia.

Needing round-the-clock care is a huge task for the caregiver, and should not be done alone. Studies have shown that even caregivers who want to provide care themselves 24 hours a day/7 days a week invariably "burn out" faster than if they had shared the care of the patient. Some families, particularly if large and/or close-knit, can do well sharing caregiving duties, giving the primary caregiver needed time alone. Note that if there are a number of different family members helping out, it is usually better for the patient if the family comes to the patient's house, rather than the patient to the family's house, although we have seen it work well both ways.

Sooner or later, most families greatly benefit from additional help taking care of the patient. Home health aides, day programs, assisted living, and long-term care are some of the commonly used options.

(See Chapter 20: *Caring for and educating the caregiver*, for more on these important topics.)

Home health aides and homemakers

Home health aides can provide assistance to caregivers by helping with activities of daily living such as showering, shaving, and brushing teeth. Homemakers do not provide personal care to the patient but help with laundry, cooking, light cleaning, and other tasks. In each case these individuals also provide much needed time for the caregiver to pay the bills, do household chores, go out with friends, or simply spend a few minutes by themselves.

Day programs

Day programs can provide much needed respite for the caregiver, and also a nice routine for the patient. Many of our patients truly look forward to the "bus" (really a van) that comes to take them to their "club" (really the day program). We recommend that patients go to the day program at least 2 days a week to allow them to develop a routine; 3 or 4 days a week are probably ideal early on, and can be increased as the need arises and/or the caregiving duties become more difficult. Day programs provide appropriate activities for the patients, and some will also help with hygiene issues such as showering a patient when they are there. We also find that patients who attend day programs do better in the evening when they return home.

Assisted living facilities

Assisted living is ideal for patients who need more care than can be provided for them in their home for a number of reasons:

- patients may have been living alone without family members in the area
- the caregiver may not be able to provide adequate care because of their own medical problems

- family members may be busy with their own families or jobs and unable to provide care to the patient.

Unlike long-term care services for those with more severe dementia, health insurance does not usually pay for assisted living, greatly reducing the numbers of individuals who would otherwise benefit from assisted living. Some states (e.g., Vermont), however, have now recognized that assisted living is a less expensive and more appropriate alternative to nursing home care (which is often paid for by state-funded Medicaid programs) for many patients and will contribute substantially to the cost. The local council on aging or similar agency can often facilitate this type of placement.

There is a huge variety of services which assisted living facilities can provide, with some providing more services and some less. All will provide residents with their own room, as well as common areas for activities and dining. Most have additional services available, such as nurses to administer medications and aides to help with personal hygiene. Often these additional services are available "à la carte," with additional cost for each additional service. Some assisted living residences are part of a larger facility that includes long-term care residences, whereas patients in other facilities will need to move to a different long-term care residence when the severity of their dementia is more than can be handled in assisted living.

Long-term care facilities

When patients can no longer be managed at home or in assisted living, a long-term care facility is necessary. Ideally the move to long-term care should be done with a certain amount of planning. Unfortunately, patients frequently end up at a long-term care facility in a time of crisis, often after a medical illness. The typical scenario is that the patient is admitted to an acute care facility after a fall, urinary tract infection, pneumonia, or even dehydration, and it is determined that they are not safe to return home. In either situation, families should look for a facility that they are comfortable with and is close to home. Some facilities accept patients with a wide range of cognitive and physical impairments, whereas others specialize in one type or severity of impairment.

If possible, we recommend considering a special unit that focuses on patients with Alzheimer's disease and other types of dementia. These units are often inside a more general nursing home, consisting of a floor or a wing. These are often referred to as Alzheimer's Special Care Units, Dementia Special Care Units, or Memory Care Units. In 2010, 27 states had legislation requiring such units to have special standards regarding the services provided, training of the staff, activities offered, ability of the staff to care for residents with behavioral and psychological symptoms of dementia, and also what fees they charge.

(See also Chapter 20: *Caring for and educating the caregiver*, for additional discussion of these important issues.)

References

Dubinsky, R.M., Stein, A.C., Lyons, K., 2000. Practice parameter: risk of driving and Alzheimer's disease (an evidence-based review): report of the quality standards subcommittee of the American Academy of Neurology. Neurology 54, 2205–2211.

Iverson, D.J., Gronseth, G.S., Reger, M.A., et al., 2010. Practice parameter update: evaluation and management of driving risk in dementia. Report of the Quality Standards Subcommittee of the American Academy of Neurology. Neurology 74, 1316–1324.

Triebel, K.L., Martin, R., Griffith, H.R., et al., 2009. Declining financial capacity in mild cognitive impairment: a 1-year longitudinal study. Neurology 73, 928–934.

24 Legal and financial issues

QUICK START: LEGAL AND FINANCIAL ISSUES

- The Alzheimer's Association is an up-to-date helpful resource for families.
  - Encourage your families to visit the website (www.alz.org) or call to find their local chapter (800-272-3900).
- Legal capacity is the capacity to make decisions and judgments necessary to sign legal documents, and depends upon the answers to three questions:
  - What type of deliberation needs to be undertaken to fully understand the implications and ramifications of the document, if signed?
  - How impaired is the patient?
  - Is everyone in the family in agreement? Or are there other family members who will likely be contesting the patient's capacity to make these decisions?
- Important legal documents are:
  - Guardianship
  - Living will
  - Power of attorney
  - Power of attorney for healthcare.
- Alzheimer's disease is expensive. There are, however, a number of resources available that may assist in defraying the costs of the disease.

Many families need our assistance to know what legal and financial issues need to be addressed when their loved one develops Alzheimer's disease or another dementia. Although many social workers and some other clinicians may directly assist in these matters, knowledge of these issues is essential for all clinicians to allow us to help our families to obtain the assistance they need. A wonderful source of continuously updated information for families regarding all of these issues is the Alzheimer's Association. Encourage your families to visit the website (www.alz.org) or call to find their local chapter (800-272-3900).

LEGAL PLANNING

Important issues in legal planning include the capacity to make decisions and judgments and the preparation of legal documents.

Legal capacity: the importance of starting the process early

One issue that frequently arises in the clinic is whether it is appropriate for the patient to sign a legal document. The issue is that of "capacity," that is, does the patient have the capacity to make important decisions and judgments regarding who should have legal

Memory Loss: A Practical Guide for Clinicians.

control of himself or herself. The answer depends in turn upon the answer to several other questions:

- What type of deliberation needs to be undertaken to fully understand the implications and ramifications of the document, if signed?
- How impaired is the patient?
- Is everyone on the same page? Or are there other family members who will likely be contesting the patient's capacity to make these decisions?

If patients are diagnosed at the earliest signs of memory loss, and these issues are brought up soon afterwards, most patients will have the capacity to understand and sign legal documents related to who should have legal control of their affairs. In general, patients with mild cognitive impairment or Alzheimer's disease in the very mild or mild stage (CDR 0.5 or 1.0; MMSE >17) have the capacity to make decisions related to the control of their own legal, financial, and health decisions.

Note that, because different documents pertain to different issues that may involve a different level of complexity or require a different level of understanding, patients may have capacity for one document but not for another. However, the capacity required for the documents discussed here is similar for each document.

As the clinician, you can help determine whether the patient has capacity to sign certain documents by (1) talking with the patient, (2) working with the family, and (3) using your knowledge of the patient's cognitive status to assess whether the patient is able to understand the issue raised in the document to be signed. For example, Mr. John Jones (the patient) and his wife (primary caregiver) come to the clinic today, and Mrs. Jones asks, "Is it alright for John to sign paperwork for legal and healthcare power of attorney?" We know that Mr. Jones has mild Alzheimer's disease with a MMSE score of 23 (and a CDR of 1.0; see Chapter 3: *Alzheimer's disease*), and that he probably has cognitive ability necessary to have legal capacity to sign these documents. We ask Mr. Jones, "Do you understand what it means for you to sign these documents, the legal and healthcare power of attorney?" If he answers, "Yes, it means that Mary can make legal and medical decisions for me if I am not able to," then this answer, coupled with his cognitive status, leads us to the conclusion that he has the capacity to sign the documents. If, on the other hand, he gives the more common answer, "I don't know...what do these documents mean?" we would then need to explain each one to him:

> *Clinician:* Mr. Jones, the first document, the legal power of attorney, would allow your wife to make legal and financial decisions for you if you are having trouble making them, such as what investments to make with your retirement savings. Do you feel comfortable with her making those legal and financial decisions for you if you are not able to make them?
>
> *Patient:* Oh yes, I would want Mary to make those decisions for us.
>
> *Clinician:* The second document, the healthcare power of attorney, would allow your wife to make medical decisions for you if you are having trouble making them, such as whether you should have an elective surgery or not. Do you feel comfortable with her making those medical decisions for you if you are not able to make them?
>
> *Patient:* I hope I won't need to have surgery. But if I did, I would want Mary to help me make that decision.

In this scenario the patient understands what each document means and his answers, coupled with our knowledge of his cognitive status, lead us to conclude that he has the legal capacity necessary to sign them. The question of whether a patient has the capacity to allow a family member to take control of his or her affairs is typically contentious only when there is more than one family member vying for control. When multiple family members are involved, it is best to get them all in the room together with the patient. It typically becomes readily apparent who has the patient's best interests at heart, or who will be the most responsible with financial affairs. If a family consensus can be reached, then things go smoothly. If not, it will be up to the courts to decide.

It goes without saying that the less impaired the patient is, the greater capacity the patient will have, and the easier these types of issues and decisions become. We therefore encourage the family to start the legal planning early—before the patient becomes too impaired to make these decisions, before the patient loses capacity. Note that it is important that all family discussions regarding capacity and other legal issues be well documented in the medical record.

Legal documents

There are a number of legal documents of which the patient and family should be aware. An attorney is necessary to prepare and execute these documents. Finding the right attorney is important. If the patient has a family attorney, he or she may be able to assist the family in these matters, or refer them to an appropriate attorney. If not, one good place to start is to call either the local Alzheimer's Association office (http://www.alz.org/apps/findus.asp; 800-272-3900) or the local Agency on Aging office (or contact the Eldercare locator www.eldercare.gov; 800-677-1116).

- *Guardianship* (conservatorship in some US states) is the court-appointed individual to make decisions on the patient's behalf regarding the patient's assets and/or healthcare. Guardianship is only given by the court when it finds that the patient is legally incompetent. Note that a diagnosis of Alzheimer's disease alone does not make a patient legally incompetent.
- A *living will* is a document that indicates the medical choices the patient would wish to make if he or she is unable to make them, such as whether cardiopulmonary resuscitation (CPR) should be performed should there be a catastrophic event and his or her heart were to stop beating.
- *Power of attorney* is the document which allows the patient to name an individual to make legal and financial decisions when he or she is unable to. A "durable" power of attorney means that the power of attorney is valid after the patient can no longer make his or her own decisions. Usually the power of attorney is "durable."
- *Power of attorney for healthcare* is the document that allows the patient to name an individual to make medical and other healthcare decisions when he or she is unable to. These decisions would include choosing between different:
  - physicians and other healthcare providers
  - types of treatment (e.g., surgery versus medical versus palliative)
  - long-term care facilities.

Note that there is overlap between the living will and the power of attorney for healthcare, such that it might be possible that the living will specifies the preference for one treatment (e.g., DNR—Do Not Resuscitate), whereas the individual with the power of attorney for healthcare specifies another (e.g., CPR when appropriate). In these circumstances there is an assumption that the power of attorney for healthcare is following what the wishes of the patient would be if he or she were able to articulate them in the particular circumstance that has arisen. Given this assumption, it would be highly unlikely that physicians or attorneys would "overrule" the power of attorney for healthcare, despite an apparent contradiction with the patient's living will.

FINANCIAL PLANNING

In Chapter 23: *Life adjustments* we discussed the importance of the patient transitioning the household finances to a family member or other caregiver, including banking, bill paying, and investing. In this chapter we touch on the issue of how to help the patient and family cover the costs of Alzheimer's disease or other dementia.

Alzheimer's disease is expensive. In addition to the continuing costs that the patient has related to ongoing medical treatment and prescription drugs, new costs will likely occur related to in-home services (home health aide, homemaker, respite, and others), day programs, and eventually long-term care services (assisted living and nursing homes). Here we list a number of programs that patients or their families may be able to take advantage of to help defray some of these costs.

- *Medicare* is the federal health insurance program for those aged 65 years and older. Medicare covers:
  - inpatient hospital care
  - some outpatient care
  - some medical items
  - some prescription medications
  - some home healthcare
    - some skilled nursing care
    - some rehabilitation care.
  Medicare does not cover long-term nursing home care. See www.medicare.gov or call 800-633-4227 for more information.
- *Medigap* is additional insurance paid for out-of-pocket expenses that can fill in the "gaps" in Medicare coverage (such as co-insurance payments). There are several different options, with the more expensive policies paying for additional gaps. See http://www.medicare.gov/medigap/ for more information.
- *Medicaid* will pay for medical care and long-term care for patients with very low income and asset levels. Many individuals end up qualifying for Medicaid after using up their own money and other assets (the so-called "spend down" period). Patients must be very careful, however, regarding giving away their assets to family members; state laws typically prevent this action from allowing them to qualify. As with many aspects of financial planning, beginning early is the key to success.
- *The Department of Veterans Affairs (VA)* provides health and long-term care services for many veterans. Through its Geriatric Research Education Clinical Centers (GRECCs; http://www1.va.gov/GRECC/), the VA has become a leader in the care of individuals with Alzheimer's disease and other dementias. See www.va.gov, call 800-827-1000, or have the family contact their nearest GRECC (http://www1.va.gov/GRECC/GRECC_Demographics_ and_Profiles.asp).
- *Social security disability income (SSDI)* are benefits for those younger than age 65 who have worked during their life to obtain additional income from social security.

All patients with Alzheimer's disease or other dementia less than age 65 who have previously worked should look into this program, which is now easier to apply for (see http://www.alz.org/living_with_alzheimers_social_security_disability.asp). For more information contact Social Security at http://www.socialsecurity.gov/, or 800-772-1213.

- *Social security income (SSI)* are benefits for those aged 65 or older who are both disabled and also have limited income and assets. For more information contact Social Security at http://www.socialsecurity.gov/, or 800-772-1213.
- The *Family and Medical Leave Act* is very helpful for family members who are working while caring for an individual with dementia. See http://www.dol.gov/whd/fmla/ for more information.
- *Tax benefits* may be available, including deductions and credits, depending upon the specific circumstance of the patient and family. Programs such as the Household and Dependent Care Credit may be applicable. See www.irs.gov or call 800-829-1040.
- *Disability insurance* provides income for a worker who can no longer work because of illness or injury. Most employer-paid disability policies provide 60–70% of the individual's gross income. Personal disability policies differ in the amount of benefit that they provide.
- *Long-term care insurance* will usually pay for the cost of nursing homes and other long-term care facilities. If the patient is fortunate enough to have this insurance, it should be reviewed carefully to make sure that Alzheimer's disease (or other dementia) is covered, how long the benefits will last, and other details.
- *Life insurance* policies can sometimes loan money to the patient prior to their death (a "viatical" loan) when the patient is not expected to live beyond 6–12 months.
- *Retirement accounts* can be used, including individual retirement accounts (IRAs), and employee-funded accounts such as 401(k) and 403(b).
- *Personal savings and assets* are of course another option. These include savings and checking accounts, money-market accounts, property, and real estate.

Special issues

QUICK START: SPECIAL ISSUES

Some patients do not want to have their memory evaluated

- Help patients understand that the goal is to improve their memory and allow them to continue doing the activities that they enjoy.
- Explain that there are a number of medications available that could help them.

Some patients do not want you to talk to their family

- A few patients are able to manage the disease on their own, at least for a while.
- For the majority of patients, involvement of family or friends is a critical part of the patient's care, helping him or her to deal with and manage memory loss due to Alzheimer's disease or another dementia.

Talking to adult children of patients about their risk of Alzheimer's disease and what they can do about it

- Having one parent with the disease increases the lifetime risk of developing Alzheimer's disease by approximately twofold
  - We stress, however, that Alzheimer's disease is common: everyone is at risk.
- Activities shown to reduce the risk of Alzheimer's disease include:
  - Participating in social and cognitively stimulating activities
  - Performing aerobic exercise.

THE PATIENT WHO DOES NOT WANT TO COME TO THE APPOINTMENT

Difficulty in convincing a patient to come to an appointment to evaluate their memory can sometimes be one of the biggest obstacles faced by the family. Patients do not want to come to the appointment for a variety of reasons. Some patients may not want to come to the appointment because they are fearful of the diagnosis of Alzheimer's disease, particularly if they watched their parent, spouse, or friend suffer with this disorder. Others may not want to come to the appointment because they are afraid they will be sent to a nursing home. And some may simply not want to come to the appointment because they do not recognize a problem and cannot be bothered with coming.

We admit that we have not been able to convince every patient to come to an appointment. We have, however, been successful with a couple of strategies. The most reliable of these is to explain to the patient (typically on the phone) that our goal is to improve their memory to allow them to continue doing the activities that they enjoy, and that there are a number of medications available to help their memory, and even to delay the onset of Alzheimer's disease. Sometimes it is not even what you say, but just spending a minute and making a connection with the patient helps to make the appointment less frightening.

A number of families will grab us in the hallway prior to the appointment and say something like, "Please measure her blood pressure. . .the only way I was able to get her to you was to pretend that this was for her routine blood pressure check." Although we do not condone deception as a way to bring a patient to an appointment (in part because it may lead to mistrust, in part because of the ethical implications), patients brought in this way typically do just fine. These patients discover that a memory evaluation is quite similar to other medical evaluations, not as frightening or threatening as they had feared.

THE PATIENT WHO DOES NOT WANT YOU TO TALK TO THEIR FAMILY

Sometimes it happens that patients come to the clinic and they do not want you to tell their family about their memory difficulties. Should we agree with respecting their desire for confidentiality, despite the difficulties and potential danger in which they may be placing themselves and others? Or should we insist that their family be involved? Our answer is that it depends upon the circumstances (see patient examples below). For the vast majority of patients, the involvement of family or friends is a critical part of the patient's care, helping him or her to deal with and manage memory loss whether due to Alzheimer's disease or due to another dementia. There are a few patients, however, who are able to manage the disease on their own, at least for a while.

The first patient

A patient came to our office about 10 years ago, driving himself the 3 hours to get to our clinic, with concerns about his memory. He had noticed mild changes in his memory, and was worried that he might be at the earliest stage of Alzheimer's disease. He had watched his father go through the disease, and so he knew the signs well. After evaluating him we made a diagnosis of mild cognitive impairment, and prescribed a course of medication. He did not want us to mention anything to his children or his wife, which we thought was acceptable at the time given how mild his memory difficulties were, how responsibly he was acting, and that he was taking a medication which had the potential to improve his memory to the level which it was at the previous year.

Several years passed in this manner. His memory became worse, and he was diagnosed with very mild Alzheimer's disease. At each visit we discussed the importance of letting his family know about his difficulties, but he continued to decline our suggestion. He was able to persuade us, however, that he was taking all of his medications correctly, was driving safely, not getting lost, and not running into any serious difficulties. Finally a minor crisis occurred at home when he forgot to come home to take the dog out for a walk—a small thing, but very uncharacteristic for him—and he ended up explaining to his family about his disease and about not wanting to burden them with it. Our next visit with the patient included his wife and two anxious sons. We had a very productive meeting and learned many things we wished we had known about earlier, such as that he used many woodworking tools in the basement and was beginning to have minor injuries associated with not using the tools correctly. Overall, however, we were pleased that we were able to provide good treatment to the patient while at the same time respecting his wishes not to tell his family about his memory problems.

The second patient

Another patient came to our clinic several years ago. We knew that there were going to be some issues before she came in, because she had literally scheduled and then cancelled the appointment four times before finally coming in to see us. It had also been clear to us ahead of time that she did not want her family involved, because when our secretary scheduled the visit and mentioned to the patient that she should bring someone close to her to the appointment, such as a family member or close friend, she adamantly refused to do so.

During the appointment she was incredibly anxious. We were sympathetic to her. It was perfectly clear that she was absolutely terrified that she might have Alzheimer's disease. Her mother had recently died of the disease, and we gathered that the experience of her mother's illness and death had been quite traumatizing to her. Her mother, however, first showed symptoms in her mid-80s and died at age 91. The patient herself was only 68 years old. Even before we finished interviewing her we could tell that her memory problems were significant, and we wondered whether she was really able to cover her difficulties as well as she stated.

We took an extra 10 minutes, and spoke with her about some of what we typically save for the first follow-up visit. We discussed that, if it turned out that she did have Alzheimer's disease, there are many treatments that could help her—more than were available when her mother was diagnosed. Additionally, we discussed a number of experimental treatments that were currently in clinical trials, treatments that had the possibility to significantly slow the progression of Alzheimer's disease.

We then asked about her family and, when we learned that they were supportive, we explained the importance of having her family with her. She hesitated, and we gently but firmly insisted that she involve her family and bring at least one family member with her to the follow-up appointment. We insisted because we were concerned that she needed the emotional support of family to effectively come to terms with her memory problems. Additionally, her memory was already poor enough such that she would be unable to hide it for long—assuming that it was not already apparent to those around her. Both her daughter and husband came with her to the next appointment, at which time we told her that she had mild Alzheimer's disease. Although tears were shed, with their help she was able to accept the diagnosis, and she worked to have a positive attitude.

TALKING TO ADULT CHILDREN OF PATIENTS ABOUT THEIR RISK OF ALZHEIMER'S DISEASE AND WHAT THEY CAN DO ABOUT IT

Although their first concern is always for their parent, the second concern of almost all adult children is, "So what are my risks, doc? Will I develop Alzheimer's disease too?" As we discussed in Chapter 3: *Alzheimer's disease*, compared with not having a parent with the disease, having one parent with Alzheimer's disease increases the lifetime risk of developing it by approximately twofold (Lautenschlager et al., 1996). Knowledge of this increase in risk causes many middle-aged children of patients with Alzheimer's disease to become apprehensive that they, too, will develop this disorder. We generally point out to these family members that, although the risk of Alzheimer's disease is increased with a family history of the disorder, Alzheimer's disease is unfortunately extremely common as we age, such that everyone is at risk for the disorder, with or without a family history. More importantly, if the overall risk of Alzheimer's disease is about 2.5% between ages 65 and 70, the risk without a family history is probably around 1.5% and the risk with a family history is probably around 3%. Thus, although the relative risk may be doubled, the overall risk is still quite small.

The next question asked by those at risk for Alzheimer's disease is, "So what can I do to prevent it?" Although there is no definitive answer to this question, we emphasize the activities that have been repeatedly shown to be helpful. As discussed in Chapter 18: *Non-pharmacological treatment of memory loss*, activities that can slow down memory loss and stave off Alzheimer's disease include participating in social and cognitively stimulating leisure activities (Boyke et al., 2008; Akbaraly et al., 2009; Leung et al., 2010) and performing aerobic exercise

(Scarmeas et al., 2009). These are, therefore, the activities and lifestyle changes that we recommend. If they ask us about vitamins, herbs, supplements, or diets, we share with them the information discussed in Chapters 16: *Vitamins, herbs, supplements, and anti-inflammatories* and 18: *Non-pharmacological treatment of memory loss*; in our view none of these factors has sufficient evidence that would justify a change in diet or use of vitamins, herbs, and supplements.

References

Akbaraly, T.N., Portet, F., Fustinoni, S., et al., 2009. Leisure activities and the risk of dementia in the elderly: results from the Three-City Study. Neurology 73, 854–861.

Boyke, J., Driemeyer, J., Gaser, C., et al., 2008. Training-induced brain structure changes in the elderly. J. Neurosci. 28, 7031–7035.

Lautenschlager, N.T., Cupples, L.A., Rao, V.S., et al., 1996. Risk of dementia among relatives of Alzheimer's disease patients in the MIRAGE study: what is in store for the oldest old? Neurology 46, 641–650.

Leung, G.T., Fung, A.W., Tam, C.W., et al., 2010. Examining the association between participation in late-life leisure activities and cognitive function in community-dwelling elderly Chinese in Hong Kong. Int. Psychogeriatr. 22, 2–13.

Scarmeas, N., Luchsinger, J.A., Schupf, N., et al., 2009. Physical activity, diet, and risk of Alzheimer disease. JAMA 302, 627–637.

The cases below, all actual patients from our clinic, represent some of the common causes of memory loss and other cognitive impairment (Figure 1). We would recommend that as you go through these cases and those in your own practice you first consider whether the patient has Alzheimer's disease, the most common cause of memory loss, or whether there is a reason to consider another cause of cognitive dysfunction (Figure 2).

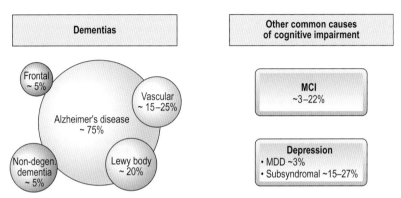

FIGURE 1 Visual representation of the prevalence of the common causes of memory loss and other cognitive impairment.

Visual representation of the prevalence of the common causes of memory loss and other cognitive impairment.

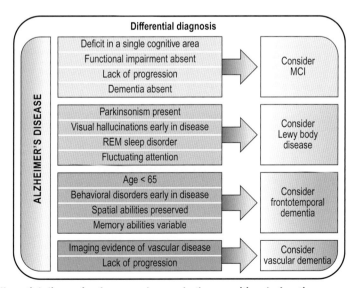

FIGURE 2 Differential diagnosis of memory loss and other cognitive dysfunction.

Starting with the assumption of Alzheimer's disease on the *left*, factors in the *middle* lead to other common diagnoses on the *right*.

PATIENT 1 (Figure 3)

An 81-year-old man was brought in by his son and daughter for memory loss. They reported that the problems started eight years ago when he became lost while driving, and repeatedly asked the same questions again and again. Around that time he lost his car in a parking lot for more than an hour. Over the ensuing eight years he became gradually worse. They knew that they should have had him evaluated earlier, but they were busy caring for their mother who had cancer. She recently died, and it became clear how much she was compensating for his memory loss. She had long since taken over all household tasks that he had performed in the past, such as balancing the checkbook and paying the bills, but they did not understand that he was unable to take his medications correctly or prepare simple meals until she was no longer there to help him with those activities. His memory became so impaired that he forgot most things within a few minutes. He no longer remembered the names of his grandchildren, all of which he used to know. What he could remember was his experience in World War II, and for the 6–12 months it seemed like that was all he could remember.

During the interview and examination it was clear that he had word-finding problems and difficulties with comprehension. He scored 13/30 on the Mini-Mental State Examination (MMSE), missing all (three out of three) of the recall items, most of the orientation

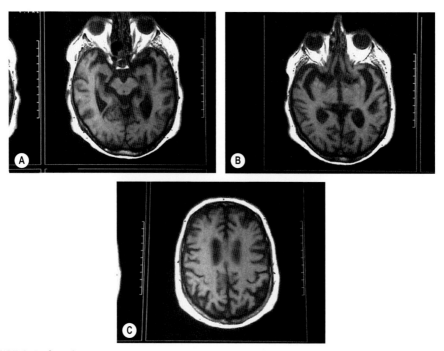

FIGURE 3 Patient 1.

Axial slices from a brain MRI showing moderate to severe hippocampal atrophy (A), anterior temporal lobe atrophy (B), and parietal lobe atrophy (C).

items to place and time, attention, calculations, and copying intersecting pentagons. On the Blessed Information, Memory, and Concentration test he made 19 errors out of a possible 37, missing all (five out of five) of the 5-minute recall items, most of the orientation items to place and time, reciting the months of the year backwards (attention), and items of non-personal history (dates of World War II, name of current President and Vice-President). His 7 Minute Screen was positive, as was his Alzheimer's Disease Caregiver Questionnaire. He scored 1 out of 15 (non-depressed) on the Geriatric Depression Scale.

What is the likely diagnosis?

Alzheimer's disease, in the moderate stage, is the most likely diagnosis. Although we do not know of other risk factors, the patient was 81 years old, a risk factor in itself. He had a gradually progressing disorder that began with memory problems and then included many other cognitive domains including language, attention, calculations, and visuospatial function. His instrumental activities of daily living were clearly impaired (see Box 2.2). He was thus demented from a progressive disorder affecting memory first and foremost, but also affecting many other cognitive domains. His MRI scan was read as showing "global atrophy," but actually showed a pattern of multifocal atrophy: a moderate to severe degree of atrophy of the hippocampi, anterior temporal lobes, and parietal lobes bilaterally, and mild to moderate atrophy of frontal lobes bilaterally; occipital lobes were normal (Figure 3). Although this pattern of atrophy is not necessary for a diagnosis of Alzheimer's disease, it is the expected pattern and therefore consistent with the disease. There was no indication of vascular disease from the history, but even if we saw mild to moderate small vessel ischemic disease—common in an 81 year old—Alzheimer's disease would still be the most likely diagnosis because mild to moderate small vessel ischemic disease would not explain the pattern or the degree of functional and cognitive impairments observed in the history and examination. The patient was treated with a cholinesterase inhibitor, followed in 2 months by memantine. See Chapter 3: *Alzheimer's disease*, for more information.

PATIENT 2 (Figure 4)

A 73-year-old woman came to the clinic complaining of word-finding difficulties. She had noticed 6–12 months of difficulty naming not only people (proper nouns) but also other items such as pocket book, hanger, and hose. She admitted that her word-finding difficulty sometimes interfered with her ability to communicate with family and friends, but what she found particularly bothersome was when she would, for example, go into a department store and was not able to think of the right word when talking with a sales person. Her son accompanied her to the appointment. When we spoke with him alone he told us that, although his mother complained only about her word-finding difficulties, he believed that she had memory problems as well. He noted that his mother used to have an excellent memory: she used to remember her calendar in her head, grocery lists in her head, etc. He continued that her memory problems had worsened to the point that she needed to write everything down to compensate or she would have been totally lost. He believed that her decline in memory had started about 5 years earlier and had become progressively worse.

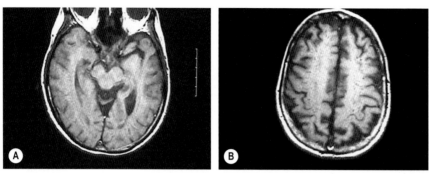

FIGURE 4 Patient 2.

Axial slices from a brain MRI showing mild, left greater than right, hippocampal and anterior temporal lobe atrophy (A), and mild bilateral parietal lobe atrophy (B).

She scored 24/30 on the Mini-mental state examination (MMSE), missing two out of three of the recall items, and several items of orientation. On the Blessed Information Memory Concentration test she made seven errors out of a possible 37, missing three out of five of the 5-minute recall items, several orientation items to place and time, and reciting the months of the year backwards (attention). Her 7 Minute Screen was positive, as was her Alzheimer's disease Caregiver Questionnaire. She scored 3 out of 15 (non-depressed) on the Geriatric Depression Scale.

What is the differential diagnosis?

Alzheimer's disease, in the mild stage, is the most likely diagnosis. Because the patient complained about word-finding, a language problem, one has to worry about a dementia that affects language primarily, such as a frontotemporal dementia (specifically progressive non-fluent aphasia or semantic dementia variants; see Chapter 7: *Frontotemporal dementia*, for more information). However, if the language problem is only word-finding, and the patient also has memory problems, Alzheimer's disease is the more likely diagnosis in a 73 year old. Her MRI scan showed mild, left greater than right, atrophy of the hippocampus and anterior temporal lobes, mild atrophy of parietal lobes bilaterally, and very mild atrophy of frontal lobes bilaterally; occipital lobes were normal (Figure 4). Although not necessary for diagnosis, this pattern of atrophy is consistent with Alzheimer's disease. She was treated with a cholinesterase inhibitor. See Chapter 3: *Alzheimer's disease*, for more information.

PATIENT 3

A 72-year-old man presented with mild memory difficulties. He was the Chief Executive Officer of a large company. He explained to us that he used to have an excellent memory, and he had noticed a definite decline. He used to remember his busy daily schedule after glancing at it in the morning; now, if his secretary did not remind him, he would miss meetings. He used to remember the important details of meetings in his head; now, he needed to take detailed notes. Although he did not have trouble with other aspects of cognition, his memory problems had worsened gradually over the last 2 years. He also pointed out, however, that he never forgot anything critically important. With the help of his secretary and the additional note-taking he was able to continue to perform his job successfully.

He was well educated, having graduated with a master's degree in business administration from a prominent university. His physical and neurological examinations were normal. On the Mini-mental state examination (MMSE) he scored 29/30, missing just one of the three recall items. On the Blessed Information Memory Concentration test he made two errors out of a possible 37, missing two of the five items of the 5-minute recall. His 7 Minute Screen was negative, as was his Alzheimer's disease Caregiver Questionnaire. He scored 2 out of 15 (non-depressed) on the Geriatric Depression Scale. Formal neuropsychological testing revealed isolated problems with memory compared with his age- and education-matched peers. His laboratory studies and MRI scan were normal.

What is the most likely diagnosis?

Amnestic mild cognitive impairment (amnestic MCI) is the best characterization for this patient, who had an isolated memory problem compared with his age- and education-matched peers but who was still highly functional (and therefore not demented). Treatment with a cholinesterase inhibitor was discussed as it would likely help his memory function, although we explained that such treatment was not approved by the US Food and Drug Administration for mild cognitive impairment and could also have repercussions regarding long-term care insurance or life insurance, as it could imply a diagnosis of Alzheimer's disease. He opted to take the cholinesterase inhibitor and he was able to continue working for another year, during which time he successfully transitioned the leadership of the company to his successor. We continued to see him every 6 months, and after another 2 years he had declined to the point that he met criteria for Alzheimer's disease. See Chapter 4: *Mild cognitive impairment*, for more information.

PATIENT 4

A 78-year-old man was brought to the clinic by his family because of his memory difficulties and inappropriate behavior. They reported that his problems began 3–4 years earlier when he had difficulty remembering things and became confused in unfamiliar places. However, the real issue was that for the past year he had been watching pornography on cable TV for hours at a time, and telling sexually explicit jokes in front of his daughters. They described him as apathetic, withdrawn, and depressed. He no longer pursued his hobbies. He often paced and moved around the house without purpose. He would lose his temper over minor things. His family noted that these behaviors were uncharacteristic for him; he often seemed like a different person.

He was being treated with paroxetine (Paxil) and trazodone for depression from his primary care physician. His family history was notable for dementia in his mother when she was in her 80s. His neurological examination was notable for increased tone and brisk reflexes throughout, including a prominent jaw jerk. He had a right-sided Babinski's sign; the left toe was equivocal. On his Mini-mental state examination (MMSE) he scored 22, missing one out of the three recall items, orientation to time of day, date, and place, as well as several items in the attention and calculation section. On the Blessed Information Memory Concentration test he made 10 errors out of a possible 37, missing two out of five of the 5-minute recall items, orientation to time of day and date, as well as attention (months of the year backwards) and non-personal memory. His 7 Minute Screen was positive, as was his Alzheimer's disease Caregiver Questionnaire. He scored 1 out of 15 (non-depressed) on the Geriatric Depression Scale. His MRI scan was unremarkable.

What is the differential diagnosis? What additional tests might you obtain to help make the correct diagnosis?

Although this patient also had memory problems, the most prominent feature of the case is the behavior and personality changes. These behavior and personality changes suggest frontal lobe dysfunction. With a normal MRI scan (ruling out anatomic pathology such as strokes or tumors), the most likely diagnosis is the behavioral variant of frontotemporal dementia. Although Alzheimer's disease can have these behavioral manifestations, they do not generally occur until the moderate to severe stage of the disease, when the MMSE and Blessed scores would be worse. Sometimes a patient can have mild Alzheimer's disease that appears more frontal because there is an additional disorder affecting the frontal lobes such as chronic alcoholism or cerebrovascular disease. However, the MRI scan did not show cerebrovascular disease, there is no suggestion of alcoholism or other factors, and the quality and degree of the disinhibition is more characteristic of a frontotemporal dementia. The brisk reflexes, including a jaw jerk, indicate hyperreflexia stemming from a brain disorder (rather than a spinal cord disorder, since the neurons that innervate the jaw muscles are above the spinal cord).

Two tests that would help to make the correct diagnosis are formal neuropsychological testing and a functional imaging study using a radionucleotide (i.e., SPECT or PET). This patient had both. The neuropsychological testing showed impairment in many areas of executive function. A simple but telling abnormal finding in his neuropsychological testing was word fluency to letters, in which patients are instructed to come up with as many words as they can in 1 minute that begin with a specific letter (usually F, A, and S). The average older adult can generate at least 10–12 such words in 1 minute. Patients with mild Alzheimer's disease do almost as well, generating around 8–10 words. This patient generated only two and three words beginning with F and A, respectively, reflecting his poor frontal lobe function. This patient's actual SPECT scan can be seen in Figure 7.6. See Chapter 7: *Frontotemporal dementia*, for more information.

PATIENT 5

A 65-year-old man came to the clinic with his friend and neighbor, complaining of cognitive difficulties. He was a Professor of English who was on medical leave for these problems. He had been forgetful for about a year, often confused, and was unable to use the television remote because he kept confusing what the different buttons were for. It also became apparent that he had less volume in his voice, less expression in his face, and his walking had slowed down. When he was asked what his biggest problem was he complained of trouble seeing, stating that "no one can get my prescription correct," despite the fact that he had been to multiple optometrists.

His medical history included diabetes mellitus type 2, hypertension, depression, insomnia, and mild sleep apnea. On neurological examination he had masked facies, mild grasp and palmomental reflexes, increased tone and "cogwheeling" with enhancing maneuvers; a rest tremor was not prominent. On the Mini-mental state examination (MMSE) he scored 29/ 30, missing only the intersecting pentagons. On the Blessed Information Memory Concentration test he made one error out of a possible 37, incorrectly stating his own age. His 7 Minute Screen was positive, as was his Alzheimer's disease Caregiver Questionnaire. He scored 3 out of 15 (non-depressed) on the Geriatric Depression Scale. His MRI scan was unremarkable.

What is the most likely diagnosis? What additional elements of the history might you ask about to help confirm the correct diagnosis?

The patient had cognitive and functional impairment, along with the signs and symptoms of Parkinsonism. He also had several cerebrovascular risk factors but his MRI scan was unremarkable. When a patient has a dementia with Parkinsonism, dementia with Lewy bodies must be considered. The visual perceptual defects that the patient complained of are another common symptom of dementia with Lewy bodies; of course no eyeglass prescription could correct the visual problem as it was from his brain, not his eyes. In addition to dementia and spontaneous features of Parkinsonism, other elements of dementia with Lewy bodies should be looked for by history, including visual hallucinations of people or animals, fluctuating levels of attention and alertness, rapid eye movement sleep behavior disorder, and neuroleptic sensitivity. When asked, this patient admitted to having visual hallucinations of both people and animals. He had not mentioned them to anyone because he feared he would be thought crazy. In this case the diagnosis was clear and no further work-up was needed. If the diagnosis was unclear, a functional imaging study using a radionucleotide (i.e., SPECT or PET) could have been obtained. He was started on a cholinesterase inhibitor with good effect. See Chapter 5: *Dementia with Lewy bodies*, for more information.

PATIENT 6

A 74-year-old man presented to the clinic with a 6-year history of cognitive and functional decline. His family reported that his problems began with "small TIAs." When we asked them what they meant, they explained that he appeared to be suffering from transient ischemic attacks, such that in 1 day he might show a sudden decline in his speech, handwriting, and gait, which would subsequently improve, although not back to his baseline. Despite earning a Ph.D. from MIT, he had difficulty at that time with simple calculations, such as calculating the tip in a restaurant. He also had difficulty remembering a short list of items, and finding his way around a familiar street. His family also reported that he would often cry or laugh either inappropriately or with the least provocation.

His medical history included diabetes mellitus type 2 and hypertension. His review of systems was notable for frequent urinary and occasional fecal incontinence. His neurological examination was notable for brisk reflexes throughout, including a jaw jerk. He had bilateral Babinski responses. He also had diminished joint position sense, graphesthesia (ability to distinguish numbers drawn on the hand with eyes closed), and stereognosis (ability to distinguish objects placed in the hand with eyes closed). On his Mini-mental state examination (MMSE) he scored 28, missing two of the three recall items. On the Blessed Information test he made two errors out of a possible 37, missing two out of five of the 5-minute recall items. His 7 Minute Screen was negative; his Alzheimer's disease Caregiver Questionnaire was positive. He scored 2 out of 15 (non-depressed) on the Geriatric Depression Scale.

What is the most likely diagnosis? What additional information would you need to make the correct diagnosis?

The differential diagnosis is broad and could include consideration of many disorders. Several features of this case are notable, and when put together suggest a possible diagnosis. He is an elderly man with diabetes and hypertension whose family reports that he suffers "transient ischemic attacks," but, since the effects of the "transient ischemic attacks" do not resolve completely (i.e., they are not transient), they are actually more likely to be small strokes. His neurological examination shows brisk reflexes and bilateral Babinski responses; that he had a jaw jerk suggests that spinal cord disease alone cannot account for these signs. All of these features suggest a vascular etiology. Other features are supportive of this diagnosis as well. His crying and laughing inappropriately or with little provocation are signs of pseudobulbar affect, commonly seen in disorders of frontal subcortical white matter, including vascular dementia (see Box 6.3: *Pseudobulbar affect*). His being incontinent of both urine and feces while scoring in the normal range on both the Mini mental state examination (MMSE) and the Blessed is suggestive of specific damage to the parts of the nervous system that control continence, rather than a general decline due to dementia. In other words, although patients with Alzheimer's disease (and almost any dementia) eventually become doubly incontinent, the incontinence develops when they are in the moderate or severe stage of the disease, never when screening cognitive test scores are in the normal range. The impairment of joint position sense, graphesthesia, and stereognosis may be together thought of as signs of "cortical sensory loss," meaning that there is a brain problem resulting in impairment of high-level sensory processing, common in disorders that affect the cortex or the underlying cerebral white matter.

The additional information needed is an anatomical imaging study. His actual MRI scan is shown in Figure 6.4: the innumerable small strokes are clearly seen. Frontal subcortical white matter pathways are important for the control of emotional output as well as for continence and walking. Although he showed some impairment in memory in his screening cognitive tests, a more detailed neuropsychological evaluation revealed frontal memory problems—memory problems due to poor encoding and retrieval (consistent with frontal systems dysfunction), and not poor storage (as would be expected with hippocampal dysfunction) (see Appendix C). He was prescribed a cholinesterase inhibitor and then memantine (Namenda) 3 months later; he showed improvement with both medications.

PATIENT 7

A 76-year-old woman presented to the clinic with poor cognition over 6–12 months. Her family noted that she had poor memory and that she was easily distracted. After finding several bills unpaid, her daughter had taken over the management of her finances. She was also forgetting to take her pills, and her daughter needed to call to remind her twice each day to look in her pillbox and take her pills. Her daughter also remarked upon her walking; the patient used to walk for several miles each day but now she would tire walking more than a block or two.

Review of systems was remarkable for urinary incontinence. Her physical examination was notable for a frontal or "magnetic" gait disorder with stiff legs and short steps, brisk reflexes, as well as grasp and palmomental reflexes bilaterally. Her ability to pay attention was so impaired that she was frequently distracted during our interview and examination. She scored 24 out of 30 on the Mini-mental state examination (MMSE), missing two out of three of the recall items, and four out of five points for attention and calculations. She made seven errors out of a possible 37 on the Blessed Information Memory Concentration test, missing three out of five items of the 5-minute recall, reciting the months of the year backwards, and counting backwards from 20 to 1. Her 7 Minute Screen was positive, as was her Alzheimer's disease Caregiver Questionnaire. She scored 1 out of 15 (non-depressed) on the Geriatric Depression Scale.

What is the differential diagnosis? What additional information would you need to make the correct diagnosis?

This constellation of symptoms and signs that include impaired cognition, incontinence, and a gait disorder (particularly a frontal gait disorder) are commonly seen with frontal sub-cortical white matter dysfunction. Vascular disease, multiple sclerosis, and normal pressure hydrocephalus are three possible causes of frontal subcortical white matter dysfunction that would be consistent with the history above.

The additional information needed to distinguish between these possibilities is an anatomical imaging study. Although one might hope that the history would be sufficient, in our experience it sometimes is (as in Patient 6), but often it is not. The actual imaging study for this patient is shown in Figure 10.2. The imaging study clearly points to normal pressure hydrocephalus, a rare disorder but important to identify. After receiving a ventriculoperitoneal shunt her walking improved significantly and her incontinence resolved. Her cognition improved more modestly. See Chapter 10: *Normal pressure hydrocephalus*, for more information.

PATIENT 8 (Figure 5)

An 88-year-old woman was brought to clinic by her children for a 3-year history of memory and other cognitive problems. Her children reported that she would repeat questions multiple times within the same conversation, rapidly forgetting the answers as soon as she was told. They had to take over paying her bills and other aspects of her finances. In addition to filling her pillbox each week, her son also needed to call her to remind her to take her medications. She had prominent word-finding difficulty as well.

Her medical history included hypothyroidism, for which she was taking levothyroxine, mild anemia, and mild arthritis. She had 19 years of education, and had previously taught at college level. Her physical and neurological examinations were unremarkable. She scored 24/30 on the Mini-mental state examination (MMSE), missing three out of three of the recall items, and several items of orientation. On the Blessed Information Memory Concentration test she made nine errors out of a possible 37, missing all five of the 5-minute recall items as well as several orientation items. Her 7 Minute Screen was positive, as was her Alzheimer's disease Caregiver Questionnaire (owing to endorsement of forgetting conversations and deficits in executive function). She scored 2 out of 15 (non-depressed) on the Geriatric Depression Scale.

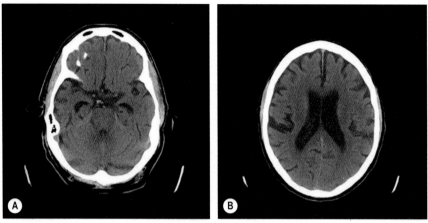

FIGURE 5 Patient 8.

Axial slices from a head CT showing moderate hippocampal atrophy (A), and milder frontal lobe atrophy (B).

What is the most likely diagnosis?

In an 88-year-old woman with memory problems characterized by rapid forgetting, word-finding difficulties, and executive dysfunction, Alzheimer's disease is the most likely diagnosis. This diagnosis is supported by the results of the cognitive tests and the questionnaire. Her CT scan showed moderate hippocampal and milder cortical (parietal and frontal lobe) atrophy (Figure 5), consistent with Alzheimer's disease. She was treated with a cholinesterase inhibitor. See Chapter 3: *Alzheimer's disease*, for more information.

PATIENT 9 (Figure 6)

An 87-year-old woman came to the clinic with her husband with complaints of mild memory problems. Approximately 1.5 years previously she had begun to repeat stories and questions. For the last year she had been forgetting phone messages, hair appointments, and invitations to social functions. There were no issues with other areas of cognition. Of note, her daughter-in-law had been killed in an automobile accident 3 years earlier, and the patient had had intermittent issues with depression since then.

Her medical history included hypertension, bilateral hip replacements, and intermittent incontinence for which she was taking Ditropan (oxybutynin) XL 5 mg QD. She had 14 years of education. She was a homemaker and philanthropist. Her physical and neurological examinations were unremarkable. She scored 28 out of 30 on the Mini-mental state examination (MMSE), missing two out of the three recall items. On the Blessed Information Memory Concentration test she made three errors out of a possible 37, missing three out of five of the 5-minute recall items. Her 7 Minute Screen was negative, as was her Alzheimer's disease Caregiver Questionnaire. She scored 1 out of 15 (non-depressed) on the Geriatric Depression Scale.

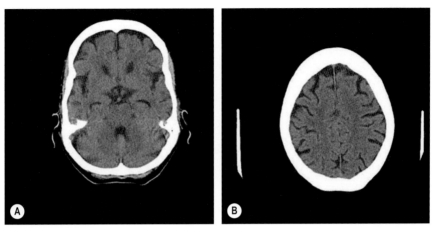

FIGURE 6 Patient 9.

(A and B) Axial slices from a head CT showing only mild, age-related atrophy in this 87-year-old patient.

What is the differential diagnosis?

The differential diagnosis is broad and includes early Alzheimer's disease, amnestic mild cognitive impairment, depression, medication side-effects, and causes of frontal subcortical dysfunction (to explain the incontinence). Alzheimer's disease can be excluded because the patient is not demented; i.e., her function is only slightly affected by her cognitive dysfunction, and the vast majority of instrumental activities of daily living were intact. Depression is unlikely because she did not currently endorse a depressed mood, scoring well in the non-depressed range of the Geriatric Depression scale. Medication side-effects, in particular the Ditropan (oxybutynin), is a possibility to be seriously considered because of its anticholinergic effects. However, her symptoms developed and worsened while she was on a stable dose of the medication, making it somewhat less likely. Although one always must consider causes of frontal subcortical dysfunction when incontinence is present, there was no suggestion of cognitive complaints or impairment on testing to indicate frontal subcortical dysfunction.

The best characterization of her cognitive dysfunction was amnestic mild cognitive impairment. Her CT scan showed only mild, age-related atrophy (Figure 6). She was treated with a cholinesterase inhibitor. See Chapter 4: *Mild cognitive impairment*, for more information.

PATIENT 10 (Figure 7)

A 71-year-old woman presented to the clinic with her family because of difficulty living at home after the death of her husband. Her family reported a 2- to 3-year gradual progression of cognitive deficits. She rapidly forgot conversations. She was unable to manage her checkbook or medications without the help of her family. She had prominent word-finding difficulties. She had difficulty dressing correctly, and she was unable to use the television remote. She also had fluctuations in her alertness and attention such that she would sometimes

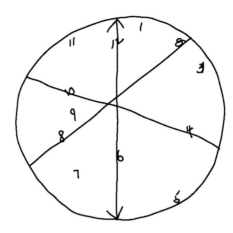

FIGURE 7 Patient 10.

Clock drawing demonstrating both disorganization and visuospatial dysfunction.

not pay attention to those talking to her, and would even occasionally fall asleep in the middle of a conversation!

Her medical history included hypercholesterolemia and arthritis. She had 12 years of education, and previously worked as a home health aide. Her neurological examination revealed Parkinsonism, including masked facies and increased tone in her extremities. Her head CT was unremarkable. She scored 25 out of 30 on the Mini-mental state examination (MMSE) missing points for disorientation to time and place, and poor figure copy. Clock drawing was also impaired (Figure 7). On the Blessed Information Memory Concentration test she made eight errors out of a possible 37, again missing points for orientation. Her 7 Minute Screen was positive, as was her Alzheimer's disease Caregiver Questionnaire. She scored 3 out of 15 (non-depressed) on the Geriatric Depression Scale.

What is the most likely diagnosis? What additional information would you need to make the correct diagnosis?

As mentioned in the discussion of Patient 5, whenever there is a patient with dementia and Parkinsonism, dementia with Lewy bodies must be considered. This patient met criteria for probable dementia with Lewy bodies because she had dementia, spontaneous features of Parkinsonism, and fluctuating cognition. The patient's review of systems revealed visual hallucinations of little men dancing on the walls, which she knew could not be real. Note that, as in this case, it frequently happens that families understand that parents are impaired when spouses and friends can no longer support them. She was started on a cholinesterase inhibitor with good effect. See Chapter 5: *Dementia with Lewy bodies*, for more information.

PATIENT 11 (Figure 8)

A 67-year-old man was brought to the clinic by his wife. Over the past year she noted that he had developed problems with forgetfulness and word-finding difficulty. About 2 years previously she had had to take over the household finances and projects that her husband used to do. A number of behavioral symptoms had started 9 years earlier, including making embarrassing comments in social situations and developing an unusually high sex drive. He became paranoid, thinking that items he misplaced were actually stolen by other people. He believed that people on television were speaking directly to him. He wanted to eat whenever anyone else was eating.

His medical history included hypertension and hypercholesterolemia. For his cognitive problems he had been prescribed Aricept (donepezil) 10 mg QD several years earlier. He was a retired truck driver with 12 years of education. His physical and neurological examinations were unremarkable. He scored 28 out of 30 on the Mini-mental state examination (MMSE), missing points for attention and calculations. On the Blessed Information Memory Concentration test he made six errors out of a possible 37, again missing points for concentration and attention. His 7 Minute Screen was positive, as was his Alzheimer's disease Caregiver Questionnaire. He scored 2 out of 15 (non-depressed) on the Geriatric Depression Scale. Both his instrumental and basic activities of daily living were impaired. His MRI scan showed scattered T2 hyperintensities and mild cortical atrophy.

What is the differential diagnosis? What additional information would you need to make the correct diagnosis?

This patient had a combination of cognitive, behavioral, and psychiatric signs and symptoms. The main differential diagnoses are a frontotemporal dementia, Alzheimer's disease, vascular dementia, a primary psychiatric disease, and some combination of these disorders. Regarding the possibility of a vascular dementia, scattered T2 hyperintensities are often seen in patients over 65 years of age, particularly in those with hypertension and hypercholesterolemia. Scattered T2 hyperintensities are not sufficient to cause the symptoms and signs described above. To differentiate among the other possibilities it is important to evaluate the functions of the regions of the brain that are affected by Alzheimer's disease compared with those of the regions affected by frontotemporal dementia. We already have a clue from the screening testing with the Mini-mental state examination (MMSE) and the Blessed: these measures both showed problems with attention and calculations, not with memory. Formal neuropsychological testing and a functional imaging study using a radionucleotide (i.e., SPECT or PET) use different methods to evaluate the regions impaired by a dementia. This patient's neuropsychological examination was notable for very impaired executive function including perseveration, poor organization, inability to properly carry out Luria's hand motor sequence (palm, fist, side; see Figure 8A), and impaired working memory (ability to keep information in one's head and manipulate it). His episodic memory problems appeared secondary to his executive dysfunction; in other words, his recent memory was impaired because he had difficulties encoding and retrieving information, but storage of information appeared normal (see Appendix C). His PET scan showed clear hypometabolism of the frontal lobes bilaterally (Figure 8B). A diagnosis of the behavioral variant of frontotemporal dementia was made. A trial taking him off the cholinesterase inhibitor was made; no differences were observed after 1 month and the medication was not restarted. Treatment was supportive.

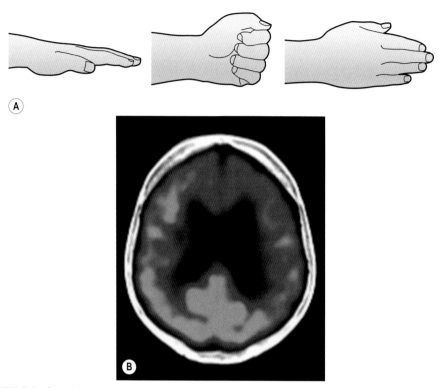

FIGURE 8 Patient 11.

(A) The proper order of Luria's hand motor sequence, a task that is sensitive to executive dysfunction. (B) An axial PET scan slice demonstrating frontal hypometabolism.

Index

Note: Page numbers followed by *b* indicate boxes, *f* indicate figures, *t* indicate tables and *vs.* indicates a comparison or differential diagnosis

dementia with Lewy bodies 86
frontal release signs 18–19
frontotemporal dementia 112–113
gait 18
mild cognitive impairment 76
normal pressure hydrocephalus 139
progressive supranuclear palsy 122
rigidity 17–18
tremor 17
vascular dementia 99
see also specific tests
Neurological symptoms, Creutzfeldt–Jakob disease 143*b*
Neuropil threads 120–121
Neuropsychiatry Inventory (NPI) 28–29, 29*b*, 224*t*
behavioral/psychological symptom
evaluation 223
Neuropsychological evaluation 27
Neurosyphilis 31–32
Neurotransmitters, Alzheimer's disease treatment,
200, 200*t*
NINCDS-ARDRA (National Institutes of
Neurological and Communicative Disorders
and Stroke-Alzheimer's Disease and Related
Disorders Association) 50–52, 51*b*
Diagnostic and Statistical Manual of Mental
Disorders *vs.* 52*b*
NINDS-AIREN, vascular dementia 94
NMDA receptor, memantine 185, 186*f*
Nomenclature, mild cognitive impairment 75
Non-pharmacological treatment, memory
loss 214–219
see also specific methods
Non-steroidal anti-inflammatories (NSAIDs)
196–197
Normal pressure hydrocephalus (NPH) 136–142
criteria 137, 138*b*
definition 136*b*, 137
diagnostic criteria 136*b*
cognitive tests 140
history 139
laboratory studies 140
lumbar puncture 141
neurologic exam 139
physical exam 139
structural imaging 140–141, 140*f*
differential diagnosis 136*b*, 141–142
multiple sclerosis 141–142
vascular dementia 141–142
genetic risk 136*b*
pathogenesis 137
pathology 137, 139*f*
prevalence 136*b*, 137
prognosis 137
risk factors 137
signs and symptoms 137–139
behavioral symptoms 136*b*

cognitive symptoms 136*b*
treatment 136*b*, 142
NPH *see* Normal pressure hydrocephalus (NPH)
NPI *see* Neuropsychiatry Inventory (NPI)
NSAIDs (non-steroidal anti-inflammatories)
196–197

O

Occupation, memory loss evaluation 15
Off label use
cholinesterase inhibitors 166*b*
memantine 184*b*
Olanzapine 251*b*
frontotemporal dementia treatment 116–117

P

Palmomental reflex 19
Paranoia 12
non-pharmacological treatment 243
Paraphrasic errors 10–11
Parkinsonian gait 18
Parkinsonian tremor 17
Parkinson's disease dementia (PDD) 80
Partial complex seizures 161
Passive immunotherapy, Alzheimer's disease
treatment 207
Pathology, history taking 7–8, 9*f*
Patient, helping of 1–2
Paying bills 260–262
PDD (Parkinson's disease dementia) 80
Periodic limb movements of sleep (PLMS) 254
Periventricular abnormalities, normal pressure
hydrocephalus 140–141
Personality changes, alcohol abuse 155
Personal savings 270
PET *see* Positron emission tomography (PET)
Phosphatidylcholine docosahexaenoic acid
see DHA (phosphatidylcholine
docosahexaenoic acid)
Physical examination 16–19, 17*b*
Alzheimer's disease 62
corticobasal degeneration 133
dementia with Lewy bodies 86
frontotemporal dementia 112–113
general 16
mild cognitive impairment 76
neurological exam *see* Neurological exam
normal pressure hydrocephalus 139
progressive supranuclear palsy 122, 123*f*
vascular dementia 99
Physiologic tremor 17
Pick's disease 107
pathology 108*f*
Pittsburgh compound B 38–39
PLMS (periodic limb movements of sleep) 254